AF620145

Urinary Stones

Urinary Stones

Medical and Surgical Management

EDITED BY

Michael Grasso, MD
Professor and Vice Chairman
Department of Urology
New York Medical College
Valhalla, NY, USA

David S. Goldfarb, MD, FASN
Clinical Chief, Nephrology Division
NYU Langone Medical Center;
Professor of Medicine and Physiology
New York University School of Medicine
New York, NY, USA

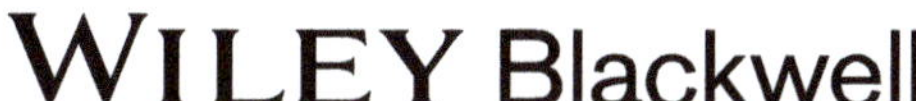

Registered Office
John Wiley & Sons, Ltd, The Atrium, Southern Gate, Chichester, West Sussex, PO19 8SQ, UK

Editorial Offices
9600 Garsington Road, Oxford, OX4 2DQ, UK
The Atrium, Southern Gate, Chichester, West Sussex, PO19 8SQ, UK
111 River Street, Hoboken, NJ 07030-5774, USA

For details of our global editorial offices, for customer services and for information about how to apply for permission to reuse the copyright material in this book please see our website at www.wiley.com/wiley-blackwell.

Library of Congress Cataloging-in-Publication Data

Urinary stones : medical and surgical management / edited by Michael Grasso III, David S. Goldfarb.
p. ; cm.
Includes bibliographical references and index.
ISBN 978-1-118-40543-7 (cloth)
I. Grasso, Michael, III, editor of compilation. II. Goldfarb, David S., editor of compilation.
[DNLM: 1. Urinary Calculi–therapy. 2. Urinary Calculi–prevention & control. WJ 140]
RC916
616.6′22–dc23

2013041992

A catalogue record for this book is available from the British Library.

Wiley also publishes its books in a variety of electronic formats. Some content that appears in print may not be available in electronic books.

Cover image: Courtesy of Dr Michael Grasso
Cover design by Meaden Creative

Set in 9.5/11.5pt Meridien by SPi Publisher Services, Pondicherry, India

1 2014

Contents

Part 2: Surgical Management of Urinary Stones

List of Contributors

Sachin Abrol, MS
Resident in Urology
Muljibhai Patel Urological Hospital
Nadiad, Gujarat, India

Ahmed Alasker, MD, FRCS(C)
Endourology, Robotic and Laparoscopy Fellow
Albert Einstein College of Medicine
Montefiore Medical Center
Bronx, NY, USA

Bobby Alexander, MD
Fellow
Division of Endourology
Lenox Hill Hospital
New York, NY, USA

John R. Asplin, MD, FASN
Medical Director, Litholink Corporation;
Clinical Associate
Department of Medicine
University of Chicago
Chicago, IL, USA

Demetrius H. Bagley, MD, FACS
The Nathan Lewis Hatfield Professor of Urology
Professor of Radiology
Department of Urology
Thomas Jefferson University
Philadelphia, PA, USA

Michael S. Borofsky, MD
Chief Resident in Urology
New York University Langone Medical Center
New York, NY, USA

Kai-wen Chuan, MD
Chief Resident
The Arthur Smith Institute for Urology
North Shore-Long Island Jewish Health System
New Hyde Park, NY, USA

Michael J. Conlin, MD
Associate Professor
Portland VA Medical Center;
Department of Urology
Oregon Health & Science University/Portland VA Medical Center
Portland, OR, USA

Angela M. Cottrell, FRCS (Urol), MBBS, BSc, Dip Clin Ed
Specialist Registrar, Urology
Derriford Hospital
Plymouth Hospitals NHS Trust
Plymouth, UK

Michel Daudon, PhD
Chief of the Stone Laboratory
Department of Clinical Physiology
APHP, Tenon Hospital
Paris, France

Michael Degen, MD
Fellow
Division of Endourology and Minimally Invasive Urology
Westchester Medical Center;
Department of Urology
New York Medical College
Valhalla, NY, USA

Mahesh R. Desai, MS, FRCS
Medical Director
Muljibhai Patel Urological Hospital
Nadiad, Gujarat, India

Sameer M. Deshmukh, MD
Resident in Urology
Department of Urologic Sciences
Stone Centre at Vancouver General Hospital
Vancouver, BC, Canada

Andrew J. Dickinson, MD, FRCSUrol, FRCSEd
Consultant Urologist
Derriford Hospital
Plymouth Hospitals NHS Trust
Plymouth, UK

Christopher M. Dixon, MD
Associate
Division of Endourology
Lenox Hill Hospital
New York, NY, USA

Brian D. Duty, MD
Assistant Professor
Department of Urology
Oregon Health & Science University/Portland VA Medical Center
Portland, OR, USA

Vidar O. Edvardsson, MD
Director of Pediatric Nephrology
Children's Medical Center
Landspitali – The National University Hospital of Iceland;
Faculty of Medicine, School of Health Sciences
University of Iceland
Reykjavik, Iceland

Brian H. Eisner, MD
Co-Director of Kidney Stone Program
Department of Urology
Massachusetts General Hospital
Harvard Medical School
Boston, MA, USA

Majid Eshghi, MD, FACS
Division of Endourology and Minimally Invasive Urology
Westchester Medical Center;
Department of Urology
New York Medical College
Valhalla, NY, USA

Andrew I. Fishman, MD
Assistant Professor of Urology
Department of Urology
New York Medical College
Valhalla, NY, USA

Israel Franco, MD
Director of Pediatric Urology
Maria Fareri Children's Hospital
Professor of Urology
New York Medical College
Valhalla, NY, USA

Sean Fullerton, MD
Assistant Professor
Department of Urology
New York Medical College
Valhalla, NY, USA

Arvind P. Ganpule, MS, DNB
Vice-Chairman
Department of Urology
Muljibhai Patel Urological Hospital
Nadiad, Gujarat, India

Reza Ghavamian, MD
Professor of Clinical Urology
Chairman of Urology
Albert Einstein College of Medicine
Montefiore Medical Center
Bronx, NY, USA

Jordan Gitlin, MD
Attending Pediatric Urologist
Cohen Children's Medical Center of New York;
The Arthur Smith Institute for Urology
North Shore-Long Island Jewish Health System
New Hyde Park, NY, USA

David S. Goldfarb, MD, FASN
Clinical Chief, Nephrology Division
NYU Langone Medical Center;
Professor of Medicine and Physiology
New York University School of Medicine
New York, NY, USA

Michael Grasso, MD
Professor and Vice Chairman
Department of Urology
New York Medical College
Valhalla, NY, USA

Kelly A. Healy, MD
Assistant Professor
Department of Urology
Thomas Jefferson University
Philadelphia, PA, USA

Nicole Hindman, MD
Assistant Professor of Radiology
Department of Radiology
New York University Lagone Medical Center
New York, NY, USA

David Hoenig, MD
Associate Professor of Clinical Urology
Albert Einstein College of Medicine
Montefiore Medical Center
Bronx, NY, USA

Paul Jungers, MD
Emeritus Professor of Nephrology
Paris V University;
APHP, Department of Nephrology
Necker Hospital
Paris, France

Francis X. Keeley Jr, MD, FRCS(Urol)
Consultant Urologist
Bristol Urological Institute
Bristol, UK

Nir Kleinmann, MD
Attending Urologist
Department of Urology
Sheba Medical Center
Tel Hashomer, Israel

Abhishek Laddha, MS
Resident in Urology
Muljibhai Patel Urological Hospital
Nadiad, Gujarat, India

Dirk Lange, BSc, PhD
Assistant Professor
Department of Urologic Sciences
University of British Columbia
Vancouver, BC, Canada

Julien Letendre, MD, FRCSC
Fellow of Endourology
Department of Urology
Tenon Hospital, Assistance Publique –
Hôpitaux de Paris
Pierre et Marie Curie University
Paris, France

John C. Lieske, MD
Professor of Medicine
Division of Nephrology and Hypertension
Mayo Clinic
Rochester, MN, USA

James E. Lingeman, MD
Professor
Department of Urology
Indiana University School of Medicine
Indianapolis, IN, USA

Naim M. Maalouf, MD
Assistant Professor of Medicine
Department of Internal Medicine and
Charles and Jane Pak Center for Mineral
Metabolism and Clinical Research
University of Texas Southwestern
Medical Center
Dallas, TX, USA

Sunil Mathur, MD, FRCS (Urol)
Consultant Urologist
Great Western Hospital
Swindon, UK

Lesli Nicolay, MD
Assistant Professor
Division of Pediatric Urology
Loma Linda University Medical Center
Loma Linda, CA, USA

Runolfur Palsson, MD
Chief, Division of Nephrology
Landspitali – The National University
Hospital of Iceland;
Associate Professor of Medicine
Faculty of Medicine, School of Health Sciences
University of Iceland
Reykjavik, Iceland

Jessica E. Paonessa, MD
Endourology Fellow
Department of Urology
Indiana University School of Medicine
Indianapolis, IN, USA

Sherry S. Ross, MD
Director of Pediatric Urology Stone Clinic
Department of Surgery
Division of Urology
Section of Pediatric Urology
Duke University Medical Center
Durham, NC, USA

Ojas Shah, MD
Associate Professor, Director of Endourology
and Stone Disease
New York University Langone Medical Center
New York, NY, USA

Shonni J. Silverberg, MD
Professor of Medicine
Columbia University
College of Physicians and Surgeons
New York, NY, USA

Olivier Traxer, MD, PhD
Professor of Urology
Department of Urology
Tenon Hospital, Assistance Publique – Hôpitaux de Paris
Pierre et Marie Curie University
Paris, France

Robert J. Unwin, PhD, FRCP, FSB, CBiol
Professor of Nephrology and Physiology
Head of Centre and Research Department of Internal Medicine UCL
UCL Centre for Nephrology
University College London Medical School
London, UK

Marcella Donovan Walker, MD, MS
Assistant Professor of Medicine
Columbia University
College of Physicians and Surgeons
New York, NY, USA

Stephen B. Walsh, PhD, MRCP
Clinical Senior Lecturer in Experimental Medicine/Honorary Consultant Nephrologist
UCL Centre for Nephrology
University College London Medical School
London, UK

Oliver M. Wrong, DM, FRCP
Former Emeritus Professor of Medicine
UCL Centre for Nephrology
University College London Medical School
London, UK

Preface

The natural history of urinary calculi reflects a spectrum of clinical presentations, some with a benign course but many others with the potential for severe and often catastrophic outcomes. Urinary calculi frequently are the sequelae of major underlying metabolic disorders, which if left untreated are regularly associated with recurrent stone events with the ultimate potential for renal parenchymal loss. It is the co-ordination of both surgical intervention to remove obstructing concretions and improve drainage, and the simultaneous application of novel medical therapies employed to alter the underlying hypermetabolic disorder that ultimately changes the natural history of this morbid ailment.

As Editors of this book we represent varied perspectives on stone management, with 18 years of daily collaboration treating the most complex hypermetabolic stone formers. We created the first multimodality stone center in New York and continue to regularly care for patients together. This collaborative spirit of endourology and nephrology has led to a broad spectrum of innovative therapies, many of which will be presented in this text. Our chapter authors reflect international thought leaders in urinary stone management, each offering unique insight into patient evaluation and specific therapies.

We, the editors and authors, are fundamentally committed to improving patient care by developing and employing new treatments, and by encouraging and nurturing the next generation of providers through fellowship training and scholarly efforts. We have always believed and taught that nephrologists need to more fully understand the surgical management of stone disease in order to counsel their patients, and urologists who understand metabolic stone disorders will offer their patients a higher and more attractive level of service.

This text is designed to be a resource for the practitioner when confronted with a challenging clinical presentation. There is an orderly division of chapters: patient assessment, imaging, surgical interventions, and medical therapies. The underlying theme, however, is collaboration of implementation – mixing and matching therapies as required by the presented clinical variables. For example, a patient who presents with urinary tract obstruction and with urosepsis during systemic chemotherapy for acute leukemia requires input from many areas to craft a comprehensive treatment plan. The emergency renal drainage algorithm in the surgical section is promptly applied. Varied interventions as necessary are employed next to clear the stone burden, with subsequent additional medical therapies to treat the underlying hyperuricosuria and minimize future episodes.

It is our intention to offer a user-friendly resource to the clinician. Various treatments are presented with regard to indications, technical nuances, complications, continuity of care, and preventive measures. It is our hope that through efforts like this text, comprehensive collaborative treatment centers will grow, employing many of the tenets described herein.

Michael Grasso
David S. Goldfarb

PART 1

Types of Urinary Stones and Their Medical Management

CHAPTER 1

How to Build a Kidney Stone Prevention Clinic

David S. Goldfarb
New York University School of Medicine, New York, NY, USA

"It's the right thing to do" (Edward Goldfarb, DDS, 1968)
"It's the right thing to do" (Michael Grasso, MD, 1996)

Introduction

Those identical, ethical mandates were told to me on two occasions: first, when as a preteen I objected to my father, a dentist, fluoridating the teeth of his young patients, suggesting that he was sacrificing his income (and my future college tuition) by the prevention of caries; second, when as a proto-lithologist, Michael Grasso and I discussed the founding of a kidney stone clinic and I asked Michael if he was worried that I would reduce the number of ureteroscopies and lithotripsies he would perform.

Kidney stones are common and preventable, but not commonly prevented. Instead, our experience has been that most patients, despite their interest, have not received any serious recommendations about how to avoid kidney stone recurrence. Stone formers seek advice regarding their disorder, whether that is about the choices for urological intervention or strategies and regimens for prevention. Bringing these two components of kidney stone practice together into a single setting is the goal of a kidney stone clinic.

Like any other disorder, expertise among practitioners develops with exposure and repetition. A kidney stone clinic offers these assets to its personnel while offering patients the confidence that develops when expertise is demonstrated. Simply titling one's office or practice a "kidney stone clinic" may lead to some assurance that the disorder is seen repeatedly there, but developing a real integration of diverse skills and mastery will be even more convincing.

This book arises from the partnership that Michael Grasso and I began in 1996 when we first formed a kidney stone clinic. Michael brought his vast experience in endourology and urological intervention for kidney stones to our enterprise. My contribution, as a nephrologist and physiologist, was

---

Urinary Stones: Medical and Surgical Management, First Edition. Edited by Michael Grasso and David S. Goldfarb.

to specialize in the metabolic evaluation and prevention of stone disease. Thousands of patients later, we have exchanged enormous amounts of information and experience, so that our patients can be certain that together we can approach any problem related to nephrolithiasis.

The urological management of kidney stones is extensively described elsewhere in this book. In this chapter I will focus on the other components of a kidney stone clinic. There are some data regarding the performance of a kidney stone clinic but inevitably what I write here includes much opinion.

Personnel

The kidney stone clinic starts with a urologist interested in kidney stones. That urologist may be an endourologist with further postresidency training in the appropriate techniques but in many settings, such a subspecialist may not be available. No matter. Patients with stones are referred to urologists first, and infrequently to nephrologists or internists. In a smaller community where an endourologist is not available, a general urologist presumably has ample experience in the management of most stones, perhaps referring to an endourologist in only more complex cases. Referral may be appropriate for larger stones, stones associated with infection, cystine stones, and anatomically abnormal or solitary kidneys.

There are urologists who can constitute a kidney stone clinic by themselves, with no other personnel required. Such urologists are widely knowledgeable about urine chemistry and how to modify it and reduce stone recurrence risk with diet and medications. They are happy to discuss the relevant variables with their patients and answer questions about appropriate preventive regimens. There are also urologists who understandably are less interested in performing such duties. After all, urology residency training often does not emphasize such skills. Compensation for urologists has a procedure-based emphasis which necessitates a shorter office visit that may not lead interested patients to feel that their concerns have been adequately addressed.

In that case, the addition of a nephrologist or internist makes an important contribution to the prevention component of a kidney stone clinic. This person, interpreting results of diagnostic tests and prescribing dietary modification or medications, does not have to be a nephrologist. An internist can learn the syllabus quickly, as internists have been trained to pay attention to these sorts of preventive modalities. In recent years, we have had a general internist doing kidney stone prevention at Bellevue Hospital, a large public facility in New York City. Two general internists oriented towards preventive care, in consultation with me, learned the field, recognizing it as similar to addressing cardiovascular risk factors. The frequency of a clinic's occurrence can be variable and obviously would depend on the volume of appropriate cases. Even a monthly clinic would offer an important service.

I note, however, that a nephrologist or internist will not easily constitute a kidney stone clinic without the involvement or endorsement of a urologist. In my experience, it takes a long while before any volume of referrals can come from anyone other than the kidney stone clinic's urologist. First, kidney stones are often not given the serious attention they deserve; family practitioners and general internists may not recognize that any preventive regimen is appropriate until significant recurrences have occurred. Second, as stated previously, most patients are seen only by urologists, who, if not specializing in stone treatment, may give prevention little heed and are unwilling to refer their patients to specialists outside their own practice. Third, most patients are unaware that anyone specializes in kidney stone prevention and find a kidney stone clinic only after the frustration of recurrence. And fourth, while most nephrologists also have little to no training in stone prevention during their fellowships, they dabble in the field and are also reluctant to give to their patients another nephrologist's name. I therefore think that a kidney stone clinic must be based on the keystone of a high-volume endourologist.

The kidney stone clinic's nephrologist or internist cannot perform procedures, but can become expert in diagnosing and managing renal colic and knowing when referral to the urologist is appropriate. He or she can also be useful and offer a second opinion to patients deciding about treatment of symptomatic or asymptomatic stones, and in choosing between urological interventions. In addition, patients with kidney stones have a host of co-morbidities including diabetes, hypertension, gout, coronary artery disease and chronic kidney disease, all of which can be favorably influenced by the involvement of an internist. Urologists may be less at ease treating such patients, dealing with underlying electrolyte disturbances or those resulting from prescribed medications and changes in kidney function that result from obstruction and its reversal. While the prevalence of chronic kidney disease in the average endourology practice has not been quantified, a nephrologist can offer a different, medical perspective to such patients, addressing mineral and bone disorders, osteoporosis, hyperparathyroidism, kidney transplants, resistant hypertension and, rarely, management of and preparation for end-stage kidney disease.

It is highly desirable to have a dietician as part of the program [1]. Patients seek dietary advice, which often is confusing. Dietary prescriptions are preferable particularly for younger people who often are more reluctant than older adults to take medications like citrate supplements or thiazides. Older people often have co-morbidities such as diabetes and cardiovascular disease and feel they have "nothing left to eat" when vegetables like spinach, which they considered "healthy," turn out to be high in oxalate.

Dieticians are most likely to be accessible in a university or Department of Veterans Affairs setting because many health insurers in the United States will not pay adequately for visits with dieticians. In such cases, patients may be reluctant to pay for such advice themselves. There are many sources of online dietary education for kidney stone prevention online. There is also a useful book, co-authored by a nephrologist, a urologist and a dietician [2].

In many urology practices, nurse practitioners play important roles in preparing patients for procedures and their aftermath and could easily help in interpreting results of 24-h urine collections and offering preventive regimens.

The final human component of the kidney stone clinic is the patient. One should not minimize the interest that patients have in understanding and preventing the disorder [3]. Medical practitioners are more likely than patients to consider kidney stones a transient condition that "passes" readily and has no consequences. In fact, as patients know, kidney stones are not just painful, but also costly and humiliating and lead to significant disruptions of quality of life [4]. As they affect a younger population than, for instance, end-stage kidney disease, each year 1% of American workers will miss some work time for this reason [5].

When surveyed, most patients with kidney stones express a desire for information regarding what to eat and drink [6]. Adherence to prescribed regimens varies, of course; we are all only human after all. It is true that patients' interest in adhering to recommendations regarding fluid intake, dietary modification, or pharmacotherapy may vary from little, early in their course, to more intense, with progressive recurrence. Adherence may also be greater the more recent the episode of renal colic. At whatever stage they are encountered, patients deserve and desire advice regarding their condition.

Evaluation

24-hour urine collections

Ideally, 24-h urine collections are done by a laboratory specializing in assessment of kidney stone risk. The epitome of such a laboratory today is Litholink Corp. (Chicago, IL), the lab doing the most such analyses in the world today [7]. The patient is mailed a kit, does the collection, records the urine volume and returns a 50 mL aliquot via Fedex to the lab. Detailed instructions are included and lab personnel are available by phone to answer questions. This process is extremely user friendly and convenient, permitting the collection to be done at home without the patient making a visit to the hospital or lab. All analytes are measured on the same collection, with one part of the aliquot acidified in order to fully dissolve calcium salts, and another part alkalinized in order to ensure full dissolution of uric acid. In other words, the patient does not have to do two separate collections into acidified and alkalinized containers. The lab then reports the data in a cumulative fashion so that all prior data are presented in a useful fashion to the clinician. In addition, supersaturation of calcium oxalate, calcium phosphate and uric acid is calculated and recorded.

The importance of supersaturation is that it gives a single number to integrate the results of the various urinary analytes. It can be shown to patients to demonstrate the net effects of changes in urine calcium, oxalate, citrate excretion, urine volume, pH, and uric acid excretion. Patients today usually know the results of testing for cholesterol and low density lipoprotein, prostate-specific antigen, and glycosylated hemoglobin. Supersaturation can have the same intuitive value: higher values are bad, lower values are good. Supersaturation values correlate with stone composition and although it is likely to be true, they have not been shown to correlate with recurrence rates [8]. Reduction of supersaturation has also been used to judge stone clinic efficacy. In one study, a group of kidney stone clinics was nearly as effective in lowering supersaturation as an academic, university-based stone clinic [7].

Writers have addressed whether first-time stone formers should do 24-h collections or whether this test should be reserved for recurrent stone formers [9]. The argument that first-time stone formers may be mostly uncomplicated with low rates of recurrence or lack motivation to adhere to prescribed regimens has merit. Sometimes first-time stone formers are older people who think they are likely to die before having a stone recurrence. On the other hand, some first-time stone formers have large and consequential stones or have co-mordibities, making stone prevention that much more important. I recommend leaving the choice to the patient, with many preferring the detailed and specific recommendations that derive from 24-h urine analysis, and others being satisfied with generic, non-individualized advice. Interpretation of 24-h urine data is detailed elsewhere in this volume.

There has long been discussion about the optimal number of 24-h urines to collect, with more collections (2–3) yielding more diagnoses of urinary risk factors than one [10]. However, there are no data demonstrating that making more diagnoses leads to better therapeutic outcomes. My practice is to do two collections before prescribing treatment and then one at intervals following patient adherence to the prescription(s) and any changes in the regimen.

Radiology

Appropriate intervals for radiological follow-up have not been established. One question that needs to be answered by physician and patient is what to do with evidence of asymptomatic, new stones or stone growth. Such findings might constitute an indication to review the adequacy of improved 24-h urine results. Some patients might want urological intervention for asymptomatic stones for a variety of reasons, while others prefer to leave well enough alone, depending on their experiences [11]. My usual practice is to repeat ultrasound of the kidneys at yearly intervals for a few years, and if metabolic activity appears quiescent, desist. The interval might decrease to 4 or 6 months for patients with particularly active disease, such as cystinuria or those suffering more frequent recurrences.

Bone mineral density

Patients with calcium stones and hypercalciuria often have decreased bone mineral density (BMD) [12]. For many, this may reflect disordered calcium metabolism and for others it is attributable as well to misguided restricted dietary calcium. A proportion of women stone formers find their way to the stone clinic because they have been found by their internists or gynecologists to have reduced BMD and are concerned about recommendations to increase dietary calcium or take calcium supplements. It is therefore frequently useful to order dual emission X-ray absorptiometry (DEXA) to measure and follow BMD and to develop expertise in assessing and treating osteoporosis. FRAX, software developed by the World Health Organization, assesses the likelihood of experiencing a fracture in the next 10 years and can aid in making decisions about when to initiate bisphosphonate therapy [13].

Treatment

Elsewhere in this volume specific recommendations for management of the various stone compositions are offered. The unfortunately limited number of randomized controlled trials that provide some of the evidence for successful stone prevention have recently been reviewed [14]. Some more general comments can be made here.

Although I endorse the performance of 24-h urine collections, and use them regularly, in fact, prescribing either dietary or pharmacological therapies based on the results has not been proven superior to making generic recommendations. Most lithologists believe that patients are interested, informed, and motivated by knowing their specific risk factors. For example, it seems illogical and counterproductive to counsel people with low sodium excretion to limit their sodium intake. It is important to note that stone preventive regimens can be prescribed for those who do not perform 24-h urine collections, either because of preference or because of limitations of insurance coverage and cost.

For people who do or do not perform 24-h urines, the most important requirement is an increase in urine volume, a manipulation proven by randomized controlled trials to be effective [15]. Many practitioners say "drink more" without being quantitative and detailed; many people think that they do drink "a lot" without having any idea what that means. A lengthy discussion about fluid intake and a handout detailing the prescribed regimen is essential. The optimal goal is a urine volume of at least 2.5 L, requiring a fluid intake of 3 L per day to account for the insensible losses of sweat and respiration. It is useful to model what 3 L looks like and have varying serving sizes available. In the US, 3 L is 96 ounces, or 8 × 12 oz (a can of soda), or 12 × 8 oz (a small coffee cup). On many occasions I have taken out a prescription pad and written "WATER, 3 L per day" on it to emphasize that this is a serious protocol, with efficacy demonstrated by a randomized controlled diet.

Fluid intake should be spaced throughout the day and include a serving before bed, with hopes to disrupt sleep minimally. There should be recognition of the need for planning to avoid the urge to void when bathroom facilities are unavailable. An occupational history should focus on whether working conditions preclude fluid intake and voiding; for instance, teachers and anesthesiologists may have limitations imposed by work schedules. Athletes, beach goers, inhabitants of more tropical climates, and outdoor workers may need to significantly increase input to account for increased extrarenal fluid losses. Measuring fluid intake in a more exacting way may be useful to help people understand what a daily, lifelong habit necessitates. I limit cola intake or other sweetened sodas to one can per day; "clear" diet sodas (e.g. 7-Up) are not limited. Coffee and alcohol are consistently associated with fewer kidney stones in epidemiological observational studies and are not proscribed [16]. If daily fluid intake and 24-h urine volume do not increase, dietary prescriptions and medications may be more important. Some patients are willing, and understand that measuring their urine volume themselves is easy, inexpensive, and worthwhile.

Dietary modifications may be appropriate for most stone formers. Ideally, dietary modifications are prescribed based on the results of 24-h urine collections. However, generic advice based on stone composition may be appropriate as well. The only successful study of diet for prevention of calcium stones showed that in men with hypercalciuria, limited intake of animal protein, salt and oxalate with higher intake of calcium was superior to a restricted calcium- and oxalate-containing diet [17]. The characteristics of the Dietary Approaches to Stop Hypertension (DASH) diet have been associated with fewer stones in observational studies, but it has not been tested in trials [18]. Uric acid and cystine stone formers should reduce animal protein intake to reduce uric acid excretion and increase pH; increasing fruits and vegetables will also increase urine pH [19].

Patients with calcium stones have often been told to restrict calcium intake by their friends and relatives and sometimes older practitioners. Observational studies have consistently shown that more, not less, dairy intake or calcium intake is associated with fewer stones [20]. This approach is supported by the single, small, randomized trial previously cited. However, the efficacy of that study's protocol has not been tested in women, may require a level of sodium restriction that is difficult to achieve in most first world settings, and assumes that adults are willing and able to increase dairy intake when in fact many are not or cannot. Using calcium supplements in lieu of increased dairy intake may not be a useful alternative as they have been associated with more stones, though the absolute increase in risk is quite small [21]. If felt to be necessary, the preferred calcium salt is calcium citrate as it is associated with less increase in urinary supersaturation than calcium carbonate [22]. It should be administered after meals to serve as a binder of oxalate in the intestinal lumen and possibly to reduce oxaluria.

Pharmacological prevention

Medications are frequently prescribed for stone prevention. Potassium citrate is almost universally prescribed for calcium, uric acid and cystine stone formers [23]. It can be useful for those who fail to increase urine volume, even if urine citrate excretion is normal. One could make a case that prescription of potassium citrate would be useful for prevention of all calcium stones and could be used in "unselected" cases, in other words, when 24-h urine data are not available. Such an approach is supported by observational studies and randomized controlled trials [24,25]. Sodium citrate is not preferred given the promotion of calciuria by the sodium load. I have often prescribed potassium citrate to use before athletic events, airplane flights, trips to the operating room, and at bedtime. Again, this is not an evidence-based approach but seems commonsensical.

Uric acid and cystine stones *in situ* can be dissolved if urine pH is maintained at values of 6.5 or 7.0 respectively around the clock. This approach usually requires administration of potassium citrate 10–30 mEq 2–3 times per day. Uric acid stones can be prevented by nocturnal treatment alone, once a day, but this approach would probably not suffice for cystine stones [26]. I have patients test urine pH using inexpensive test strips (see www.microessentialslab.com, item #067) rather than more expensive multitest strips. Patients test and record urine pH at least once a day at varying times and adjust doses appropriately. Prescription of allopurinol for uric acid stones is appropriate only if patients have gout or fail to adequately increase urine pH as may occur in people with chronic diarrhea or malabsorption syndromes [27].

Thiazides are probably underutilized for prevention of calcium stones, possibly because of the perception that they have metabolic side-effects. They have consistently been shown to prevent stones in randomized trials [28]. In addition, they are first-line agents for lowering blood pressure, especially systolic blood pressure. By lowering urine calcium excretion, thiazides are associated with increases in bone mineral density and reduction in fractures associated with osteoporosis, which often is found in people with hypercalciuria [29]. Administration with potassium citrate prevents hypokalemia, hyperglycemia, and hypocitraturia [30]. For prevention of calcium stones, prescription of allopurinol is currently reserved for people who do not have hypercalciuria, though the efficacy of urate-lowering therapy has not been tested in the presence of increased urine calcium excretion [31].

Management of struvite stones requires meticulous endoscopic removal of all stone fragments and usually low-dose suppressive antibiotics for at least 6 months [32]. Recalcitrant and recurrent stones and those less amenable to surgical removal may benefit from acetohydroxamic acid, though its side-effect profile does not make its use easy [33].

Conclusion

The kidney stone clinic is a concept that patients with recurrent kidney stones find attractive and sensible. A multidisciplinary approach to kidney stones leads to expertise and familiarity with urological and preventive regimens. The result is attention to the details of fluid, dietary and medical therapies that otherwise may be utilized in an haphazard and arbitrary fashion.

Understandably, the kidney stone field often seems dominated by a surgical approach: remove offending stones and move on. For a disorder that can successfully be prevented, more easily perhaps than hypertension and diabetes, incredibly little attention is given to the training of internists, nephrologists and urologists to actually implement preventive regimens for this highly prevalent disorder. There is a clear need for participation of today's trainees in a multidisciplinary kidney stone prevention program and a clear need for practitioners to offer appropriate time and expertise to our patients.

References

1. Penniston KL, Nakada SY. Diet and alternative therapies in the management of stone disease. Urol Clin North Am 2013; 40: 31–46.
2. Rodman JS, Sosa RE, Seidman C, et al. *No More Kidney Stones*. Hoboken, NJ: John Wiley, 2007.
3. Tiselius HG. Patients' attitudes on how to deal with the risk of future stone recurrences. Urol Res 2006; 34: 255–60.
4. Penniston KL, Nakada SY. Development of an instrument to assess the health related quality of life of kidney stone formers. J Urol 2013; 189: 921–30.
5. Saigal CS, Joyce G, Timilsina AR. Direct and indirect costs of nephrolithiasis in an employed population: opportunity for disease management? Kidney Int 2005; 68: 1808–14.
6. Grampsas SA, Moore M, Chandhoke PS. 10-year experience with extracorporeal shockwave lithotripsy in the state of Colorado. J Endourol 2000; 14: 711–14.
7. Lingeman J, Mardis H, Kahnoski R, et al. Medical reduction of stone risk in a network of treatment centers compared to a research clinic. J Urol 1998; 160: 1629–34.
8. Parks JH, Coward M, Coe FL. Correspondence between stone composition and urine supersaturation in nephrolithiasis. Kidney Int 1997; 51: 894–900.
9. Uribarri J, Oh MS, Carroll HJ. The first kidney stone. Ann Intern Med 1989; 111: 1006–9.
10. Parks JH, Goldfisher E, Asplin JR, et al. A single 24-hour urine collection is inadequate for the medical evaluation of nephrolithiasis. J Urol 2002; 167: 1607–12.
11. Sarkissian C, Noble M, Li J, et al. Patient decision making for asymptomatic renal calculi: balancing benefit and risk. Urology 2013; 81: 236–40.
12. Heilberg IP, Weisinger JR. Bone disease in idiopathic hypercalciuria. Curr Opin Nephrol Hypertens 2006; 15: 394–402.
13. Unnanuntana A, Gladnick BP, Donnelly E, et al. The assessment of fracture risk. J Bone Joint Surg Am 2010; 92: 743–53.
14. Fink HA, Wilt TJ, Eidman KE, et al. Medical management to prevent recurrent nephrolithiasis in adults: a systematic review for an American College of Physicians Clinical Guideline. Ann Intern Med 2013; 158: 535–43.
15. Borghi L, Meschi T, Amato F, et al. Urinary volume, water and recurrences in idiopathic calcium nephrolithiasis: a 5-year randomized prospective study. J Urol 1996; 155: 839–43.
16. Goldfarb DS, Fischer ME, Keich Y, et al. A twin study of genetic and dietary influences on nephrolithiasis: a report from the Vietnam Era Twin (VET) Registry. Kidney Int 2005; 67: 1053–61.

17. Borghi L, Schianchi T, Meschi T, et al. Comparison of two diets for the prevention of recurrent stones in idiopathic hypercalciuria. N Engl J Med 2002; 346: 77–84.
18. Taylor EN, Fung TT, Curhan GC. DASH-style diet associates with reduced risk for kidney stones. J Am Soc Nephrol 2009; 20: 2253–9.
19. Meschi T, Maggiore U, Fiaccadori E, et al. The effect of fruits and vegetables on urinary stone risk factors. Kidney Int 2004; 66: 2402–10.
20. Curhan GC, Willett WC, Rimm EB, et al. A prospective study of dietary calcium and other nutrients and the risk of symptomatic kidney stones. N Engl J Med 1993; 328: 833–8.
21. Jackson RD, LaCroix AZ, Gass M, et al. Calcium plus vitamin D supplementation and the risk of fractures. N Engl J Med 2006; 354: 669–83.
22. Levine BS, Rodman JS, Wienerman S, et al. Effect of calcium citrate supplementation on urinary calcium oxalate saturation in female stone formers: implications for prevention of osteoporosis. Am J Clin Nutr 1994; 60: 592–6.
23. Robinson MR, Leitao VA, Haleblian GE, et al. Impact of long-term potassium citrate therapy on urinary profiles and recurrent stone formation. J Urol 2009; 181: 1145–50.
24. Preminger GM, Harvey JA, Pak CY. Comparative efficacy of "specific" potassium citrate therapy versus conservative management in nephrolithiasis of mild to moderate severity. J Urol 1985; 134: 658–61.
25. Ettinger B, Pak CY, Citron JT, et al. Potassium-magnesium citrate is an effective prophylaxis against recurrent calcium oxalate nephrolithiasis. J Urol 1997; 158: 2069–73.
26. Rodman JS. Intermittent versus continuous alkaline therapy for uric acid stones and ureteral stones of uncertain composition. Urology 2002; 60: 378–82.
27. Maalouf NM, Cameron MA, Moe OW, et al. Novel insights into the pathogenesis of uric acid nephrolithiasis. Curr Opin Nephrol Hypertens 2004; 13: 181–9.
28. Pearle MS, Roehrborn CG, Pak CY. Meta-analysis of randomized trials for medical prevention of calcium oxalate nephrolithiasis. J Endourol 1999; 13: 679–85.
29. Adams JS, Song CF, Kantorovich V. Rapid recovery of bone mass in hypercalciuric, osteoporotic men treated with hydrochlorothiazide. Ann Intern Med 1999; 130: 658–60.
30. Huen SC, Goldfarb DS. Adverse metabolic side effects of thiazides: implications for patients with calcium nephrolithiasis. J Urol 2007; 177: 1238–43.
31. Ettinger B, Tang A, Citron JT, et al. Randomized trial of allopurinol in the prevention of calcium oxalate calculi. N Engl J Med 1986; 315: 1386–9.
32. Preminger GM, Assimos DG, Lingeman JE, et al. Chapter 1: AUA guideline on management of staghorn calculi: diagnosis and treatment recommendations. J Urol 2005; 173: 1991–2000.
33. Griffith DP, Gleeson MJ, Lee H, et al. Randomized, double-blind trial of Lithostat (acetohydroxamic acid) in the palliative treatment of infection-induced urinary calculi. Eur Urol 1991; 20: 243–7.

CHAPTER 2

Metabolic Evaluation: Interpretation of 24-Hour Urine Chemistries

John R. Asplin
Litholink Corporation *and* University of Chicago, Chicago, Il, USA

Introduction

The goals of metabolic evaluation are to provide a guide for treatment to reduce the risk of stone formation and to identify systemic disease presenting as kidney stone disease. As recommended by the NIH Consensus Conference, a limited work-up is appropriate for a patient with their first stone [1]. The limited work-up includes serum for electrolytes, calcium, and creatinine. Urine culture and/or urinalysis are needed to rule out urinary tract infection. If the stone is available, its composition should be determined. Radiological evaluation should be performed in all subjects presenting with their initial stone event, as a patient can only be considered a single stone former if no other stones are identified by imaging. Many patients have a non-contrast computed tomography (CT) scan when they present with their first attack of renal colic. If the symptomatic stone event resolved without radiological evaluation, a KUB X-ray or an ultrasound can be used to estimate stone burden. Ultrasound is often the preferred technique for children and pregnant women.

At the time of the initial stone event, if multiple stones are present on X-ray the patient should be considered a recurrent stone former and a full metabolic evaluation undertaken. The evaluation includes serum chemistries and 24-hurine collection(s) to identify the patient's specific risk factors for stone disease. In the case of children with stone disease, an extended evaluation should always be performed at initial presentation. Children are more likely to have inherited diseases such as cystinuria and primary hyperoxaluria as the cause of their stones [2]. The details of the laboratory evaluation of the stone patient are the focus of this chapter.

Urinary Stones: Medical and Surgical Management, First Edition. Edited by Michael Grasso and David S. Goldfarb.

Serum chemistries

Measurement of serum chemistries is an important part of the metabolic evaluation of the stone former. Serum creatinine provides an estimate of kidney function. Electrolytes are used to screen for renal tubular acidosis, looking for the presence of acidosis or hypokalemia. Serum calcium should be used to screen for hyperparathyroidism and other mineral disorders. Even minimal elevations of serum calcium should be evaluated with repeat testing accompanied by parathyroid hormone measurement. Serum measurements need to be repeated during active drug therapy for stone prevention to monitor for hypokalemia and hyponatremia from thiazides and hyperkalemia from potassium alkali.

Stone analysis

Stone analysis should be performed on whatever stones are passed or removed surgically at initial presentation. If a patient has not had stone analysis but has saved stones from past episodes of renal colic, those stones can be sent for analysis. Optimally, stone analysis should be performed by infra-red (IR) analysis or X-ray diffraction. Optical microscopy is often employed as an adjunct to IR or X-ray [3].

Knowledge of kidney stone composition guides prophylactic therapy in concert with urine chemistries. Less common stones such as ammonium acid urate and xanthine are usually diagnosed by stone analysis. The stone analysis is the only way to diagnose stones composed of medications or their metabolites [4]. Once prophylactic therapy has been initiated, stones that form subsequently should be analyzed. Patients can form different types of stones and in fact, may transform from one stone type to another during medical therapy [5]. If stone analysis does not match the stone type that would be expected from urine chemistries, consider the possibility that the stone may have formed years earlier and became symptomatic only recently. In such a situation a search for changes in diet, environment or other transient medical problems might reveal the cause of stones.

24-hour urine chemistries

Standard medical practice calls for 24-h urine collection(s) to identify the risk factors leading to stones. Table 2.1 provides a list of urine tests to be performed on the 24-h sample. The tests in the left-hand column are the minimum set of tests for a stone evaluation. Inclusion of the tests in the right-hand column allows better understanding of diet and physiology related to stone formation. In addition, as to what to measure, the clinician needs to decide the conditions for the collection. Most

Table 2.1 Analytes to be measured in 24-h urine collections

Minimum evaluation	Additional tests for complete evaluation
Volume	Phosphorus
Calcium	Magnesium
Oxalate	Sodium
Citrate	Potassium
Uric acid	Chloride
pH	Urea nitrogen
Creatinine	Sulfate
	Ammonium
	Supersaturations

commonly, urine collections are done with the patient consuming their normal diet and fluid intake in order to identify the factors that contributed to the formation of the stones. Whether the patient should be kept on supplements, such as calcium pills, that can alter stone risk factors is up to the individual physician. However, the clinician needs to know whether the patient was taking these kinds of pills in order to properly interpret the results. Metabolic evaluation is an outpatient process; 24-h urine collections should not be done in the hospital as a convenience for the patient. In-hospital collections should be considered only for young children who may need catheterization to get an adequate sample.

One issue that clinicians need to consider is how many 24-h urine collections should be performed. In outpatients, serum values are fairly stable day to day, but urine chemistries can vary significantly based on changes in diet and environment [6]. Table 2.2 shows data on the variability of the key stone risk factors in urine samples done on consecutive days by stone-forming patients [7]. Over one-third of urine samples showed at least a 50% variation in excretion of at least one of the critical variables. Finding such variations provides the clinician with an opportunity to identify lifestyle or dietary factors that have influenced the urine chemistries. In an optimal situation, the patient has done one collection on a work-day and the other collection when at home as one environment may be particularly conducive to stone formation.

A common question is whether a random, untimed urine specimen can be used in place of a 24-h collection as a convenience for the patient, expressing all results as a ratio with creatinine to adjust for the level of urine concentration. There are no studies which show sufficiently good correlations between spot urines and 24-h excretion rates for the main stone risk factors to recommend routine use of spot urines. In some situations, as in children who are not toilet trained, spot urines are used out of necessity.

Table 2.2 Variability of 24-h urine chemistries between two consecutive collections

	Greater than 25% variability	Greater than 50% variability
Volume	36%	15%
Calcium	20%	12%
Oxalate	20%	6%
Citrate	24%	10%
Uric acid	15%	3%
Any of the above	67%	36%

Calculated from 17,150 paired urine collections. Only sample pairs with creatinine excretion within 10% were included in the analysis. Source: Asplin 2008 [7]. Reproduced with permission of Elsevier.

Normal ranges and stone risk levels for excretion rates in children are usually defined in relation to body size or urine creatinine, which is beyond the scope of this chapter. When values are presented, they are for an adult population. When interpreting urine chemistries, it is wise to remember that definitions of abnormal in the literature are for research purposes. Urine chemistries are continuous variables and strict cut-points of normal and abnormal are somewhat arbitrary. The risk of stone formation increases as values trend toward the limit of the normal range for lithogenic factors such as calcium, oxalate, citrate,and uric acid [8].

Volume and creatinine

The volume of urine excreted per day is a critical measurement for the management of stone patients. Low urine flow is a major risk factor for stones, raising the supersaturation of all stone-forming salts. Borghi's prospective trial of high fluid intake provides a reasonable goal for stone-forming patients, as the intervention group in that study increased their urine volume to approximately 2.5 L per day [9]. Urine volumes above 2.5 L per day provide even greater benefit, but many patients have trouble maintaining such a high urine flow. Urine flow will be determined by the amount of fluid consumed and the amount lost from perspiration and the gut. It is best to give the patient a goal of urine flow rather than a set fluid intake, since non-renal fluid losses are difficult to quantify.

Urine volume should not be used to estimate the completeness of a urine collection but rather adequacy of collection should be judged by creatinine excretion. Creatinine is a waste product of muscle metabolism; production of creatinine remains stable over time as long as muscle mass does not change. For the initial 24-h urine collection, one can estimate the

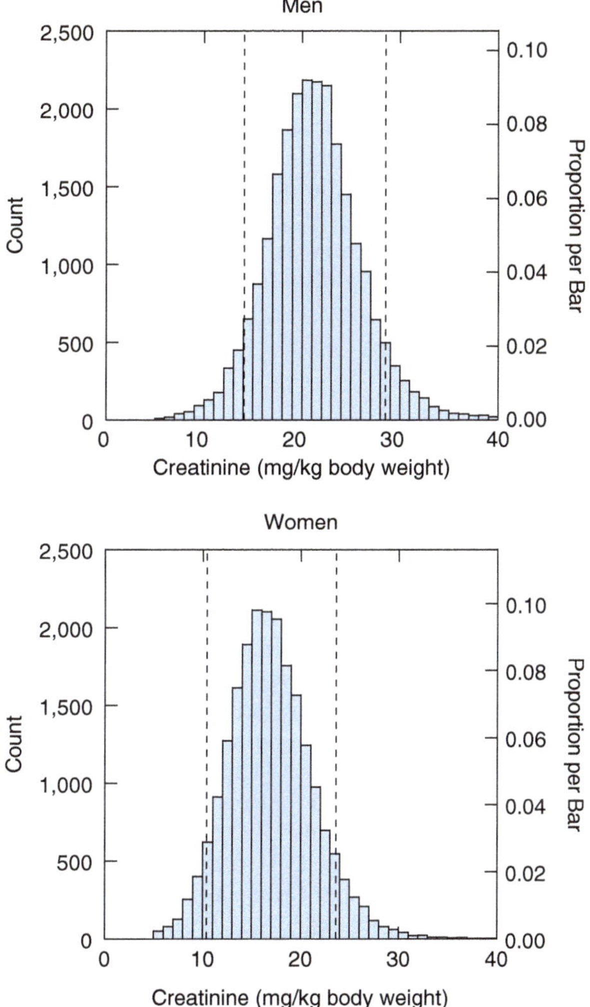

Figure 2.1 Histograms of creatinine/kg body weight ratios for male (n = 24,006) and female (n = 21,924) patients with urolithiasis. The vertical lines identify 1.5 standard deviations from the mean.

expected creatinine excretion from the subject's weight, with men having a higher creatinine/kg than women on average. Figure 2.1 shows creatinine/kg ratios of 45,930 patients from Litholink® Corporation. The vertical lines in the figures encompass 1.5 standard deviations (SD) from the mean, providing a range to use clinically. Of course, expectations for creatinine/kg values should be adjusted by the patient's body habitus; a muscular young man would be expected to have a higher level than an obese older man. If multiple urines are collected during the initial evaluation, then comparison of creatinine from day to day provides an even better guide of collection quality as the creatinine excretion should be the same on both days. The same is true of urine collections done in follow-up; creatinine excretion should be within 20% of the baseline samples. Some patients have urine volumes less than 0.5 L/day but the urine collection is complete as judged by the quantity of creatinine excreted. To discount such urines as inadequate would miss a major contributor to the patient's stone disease.

Calcium

Hypercalciuria is found in approximately 50% of calcium stone formers, making it the most common metabolic abnormality in stone patients. Hypercalciuria is generally defined as 300 mg/day in men and >250 mg/day in women. When interpreting urine calcium excretion, it is important to take into account dietary intake of calcium which can be assessed by the amount of dairy product consumed per day and intake of calcium supplements. Dietary intake of sodium and protein can also influence calcium excretion [10,11]. Urine sodium and urea excretion can be used to estimate the dietary intake of these substances (see below). Before considering pharmacological intervention for hypercalciuria, it is best to determine if dietary intervention (sodium or protein restriction) may be sufficient to resolve the hypercalciuria [12].

Since calcium excretion is dependent on diet, some investigators have proposed evaluating patients on controlled diets to better define the pathophysiology of the hypercalciuria [13]. Typically a patient is put on a restricted calcium and sodium diet for a week, collects a 24-h urine and then has an acute calcium load test. The premise of this evaluation is to differentiate patients who have intestinal hyperabsorption of calcium from those with hypercalciuria due to renal leak of calcium or excessive bone resorption. Such an evaluation is cumbersome and the benefit of this classification in routine clinical care is unclear. It had been promoted as a way to identify patients who could safely be managed with low calcium diet. However, with the recognition that many patients classified as having "absorptive hypercalciuria" actually have reduced bone mineral density and epidemiological studies linking low calcium diet to increased risk of incident stone formation, low calcium diets are seldom if ever used to treat hypercalciuria, rendering this classification scheme a moot point in clinical care [14,15].

At times, urine calcium will be found to be low in a kidney stone patient. Though not a risk factor for kidney stones, it often heralds significant disease that can affect stone risk. Most commonly, low urine calcium is due to bowel disease with malabsorption, chronic kidney disease, or severe vitamin

D deficiency. A low dietary intake of calcium or the use of thiazide diuretics lowers urine calcium but seldom into the pathologically low range.

Oxalate

Oxalate in the urine originates from diet and endogenous metabolism [16]. Oxalate salts are poorly soluble, accounting for the observation that calcium oxalate is the most common component of kidney stones. Hyperoxaluria is found in 30% of stone patients. The common upper limit of normal for oxalate excretion is 45 mg/day (0.5 mmol/day), though risk of stone formation increases even as oxalate increases within the normal range [8]. Because of the high calcium to oxalate ratio in urine, small increases in urine oxalate excretion have a significant influence on calcium oxalate supersaturation.

Mild elevations of urine oxalate are usually due to high dietary intake of oxalate or oxalate precursors. Common foods with high oxalate content include spinach, rhubarb, nuts, tea, and chocolate, though high intake of foods with even moderate oxalate content can lead to hyperoxaluria. Use of vitamin C supplements can lead to hyperoxaluria, though issues with *in vitro* conversion of vitamin C to oxalate when urine pH is high make interpretation of oxalate values difficult [17,18]. It is best to have patients stop vitamin C supplements during urine collection to avoid assay problems and overestimation of oxalate excretion due to *in vitro* conversion. When oxalate excretion exceeds 88 mg/day (1 mmol/day), the clinician should consider primary hyperoxaluria or enteric hyperoxaluria as possible causes. Most cases of enteric hyperoxaluria are accompanied by obvious bowel disease such as Crohn's disease or have had significant intestinal surgery, including bariatric surgery such as Roux-en-Y gastric bypass [19]. However, for unexplained persistent hyperoxaluria, more subtle forms of bowel disease should be considered such as celiac disease [20].

Citrate

Citrate is an organic anion present in the urine that reduces the risk of calcium stone formation. Citrate complexes calcium, reducing the amount of calcium free to bind with oxalate or phosphate. In addition, citrate has direct inhibitory effects on crystal growth. Therefore, low urine citrate is a risk factor for calcium stone formation. Hypocitraturia is found in approximately 30% of stone patients. Citrate levels tend to be higher in women than in men.

Low urine citrate may be either idiopathic or secondary to acidosis or hypokalemia [21]. The finding of hypocitraturia with a urine pH greater than 6.0 raises the possibility of distal renal tubular acidosis. A fall in urine citrate when treating hypercalciuria with thiazide could represent potassium depletion. Hypocitraturia can be treated by administration of alkali salts, though results of such therapy should be monitored with 24-h urine collections to be sure the patient is responding with an appropriate increase in urine citrate and not just an isolated increase in urine pH, which could increase the risk of calcium phosphate stones.

Uric acid

Uric acid is the end-product of purine metabolism in humans. Uric acid can crystallize into stones itself or can promote the formation of calcium oxalate stones, so measurement of uric acid excretion is a critical component of the metabolic evaluation. The pKa of uric acid in urine is 5.4. The fully protonated form of uric acid is poorly soluble so acidic urine is a more important determinant of uric acid stone risk than uric acid excretion [22]. However, at very high levels of uric acid excretion, stones may form even in the absence of an acidic urine or low urine flow rate. Severe hyperuricosuria may indicate the presence of an inborn error of purine metabolism, particularly if markers of protein intake are not excessive. Dietary protein and purine are from the same foods so estimating diet protein from urea excretion provides an indirect assessment of dietary purine (Figure 2.2).

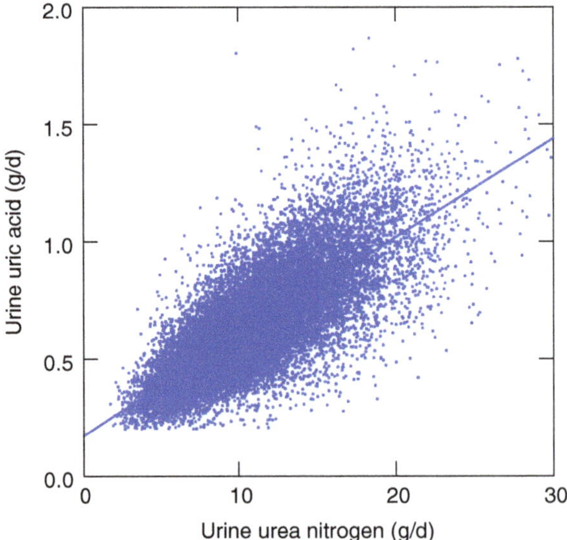

Figure 2.2 Plot of urine urea nitrogen excretion versus uric acid excretion in 45,930 patients with urolithiasis. The line is the linear regression, $r = 0.76$, $p < 0.001$.

pH

Urine pH is one of the most critical measurements in the metabolic evaluation, but is often overlooked. The formation of calcium oxalate stones is fairly independent of urine pH but the crystallization of calcium phosphate, uric acid, struvite, and cystine are all pH dependent in the range found in human urine. Human urine pH can vary from 4.5 to 8.0, but in normal healthy subjects the mean urine pH over 24 h is 5.7–6.3. Figure 2.3 shows the effect of urine pH on the supersaturation of calcium phosphate and uric acid. As can be seen, uric acid risk is greatest at urine pH below 5.5 and calcium phosphate at pH above 6.5. The mean urine pH of healthy people is in the range that would minimize the risk of crystallization of either uric acid or calcium phosphate. Common causes of low urine pH include high dietary acid from high-protein diets, loss of alkali from diarrhea, and metabolic syndrome. High urine pH is seen with vegetarian diets, use of alkali supplements, acidification disorders of the kidney such as distal renal tubular acidosis, or in urinary tract infection caused by bacteria that possess urease activity.

Urine pH is commonly available from a single spot urine specimen. This is not an adequate assessment as urine pH covers too large a range in normal subjects for any single measurement to have clinical significance. Urine pH should either be evaluated by measuring pH on multiple spot urines per day or by measuring pH of a 24-h urine collection.

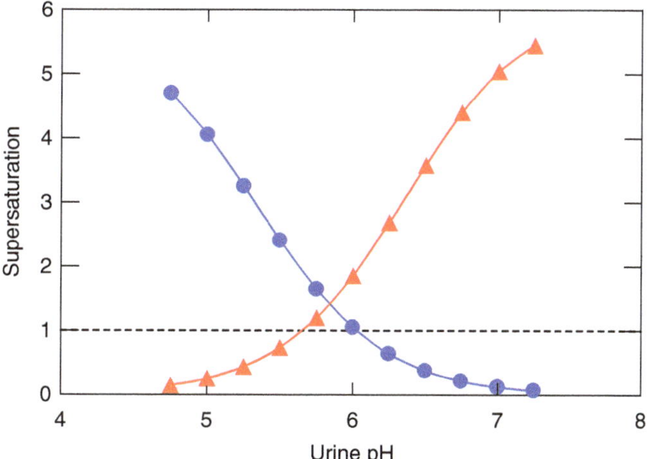

Figure 2.3 Plot of uric acid supersaturation (*circles*) and calcium phosphate supersaturation (*triangles*) versus pH. Supersaturation was calculated with Equil 2 software, using fixed urine concentrations of all chemsitries while varying urine pH. The horizontal line indicates the saturation point.

Sodium and potassium

Dietary sodium is almost completely absorbed by the intestines when gut function is normal. Therefore, in the steady state, urine sodium excretion will approximate dietary sodium intake. Volume expansion caused by high diet sodium is a key factor in driving urine calcium excretion, so management of hypercalciuria should include a reduction of dietary sodium, and therefore sodium excretion, to 100–120 mmol/day. Sodium excretion is still an accurate measure of diet sodium intake even when the patient is on diuretics, once the patient has been on a stable dose for 2 weeks. When a patient has chronic diarrhea or excess sweating from exercise or working in a hot environment, urine sodium will not match dietary sodium. However, the urine sodium excretion will reflect the volume status of the patient, which is more germane to the risk of stone formation than the dietary sodium.

Urine potassium is a marker of dietary potassium intake, assuming normal gut function. The most useful aspect of urine potassium measurement is to monitor treatment with potassium citrate. If a patient's urine potassium does not increase significantly during treatment with potassium salts, the clinician can assume the patient is not taking or is not absorbing the medication. Potassium is a more reliable estimate of compliance than changes in citrate excretion, as citrate excretion is influenced by many factors.

Phosphorus

Approximately 10–15% of calcium stones have calcium phosphate as their major component, and many calcium oxalate contain small amounts of calcium phosphate as the stone nidus [23]. The pKa for the monohydrogen/dihydrogen phosphate buffer is 6.8. As urine pH rises, the fraction of phosphate existing as monohydrogen phosphate increases, which is the form of phosphate that crystallizes with calcium. Because of this, pH is a much more important determinant of calcium phosphate stone formation than actual phosphate excretion. However, without a phosphorus measurement (all inorganic phosphorus exists as phosphate), calcium phosphate supersaturation cannot be calculated.

Magnesium

Approximately 40–50% of dietary magnesium is absorbed from the diet and in steady-state conditions is then excreted in the urine. Hypomagnesuria (<60 mg/day) is felt to be a risk factor for stone formation and usually represents inadequate dietary intake of magnesium or reduced absorption due to intestinal malabsorption [24]. Low urine magnesium is often a better indicator of body stores than serum magnesium levels. There have not been any prospective controlled trials of magnesium repletion in magnesium-deficient stone-forming patients. Very high magnesium excretion may be an indication of use of magnesium-containing laxatives, and should be noted in any patient in whom diarrhea is suspected of being a cause of stone formation.

Sulfate and urea

Urine sulfate and urea are both waste products of protein metabolism. Sulfate is generated by the metabolism of cysteine and methionine, while urea is an end-product of all amino acid metabolism [25]. These urine chemistries mark protein intake only if the patient is in protein balance, a reasonable assumption in the outpatient evaluation of a kidney stone patient.

Sulfate is only generated by metabolism of sulfur-containing amino acids, which are present in highest concentration in animal flesh and in lower concentrations in vegetable protein. Thus sulfate excretion is high when intake of animal protein is high. There may be a dissociation of urea and sulfate excretion, which suggests high intake of protein/amino acids of low biological value. However, in the vast majority of people, sulfate and urea excretion are highly correlated. Sulfate provides an estimate of animal protein intake and is an indicator of dietary acid load, as sulfur amino acids are oxidized to sulfuric acid, which is excreted as sulfate [25].

Protein intake is important to quantify since it influences multiple lithogenic factors. The acid load associated with high-protein diets will lower urine pH promoting uric acid stone formation, and lower urine citrate excretion promoting calcium oxalate stone formation. Since protein intake is strongly associated with purine intake, high protein intake often lead to hyperuricosuria. Finally, high protein intake increases urine calcium excretion. High-protein diets used for weight loss, such as the Atkins diet, have been associated with an increased risk of urolithiasis [26].

Ammonium

Ammonium is produced in the proximal renal tubule cells via metabolism of glutamine. Excretion of ammonium is one way in which the kidney excretes daily acid load and, as opposed to titratable acid, allows the acid load to be excreted at a higher pH, reducing the risk of uric acid stone formation. The interpretation of urine ammonium paired with urine pH provides insights into the patient's acid–base status and stone risk. When urine pH is less than 6 and ammonium excretion is high, this suggests the presence of an acid load, usually from a high-protein diet or chronic diarrhea [25]. When acidosis is of short duration, ammonium excretion may only be mildly elevated as a few days are required to reach maximal levels. When ammonium is low in the presence of a urine pH above 6, this suggests a high-alkaline diet or treatment with alkali salts. Effectiveness of alkali therapy can be monitored by changes in pH and suppression of ammonium production. When ammonium excretion is high and urine pH is above 7, consider infection or colonization with urease-producing organisms such as *Proteus* species [27].

Supersaturation of stone-forming salts

Supersaturation can be thought of as the chemical driving force for crystallization of a particular salt. As supersaturation increases, the risk of nucleation and growth of crystals increases. Clinical laboratories specializing in urolithiasis frequently offer computer calculations of supersaturation values [28]. In the initial evaluation, supersaturations act as a surrogate for a stone analysis, if none is available. Supersaturations have been shown to be highly correlated to the type of stones a patient forms [29]. The baseline supersaturation values help define the goal of therapy, which should be at least a 50% reduction of the pertinent supersaturation during therapy. Such a reduction has been shown to correlate with an 80% reduction in stone formation [29].

References

1. NIH Consensus Conference. Prevention and treatment of kidney stones. JAMA 1988; 260: 978–81.
2. Sas DJ. An update on the changing epidemiology and metabolic risk factors in pediatric kidney stone disease. Clin J Am Soc Nephrol 2011; 6(8): 2062–8.
3. Mandel G, Mandel N. Analysis of stones. In: Coe FL, Favus MJ, Pak CYC, Parks JH, Preminger GM, eds. *Kidney Stones: Medical and Surgical Management.* Philadelphia: Lippincott-Raven, 1996, pp. 323–36.
4. Daudon M, Jungers P. Drug-induced renal calculi: epidemiology, prevention and management. Drugs 2004; 64(3): 245–75.
5. Mandel N, Mandel I, Fryjoff K, Rejniak T, Mandel G. Conversion of calcium oxalate to calcium phosphate with recurrent stone episodes. J Urol 2003; 169(6): 2026–9.
6. Parks JH, Goldfisher E, Asplin JR, Coe FL. A single 24-hour urine collection is inadequate for the medical evaluation of nephrolithiasis. J Urol 2002; 167(4): 1607–12.
7. Asplin JR. Evaluation of the kidney stone patient. Semin Nephrol 2008; 28(2): 99–110.
8. Curhan GC, Willett WC, Speizer FE, Stampfer MJ. Twenty-four-hour urine chemistries and the risk of kidney stones among women and men. Kidney Int 2001; 59(6): 2290–8.
9. Borghi L, Meschi T, Amato F, Briganti A, Novarini A, Giannini A. Urinary volume, water and recurrences in idiopathic calcium nephrolithiasis: a 5-year randomized prospective study. J Urol 1996; 155(3): 839–43.

10. Sakhaee K, Harvey JA, Padalino PK, Whitson P, Pak CY. The potential role of salt abuse on the risk for kidney stone formation. J Urol 1993; 150(2 Pt 1): 310–12.
11. Licata AA, Bou E, Bartter FC, Cox J. Effects of dietary protein on urinary calcium in normal subjects and in patients with nephrolithiasis. Metabolism 1979; 28(9): 895–900.
12. Borghi L, Schianchi T, Meschi T, et al. Comparison of two diets for the prevention of recurrent stones in idiopathic hypercalciuria. N Engl J Med 2002; 346(2): 77–84.
13. Levy FL, Adams-Huet B, Pak CY. Ambulatory evaluation of nephrolithiasis: an update of a 1980 protocol. Am J Med 1995; 98(1): 50–9.
14. Pietschmann F, Breslau NA, Pak CY. Reduced vertebral bone density in hypercalciuric nephrolithiasis. J Bone Miner Res 1992; 7(12): 1383–8.
15. Curhan GC, Willett WC, Rimm EB, Stampfer MJ. A prospective study of dietary calcium and other nutrients and the risk of symptomatic kidney stones. N Engl J Med 1993; 328(12): 833–8.
16. Holmes RP, Goodman HO, Assimos DG. Contribution of dietary oxalate to urinary oxalate excretion. Kidney Int 2001; 59(1): 270–6.
17. Traxer O, Huet B, Poindexter J, Pak CY, Pearle MS. Effect of ascorbic acid consumption on urinary stone risk factors. J Urol 2003; 170(2 Pt 1): 397–401.
18. Urivetzky M, Kessaris D, Smith AD. Ascorbic acid overdosing: a risk factor for calcium oxalate nephrolithiasis. J Urol 1992; 147(5): 1215–18.
19. Patel BN, Passman CM, Fernandez A, et al. Prevalence of hyperoxaluria after bariatric surgery. J Urol 2009; 181(1): 161–6.
20. Ciacci C, Spagnuolo G, Tortora R, et al. Urinary stone disease in adults with celiac disease: prevalence, incidence and urinary determinants. J Urol 2008; 180(3): 974–9.
21. Hamm LL. Renal handling of citrate. Kidney Int 1990; 38(4): 728–35.
22. Kenny JE, Goldfarb DS. Update on the pathophysiology and management of uric acid renal stones. Curr Rheumatol Rep 2010; 12(2): 125–9.
23. Mandel NS, Mandel GS. Urinary tract stone disease in the United States veteran population. II. Geographical analysis of variations in composition. J Urol 1989; 142(6): 1516–21.
24. Preminger GM, Baker S, Peterson R, Poindexter J, Pak CYC. Hypomagnesiuric hypocitraturia: an apparent new entity for calcium nephrolithiasis. J Lithotripsy Stone Dis 1989; 1: 22–5.
25. Lemann J Jr, Relman AS. The relation of sulfur metabolism to acid–base balance and electrolyte excretion: the effects of dl-methionine in normal man. J Clin Invest 1959; 38: 2215–23.
26. Reddy ST, Wang CY, Sakhaee K, Brinkley L, Pak CY. Effect of low-carbohydrate high-protein diets on acid–base balance, stone-forming propensity, and calcium metabolism. Am J Kidney Dis 2002; 40(2): 265–74.
27. Healy KA, Ogan K. Pathophysiology and management of infectious staghorn calculi. Urol Clin North Am 2007; 34(3): 363–74.
28. Werness PG, Brown CM, Smith LH, Finlayson B. EQUIL 2: a basic computer program for the calculation of urinary saturation. J Urol 1985; 134: 1242–4.
29. Parks JH, Coward M, Coe FL. Correspondence between stone composition and urine supersaturation in nephrolithiasis. Kidney Int 1997; 51(3): 894–900.

CHAPTER 3

Uric Acid Stones

Naim M. Maalouf
University of Texas Southwestern Medical Center, Dallas, TX, USA

Do's and don'ts box

Do:

- send stone for analysis to confirm the diagnosis in cases of suspected uric acid urolithiasis
- have patients with uric acid stones collect a 24-h for stone risk profile (including urine pH)
- use potassium citrate as initial management for patients with uric acid stones and low urine pH.

Don't:

- use X-rays (e.g. KUB) to detect or follow uric acid stones, as they are radiolucent on plain radiographs
- start every patient with uric acid stones on urate-lowering agents (such as allopurinol)
- consider urological intervention as first-line therapy for uric acid stones

Introduction

Uric acid stones constitute around 10–20% of all urolithiasis cases, but are particularly more common among obese and diabetic stone formers, a growing segment of the population of industrialized countries. The principal abnormality responsible for uric acid precipitation and stone formation is an overly acidic urine, which makes urine pH a therapeutic target in the management of this condition. This chapter reviews the epidemiology, pathogenesis, and diagnosis of uric acid urolithiasis, and focuses on the management of uric acid stone formers.

Urinary Stones: Medical and Surgical Management, First Edition. Edited by Michael Grasso and David S. Goldfarb.

Epidemiology of uric acid stones

The prevalence of uric acid (UA) stones varies considerably between different countries. In large retrospective series, UA stones were the predominant component of 5–10% of all kidney stones analyzed in the US and the UK, 25% in Germany, and 30% in the Middle East [1]. These regional differences are in part related to environmental (climate, diet) and genetic factors. In addition to geographical variation, temporal increases in UA stones have recently been described [2], which have been ascribed to the aging population and the rising prevalence of obesity and its associated complications [2]. In fact, UA stones are significantly more common among stone formers who are diabetic [3], obese [4] or suffer from the metabolic syndrome [5]. Uric acid stones are also prevalent in individuals with gout [6] or with congenital disorders of uric acid metabolism [7]. Finally, uric acid stones have been described during a recent outbreak of kidney stones in children related to consumption of melamine-contaminated infant formula [8].

Pathogenesis of uric acid stones

The pathogenesis of UA stones is complex and diverse, and has been ascribed to acquired as well as inherited conditions [9]. In studies that have compared UA stone formers to calcium stone formers or non-stone-forming controls, three major urinary abnormalities have been described: low urine pH, low urine volume, and elevated urine uric acid [10,11].

A low urine pH is a key and major risk factor for UA crystallization and stone formation. This is due to dissociation of uric acid in urine according to the chemical equation: uric acid $\leftrightarrow$ H^+ + $urate^-$. At a urinary pH of 5.5 (the pKa of uric acid), half of the UA is in its sparingly soluble undissociated form, with the other half in the more soluble $urate^-$ form. These proportions vary widely as urine pH fluctuates in any given individual, with lower urine pH predisposing to greater UA precipitation. At a urine pH of 6.0, UA solubility is around 600 mg/L. Therefore 2 L of urine output at a urinary pH of 6.0 are needed to maintain a typical daily uric acid excretion of 1200 mg/day in solution and prevent uric acid crystallization and stone formation (Figure 3.1).

The vast majority of UA stone formers exhibit a urine pH less than 5.5 on 24-h urine collection [10,11], with persistently lower urine pH compared to non-stone-forming volunteers despite significant diurnal variation [12]. This overly acidic urine may be caused by chronic diarrheal states [13], excessive dietary animal protein intake [14], or strenuous exercise [15]. However, the majority of UA stone formers exhibit low urine pH despite the absence of these risk factors, and are therefore said to have idiopathic UA stone formation. In this subgroup, the overly acidic urine has been ascribed to two main pathophysiological abnormalities: greater

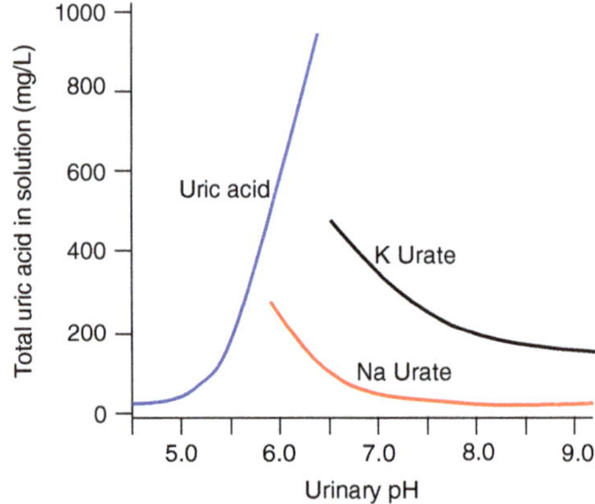

Figure 3.1 Solubility of uric acid and its sodium and potassium salts in urine according to ambient pH. Source: Data from Pak et al. J Clin Invest 1977; 59: 426–31, and reproduced from Moe et al. 2002 [1]. Reproduced with permission of Elsevier.
Note that:
1. *uric acid is relatively insoluble at low urine pH (below 5.5)*
2. *at a urine pH of 6.0, uric acid solubility is around 600 mg/L. Therefore 2 L of urine output at a urinary pH of 6.0 are needed to maintain a typical daily uric acid excretion of 1200 mg/day in solution and prevent uric acid crystallization/ stone formation*
3. *potassium urate is more soluble than sodium urate at a given urine pH, hence the preferred use of potassium salts (e.g. potassium citrate) over sodium salts (e.g. sodium bicarbonate) to alkalinize the urine of uric acid stone formers.*

net acid excretion and inadequate urinary buffering of this excessive acid due to impaired ammonium excretion [11,12].

Excessive urinary UA excretion (hyperuricosuria) may predispose to UA stones, but is only observed in a minority of UA stone formers. Hyperuricosuria may be related to excessive UA production as in gout, lymphoproliferative or myeloproliferative disorders (leukemias, polycythemia, hemolytic disorders, hemoglobinopathies), or inherited disorders of UA metabolism (such as Lesch–Nyhan syndrome, hypoxanthine-guanine phosphoribosyltransferase deficiency, and some glycogen storage diseases). Alternatively, hyperuricosuria may result from impaired renal UA reabsorption, due to either congenital conditions [16] or acquired states such as intake of uricosuric medications (probenecid, losartan, and high-dose aspirin).

A low urine volume increases the urinary concentration of UA, predisposing to UA stone formation. Low urine volume can be seen in patients with chronic diarrhea or excessive perspiration. While low urine volume alone is unlikely to result in UA nephrolithiasis, it can contribute to this condition in patients with other predisposing factors.

Diagnosis of uric acid stones

Patients with UA stones may present with typical symptoms of renal colic (colicky flank pain radiating to the groin, at times associated with nausea and vomiting), dysuria or hematuria. Stones may be asymptomatic and discovered incidentally on imaging studies. Some patients report passage of orange-colored gravel in their urine.

Unlike the more common calcium-containing stones, UA stones are radiolucent and may not be visualized on plain abdominal radiographs (KUB), at times delaying the diagnosis. However, UA stones are readily visualized on computed tomography (CT) and are recognized as filling defects on intravenous urography (IVP). Because of lower cost and radiation exposure, ultrasound may be a better imaging modality than CT scan to follow stone burden in UA stone formers.

The definitive diagnosis of UA stones is made by stone analysis. Whenever possible, stone analysis should be obtained in first-time stone formers, and in stone formers who are more likely to present with UA stones (such stone formers who are obese, who suffer from gout or diabetes, or have chronic diarrhea). Recent studies have suggested that UA stones may be differentiated from calcium stones on CT scan due to differences in attenuation [17], although this modality for identifying UA stones in patients with suspected renal colic remains a research tool at this time [18,19].

Management of uric acid stone formers

Metabolic evaluation

In view of the high rate of stone recurrence and the significant morbidity associated with recurrent stone episodes, a metabolic evaluation is recommended to guide the management of UA stone formers. As part of this evaluation, a history focused on identifying factors contributing to UA stone formation is recommended. This includes past medical history (e.g. gout, chronic diarrhea), medication use (e.g. uricosuric drugs, allopurinol), environmental exposure (excessive heat, profuse sweating), and dietary history (animal protein intake, fluid intake). Laboratory studies recommended in all UA stone formers include serum chemistry profile (electrolytes, renal function, serum UA) and 24-h urine stone risk profile (including urine volume, pH, uric acid, sulfate, sodium, potassium, and others). Urine pH measurement by pH electrode (rather than by the less accurate and reproducible measurement by dipstick) is a key component of metabolic evaluation of UA stone formers. Subsequent management is directed at correcting the underlying metabolic abnormalities that lead to UA stone formation, with a particular focus on low urine pH, hyperuricosuria and low urine volume (Figure 3.2).

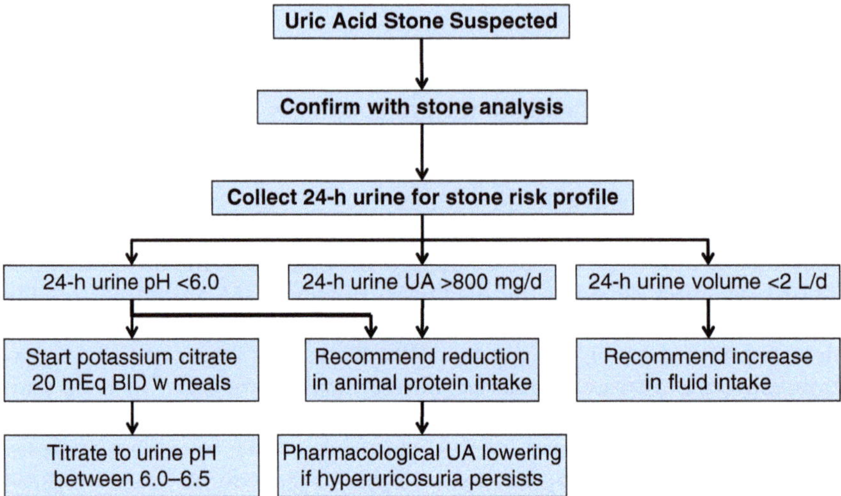

Figure 3.2 Evaluation and management of uric acid nephrolithiasis.

Lifestyle interventions

Correction of low urine pH is the cornerstone of therapy in uric acid nephrolithiasis. Dietary intake of animal proteins confers an acid load and lowers urine pH, due to the generation of protons during the oxidation of sulfur-containing amino acids in animal proteins to sulfuric acid [20]. Reduction in dietary intake of animal proteins should therefore be recommended to all UA stone formers (see Figure 3.2). Lowering animal protein intake is associated with a rise in urine pH and a decline in urine UA excretion, further reducing urinary saturation with respect to uric acid [21]. Increasing fluid intake should be recommended to reduce urinary saturation, especially in patients with low urine volume, with a goal of maintaining a urinary volume over 2 L a day. Consumption of certain fruit juices such as orange juice and grapefruit juice provides an alkali load and increases urine pH in addition to raising urine volume [22,23,24]. Other citrus fruit juices (in particular lemonade) may not raise urine pH to a significant extent [24].

Pharmacological therapy

The initial treatment of patients with UA stones consists of medical dissolution therapy as this non-invasive approach is successful in most cases [25,26,27]. Urinary alkalinization results in dissolution of existing stones and prevents stones from recurring [28], since the total amount of UA that can be dissolved in urine increases substantially at higher urine pH (see Figure 3.1). In addition to reduction of animal protein intake, alkali therapy is the cornerstone of the management of UA stones [29]. Although no randomized clinical trials have been conducted to assess the efficacy of urinary alkalinization on stone recurrence in UA stone formers, a number of observational studies have solidified this practice [13,25,26, 27]. Potassium citrate is the preferred agent to raise urine pH in UA stone formers. The starting dose of potassium citrate is 30–60 mEq/day taken in divided doses along with meals. The daily dose is titrated to maintain urine pH between 6.0–6.5 (see Figure 3.2), since raising urine pH further may lead to the unwanted formation of calcium phosphate stones [30]. Potassium citrate is generally well tolerated, and gastrointestinal side-effects (heartburn, nausea, and diarrhea) can be minimized if this medication is taken with food. One limiting side-effect is the development of hyperkalemia, which is primarily seen in patients with underlying chronic kidney disease. Urinary alkalinization with sodium bicarbonate instead of potassium citrate is a potential alternative in such cases [31]. Nevertheless, potassium salts are preferred over sodium salts as alkalinizing agents whenever possible, because monopotassium urate is more soluble in urine than monosodium urate at any given urine pH (see Figure 3.1). At times, adjunct use of carbonic anhydrase inhibitors may be needed for adequate urinary alkalinization [32,33].

Besides alkali therapy, UA lowering is another target for therapy in UA stone formers. Pharmacological lowering of urinary UA is reserved for stone formers with hyperuricosuria, when urinary alkalinization cannot be achieved, or when stones recur despite urinary alkalinization [34]. No randomized clinical trials have been conducted specifically in UA stone formers, but xanthine oxidase inhibition with allopurinol is generally used. The starting dose is generally 300 mg daily, although a lower dose is recommended in patients with chronic kidney disease. The dose is titrated to normalize urine UA excretion. Febuxostat is a newer xanthine oxidase inhibitor that reduces urinary UA excretion [35]. A potential complication of xanthine oxidase inhibition in patients with significant hyperuricosuria is the formation of xanthine stones [36] due to xanthinuria resulting from the inhibition of xanthine to uric acid conversion. Stone analysis in UA stone formers on allopurinol is recommended to differentiate xanthine stones from recurrent uric acid nephrolithiasis.

The majority of UA stone formers achieve durable results with lifelong alkali therapy [37]. Typical causes of medical therapy failure include intolerance or non-compliance with prescribed medications [28]. In some cases, patient self-monitoring of urine pH using commercially available testing paper can help identify periods of persistently overly acidic urine during the day [34]. Periodic re-evaluation of stone size/stone burden is recommended [38], although ultrasound is preferred over non-contrast CT which is rarely indicated for follow-up.

Urological intervention

Urological intervention is seldom used in the management of UA stone disease. Indications for urological intervention include progressive renal insufficiency, intractable pain, prolonged obstruction, and/or poor response to pharmacological modalities [39]. Local irrigation of the collecting system with alkaline solutions such as sodium bicarbonate was commonly used to dissolve UA stones (by "contact chemolysis") [40]. This is no longer practiced due to the prolonged duration of hospitalization and the loss of productivity in patients treated with direct irrigation, and in view of the excellent efficacy of oral alkali therapy. Depending on stone size and location as well as patient-related factors, ureteroscopic or percutaneous retrieval may be indicated [38]. Shock wave lithotripsy and laser lithotripsy are also effective, although radiocontrast material is needed for stone visualization [41,42]. UA stone fragmentation by extracorporeal, electrohydraulic, and pulsed-dye laser lithotripsy is relatively easily achievable [43]. While *in vitro* studies have documented cyanide production during fragmentation of UA stones with holmium:YAG lasers [44], there are no reported cases of cyanide toxicity with this modality [42].

Ammonium urate stones

Ammonium urate stones (also described as ammonium acid urate stones) are a rare cause of nephrolithiasis in industrialized countries but are endemic in some countries, particularly in Asia [45]. In endemic areas, they are more likely to present as bladder stones in the setting of urinary tract infection with urease-producing bacteria [45]. In the absence of infection, ammonium urate may appear either as the major component or, along with uric acid, as a mixed component of stones in the upper urinary tract [46]. In sporadic cases, ammonium urate stones typically occur in the setting of a chronic diarrheal state (inflammatory bowel disease, laxative abuse). The gastrointestinal losses of fluids, sodium and potassium result in concentrated urine with low urinary sodium and potassium content, leaving ammonium (excreted in response to gastrointestinal alkali loss) as the major cation in urine to bind urate and precipitate as ammonium urate. Ammonium urate stones can be distinguished from UA stones by stone analysis. Treatment should be directed at the underlying pathophysiology (antibiotics in the case of urinary tract infection, discontinuation of offending agent in cases of laxative abuse, volume repletion and potassium supplementation as needed) [46].

Summary and conclusions

Uric acid stones contribute significantly to the burden of urolithiasis, in particular in stone formers with diabetes, gout or the metabolic syndrome. Uric acid stones are radiolucent on plain radiograph and are generally visualized on CT scan or ultrasound. An overly acidic urine is the key pathogenetic factor in the genesis of uric acid stones, and the major target of therapy. Urinary alkalinization with potassium citrate results in the dissolution of most uric acid stones, and is considered the first line of therapy.

Key points

- The metabolic syndrome and its individual features including diabetes and obesity are associated with an increased risk of uric acid stone formation.
- Stone analysis is essential for making the diagnosis of uric acid stone disease.
- An overly acidic urine (urine pH <5.5) is the principal risk factor for the formation of uric acid stones.
- The initial treatment of patients with uric acid stones consists of medical dissolution therapy with alkalinizing agents.
- In patients with uric acid stones, urological intervention is reserved for cases of severe obstruction, progressive decline in renal function, infection or intractable pain.

References

1. Moe OW, Abate N, Sakhaee K. Pathophysiology of uric acid nephrolithiasis. Endocrinol Metab Clin North Am 2002; 31: 895–914.
2. Daudon M, Knebelmann B. Epidemiology of urolithiasis. Rev Prat 2011; 61: 372–8.
3. Pak CY, Sakhaee K, Moe O, et al. Biochemical profile of stone-forming patients with diabetes mellitus. Urology 2003; 61: 523–7.
4. Daudon M, Lacour B, Jungers P. Influence of body size on urinary stone composition in men and women. Urol Res 2006; 34: 193–9.
5. Kadlec AO, Greco K, Fridirici ZC, et al. Metabolic syndrome and urinary stone composition: what factors matter most? Urology 2012;80:805–10.
6. Marchini GS, Sarkissian C, Tian D, et al. Gout, stone composition and urinary stone risk: a matched case comparative study. J Urol 2013; 189(4): 1334–9.
7. Cochat P, Pichault V, Bacchetta J, et al. Nephrolithiasis related to inborn metabolic diseases. Pediatr Nephrol 2010; 25: 415–24.
8. Chang H, Shi X, Shen W, et al. Characterization of melamine-associated urinary stones in children with consumption of melamine-contaminated infant formula. Clin Chim Acta 2012 14; 413: 985–91.
9. Maalouf NM, Cameron MA, Moe OW, Sakhaee K. Novel insights into the pathogenesis of uric acid nephrolithiasis. Curr Opin Nephrol Hypertens 2004; 13: 181–9.
10. Pak CY, Sakhaee K, Peterson RD, et al. Biochemical profile of idiopathic uric acid nephrolithiasis. Kidney Int 2001; 60: 757–61.
11. Sakhaee K, Adams-Huet B, Moe OW, Pak CY. Pathophysiologic basis for normouricosuric uric acid nephrolithiasis. Kidney Int 2002; 62: 971–9.
12. Cameron M, Maalouf NM, Poindexter J, Adams-Huet B, Sakhaee K, Moe OW. The diurnal variation in urine acidification differs between normal individuals and uric acid stone formers. Kidney Int 2012; 81: 1123–30.
13. Worcester EM. Stones from bowel disease. Endocrinol Metab Clin North Am 2002; 31: 979–99.
14. Maalouf NM, Moe OW, Adams-Huet B, Sakhaee K. Hypercalciuria associated with high dietary protein intake is not due to acid load. J Clin Endocrinol Metab 2011; 96: 3733–40.
15. Sakhaee K, Nigam S, Snell P, et al. Assessment of the pathogenetic role of physical exercise in renal stone formation. J Clin Endocrinol Metab 1987; 65: 974–9.

16. Hirasaki S, Koide N, Fujita K, et al. Two cases of renal hypouricemia with nephrolithiasis. Intern Med 1997; 36: 201–5.
17. Nakada SY, Hoff DG, Attai S, et al. Determination of stone composition by noncontrast spiral computed tomography in the clinical setting. Urology 2000; 55: 816–19.
18. Ascenti G, Siragusa C, Racchiusa S, et al. Stone-targeted dual-energy CT: a new diagnostic approach to urinary calculosis. Am J Roentgenol 2010; 195: 953–8.
19. Thomas C, Heuschmid M, Schilling D, et al. Urinary calculi composed of uric acid, cystine, and mineral salts: differentiation with dual-energy CT at a radiation dose comparable to that of intravenous pyelography. Radiology 2010; 257: 402–9.
20. Sabry ZI, Shadarevian SB, Cowan JW, Campbell JA. Relationship of dietary intake of sulphur amino-acids to urinary excretion of inorganic sulphate in man. Nature 1965; 29; 206(987): 931–3.
21. Siener R, Hesse A. The effect of a vegetarian and different omnivorous diets on urinary risk factors for uric acid stone formation. Eur J Nutr 2003; 42: 332–7.
22. Wabner CL, Pak CY. Effect of orange juice consumption on urinary stone risk factors. J Urol 1993; 149:1405–8.
23. Goldfarb DS, Asplin JR. Effect of grapefruit juice on urinary lithogenicity. J Urol 2001; 166: 263–7.
24. Odvina CV. Comparative value of orange juice versus lemonade in reducing stone-forming risk. Clin J Am Soc Nephrol 2006; 1: 1269–74.
25. Kursh ED, Resnick MI. Dissolution of uric acid calculi with systemic alkalization. J Urol 1984; 132: 286–7.
26. Pak CY, Sakhaee K, Fuller C. Successful management of uric acid nephrolithiasis with potassium citrate. Kidney Int 1986; 30: 422–8.
27. Preminger GM. Pharmacologic treatment of uric acid calculi. Urol Clin North Am 1987; 14: 335–8.
28. Moran ME, Abrahams HM, Burday DE, Greene TD. Utility of oral dissolution therapy in the management of referred patients with secondarily treated uric acid stones. Urology 2002; 59: 206–10.
29. Cameron MA, Sakhaee K. Uric acid nephrolithiasis. Urol Clin North Am 2007; 34: 335–46.
30. Pak CY. Physicochemical basis for formation of renal stones of calcium phosphate origin: calculation of the degree of saturation of urine with respect to brushite. J Clin Invest 1969; 48: 1914–22.
31. Sakhaee K, Nicar M, Hill K, Pak CY. Contrasting effects of potassium citrate and sodium citrate therapies on urinary chemistries and crystallization of stone-forming salts. Kidney Int 1983; 24: 348–52.
32. Cameron MA, Baker LA, Maalouf NM, et al. Circadian variation in urine pH and uric acid nephrolithiasis risk. Nephrol Dial Transplant 2007; 22: 2375–8.
33. Sterrett SP, Penniston KL, Wolf JS Jr, Nakada SY. Acetazolamide is an effective adjunct for urinary alkalization in patients with uric acid and cystine stone formation recalcitrant to potassium citrate. Urology 2008; 72: 278–81.
34. Mehta TH, Goldfarb DS. Uric acid stones and hyperuricosuria. Adv Chronic Kidney Dis 2012; 19: 413–18.
35. Becker MA, Kisicki J, Khosravan R, et al. Febuxostat (TMX-67), a novel, non-purine, selective inhibitor of xanthine oxidase, is safe and decreases serum urate in healthy volunteers. Nucleosides Nucleotides Nucleic Acids 2004; 23: 1111.

36. Pais VM Jr, Lowe G, Lallas CD, et al. Xanthine urolithiasis. Urology 2006; 67: 1084.
37. Parks JH, Coe FL. Evidence for durable kidney stone prevention over several decades. BJU Int 2009; 103(9): 1238–46.
38. Ngo TC, Assimos DG. Uric acid nephrolithiasis: recent progress and future directions. Rev Urol 2007; 9: 17–27.
39. Preminger GM, Tiselius HG, Assimos DG, et al. 2007 Guidelines for the management of ureteral calculi. Eur Urol 2007; 52: 1610–31.
40. Bernardo NO, Smith AD. Chemolysis of urinary calculi. Urol Clin North Am 2000; 27: 355–65.
41. Sun XZ, Zhang ZW. Shock wave lithotripsy for uric acid stones. Asian J Surg 2006; 29: 36–9.
42. Teichman JM, Champion PC, Wollin TA, Denstedt JD. Holmium:YAG lithotripsy of uric acid calculi. J Urol 1998; 160: 2130–2.
43. Wu TT, Hsu TH, Chen MT, Chang LS. Efficacy of in vitro stone fragmentation by extracorporeal, electrohydraulic, and pulsed-dye laser lithotripsy. J Endourol 1993; 7: 391–3.
44. Zagone RL, Waldmann TM, Conlin MJ. Fragmentation of uric acid calculi with the holmium: YAG laser produces cyanide. Lasers Surg Med 2002;31:230–2.
45. Chou YH, Huang CN, Li WM, et al. Clinical study of ammonium acid urate urolithiasis. Kaohsiung J Med Sci 2012; 28: 259–64.
46. Pichette V, Bonnardeaux A, Cardinal J, et al. Ammonium acid urate crystal formation in adult North American stone-formers. Am J Kidney Dis 1997; 30: 237–42.

CHAPTER 4
Calcium Stones

John C. Lieske
Mayo Clinic, Rochester, MN, USA

Do's and don'ts box

Do:
- get all stones analyzed
- work up stone patients with 24-h urine collections on ambient diet
- develop individualized diet and drug treatment plans
- monitor effects of diet and drug interventions with follow-up urine collections.

Don't:
- perform formalized testing to differentiate between intestinal overabsorption and renal leak of calcium
- indiscriminately use citrates in calcium stone formers.

Overview

Kidney stones are very common, affecting up to 12% of men and 5% of women in industrialized countries [1], including 900,000 people in the United States each year [2]. The majority of these contain calcium oxalate (CaOx) or calcium phosphate (CaP), often admixed. Furthermore, over the last 2–3 decades the incidence around the world has increased; for example, it increased nearly three-fold in Germany (0.54% to 1.47%), with a resulting rise in prevalence from 4.0% to 4.7% within the population as a whole [3]. Many of these are recurrent stone formers (e.g. 40% of male stone formers aged 50–64 years). A recent study in Olmsted County, Minnesota, confirmed that the overall rate of symptomatic stone events also remains high in the United States [4], where the economic impact was most recently estimated at $5.3 billion per year, the majority attributed to direct medical costs [5]. Although shock wave lithotripsy can non-invasively dislodge stones after they form, it is expensive and sometimes results in renal hemorrhage [6,7], fibrosis [6], and/or hypertension [7,8]. Since the pathogenesis of most calcium stones remains undefined, it is clear that new knowledge is required to identify

Urinary Stones: Medical and Surgical Management, First Edition. Edited by Michael Grasso and David S. Goldfarb.

susceptible persons and therapeutic targets in order to prevent stones and avoid complications such as pain, infection, lost productivity, and medical costs.

The vast majority of human stones contain CaOx (70–80%), a major focus of this chapter. Urinary stone composition closely parallels urinary supersaturation (SS) [9]. A convergence of many factors appears to determine urinary SS for CaOx, most importantly urinary calcium, oxalate, uric acid (UA), and citrate excretion together with urinary volume [10]. Therefore, the regulation of each of these features is an important factor that determines CaOx stone risk. Other stone types are much less common and each has unique metabolic risk factors, e.g. low urinary pH for UA stones or high pH for CaP stones. In addition to SS, defective macromolecular urinary crystallization inhibitor function may be an important factor predisposing towards CaOx stone formation [10] (Figure 4.1).

How do stones begin?

The exact series of events that transpire within the kidney and result in renal stone formation remain unclear. Simple nucleation and growth of crystals do not seem sufficient to explain the genesis of nephrolithiasis [9]. Recent studies by Evan and colleagues highlight the role of Randall's plaques in certain idiopathic CaOx stone formers [11]. These interstitial CaP deposits initiate in the medulla around thin limbs of the loop of Henle and appear to grow and become visible below the urothelial surface of renal papillae. These suburothelial deposits can serve as anchors for CaOx stones [12]. Some evidence suggests that increased urinary SS (especially higher calcium excretion) might be an important factor driving Randall's plaque initiation and/or growth [13]. However, other evidence implicates proteins deposited in the interstitium such as the H3 chain of the inter α trypsin inhibitor [14]. Further, urinary proteins such as osteopontin or Tamm–Horsfall protein are likely to play a crucial role in CaOx deposition once plaque is exposed to the urinary space [15].

In other calcium stone-forming states, distal tubular plugs have been observed, including among patients with enteric hyperoxaluria (CaOx stones) [16], primary hyperparathyroidism (CaOx and CaP stones) [17], and those that form brushite (BR) stones, with [18] or without [19] renal tubular acidosis (RTA). In addition, recent studies document prominent plugs in a substantial portion of idiopathic CaOx patients, often co-existing with plaque [20]. Because proteins are present in both tubular fluid and the interstitium and can modulate crystal–crystal and crystal–cell interactions, they are likely to be critical mediators of these events. However, the important protein(s) are likely to differ depending on the exact pathogenesis. Recent studies suggest that decreased urinary crystal growth inhibition is observed only in stone formers with prominent plugs. Hence, to accurately study inhibitors, it becomes crucial to phenotype patients relative to stone precursor lesions.

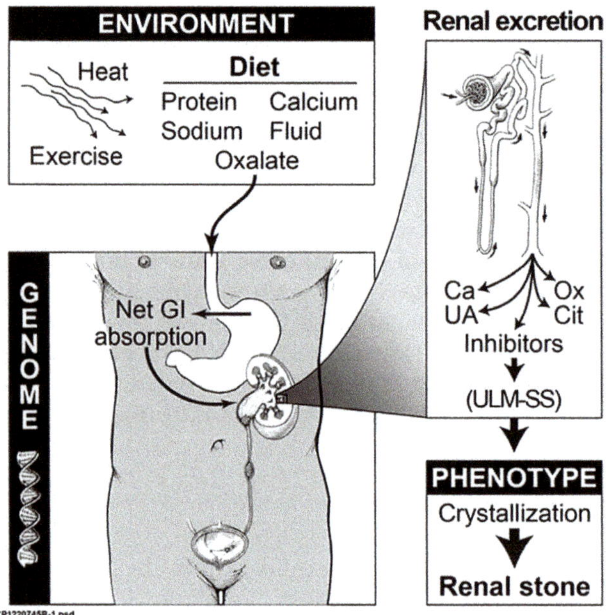

Figure 4.1 Environmental and genetic factors that contribute to calcium nephrolithiasis. Kidney stone risk is dependent on the crystallization potential of urine, which is determined by the net urinary excretion of substances that increase SS, including calcium (Ca), UA, oxalate (Ox), citrate and macromolecular inhibitors. The gap between the upper limit of metastability (ULM) and SS is a quantitative index of crystallization potential, with a lower gap indicating increased chance of crystallization. Environmental modifiers include heat, exercise, and diet. Net GI absorption and renal excretion of urinary substances are under genomic influence. Candidate genes to regulate urinary calcium excretion include, but are not limited to, the vitamin D receptor (VDR), calcium sensing receptor (CaSR), and a recently identified soluble adenylate cyclase (sAC) present in kidney. Candidate genes to regulate other urinary lithogenic factors are less well understood, but include the anion channel *SLC26A6* since it promotes intestinal oxalate secretion. Certain individuals may have functional defects in urinary inhibitor function, possibly also under genetic influence. Persons with abnormalities in two or more pathways might have a more severe outcome (i.e. more stones). Source: Copyright of Mayo Clinic, reproduced with permission.

Risk factors for calcium stones

Calcium oxalate stones are the most common variety. Their pathogenesis is also most complex, with many independent factors that seemingly increase risk of their formation. Because their pathogenesis has been so poorly understood, traditionally these have been referred to as "idiopathic" CaOx stones. However, even though many steps in the pathway from SS to stone are murky, quite a bit has been learned about key risk factors for these stones. Therefore in 2013 the term "routine" CaOx stones might be more appropriate. For example, urinary SS is a key predictor of kidney stone composition and risk [10]. Indeed, all current treatments are targeted towards reducing the SS. Thus a brief discussion of the most important factors that determine SS follows, each of which appears to be under the influence of both genes and diet.

Calcium phosphate stones are favored by a relatively alkaline urine (pH >6.5). Some individuals with CaP stones have a clear distal RTA, and cannot acidify their urine even under acid loading. Causes include genetic alterations in the apical hydrogen ion secretor (VATPase) and basolateral chloride hydrogen ion exchanger (kAE1), autoimmune processes in the medullary interstitium (most importantly Sjögren's syndrome), and exposure to certain toxins and drugs (e.g. lithium, toluene). Those with a clear distal RTA benefit from citrate to treat the systemic alkalosis and counteract daily acid production. In many calcium stone formers, the reasons for a persistently high urine pH are not as clear. Studies suggest that subtle cases of incomplete distal RTA (inability to completely acidify the urine but without systemic acidosis) might be uncovered if ammonium chloride loading was employed [21]. These individuals with so-called incomplete distal RTA might harbor a tendency towards hypocitraturia, hypercalciuria, and subclinical bone disease [21]. This is an area clearly in need of greater study.

Hypercalciuria

"Idiopathic" or genetic hypercalciuria is present in up to 50% of patients with calcium urolithiasis [22,23]. Increased intestinal absorption of calcium is often a distinguishing feature [24]. Abnormalities of vitamin D action and/or the vitamin D receptor (VDR) [25], as well as impaired renal tubular reabsorption of calcium [26,27], have all been reported. Although protocols were previously advocated to differentiate between patients that have a renal leak of calcium versus intestinal hyperabsorption, it is now appreciated that this strategy is neither clinically necessary nor useful. Overall heritability of urinary calcium excretion has been estimated at ~40% [28]. However, hypercalciuria appears to be a polygenic disorder [29] and the exact molecular defect(s) contributing to it in the majority of stone formers remain undefined.

A small subset of hypercalciuric stone formers will have primary hyperparathyroidism. A clue to this diagnosis is hypercalcemia, perhaps with hypophosphatemia. Other important diagnoses to exclude include sarcoidosis and excessive intake of vitamin D and/or calcium antacids.

Hyperoxaluria

"Mild" hyperoxaluria (40–70 mg/24 h) has been reported in up to 20–30% of idiopathic CaOx stone formers [30] although the mechanism(s) and pathogenic importance for stone formation remain unclear. Dietary oxalate, calcium, and/or the balance between the two are likely to be important determinants of gastrointestinal oxalate absorption, and hence urinary oxalate excretion [31,32]. Stone formers as a group also tend to overabsorb oxalate from food [33] and generate proportionately more oxalate from dietary protein sources (e.g. hydroxyproline) [34,35,36]. Whether hyperoxaluria could result from polymorphisms in the three genes implicated in primary hyperoxaluria (alanine glyoxylate transferase [37], glycolate reductase/hydroxypyruvate reductase [38], and 4-hydroxy-2-oxoglutarate aldolase [39]) is unknown. Familial studies suggest a genetic contribution to renal oxalate excretion, but evidence suggests this genetic variability involves absorption of oxalate from the diet, rather than hepatic oxalate synthesis or renal secretion [40]. Patients with fat malabsorption of any cause are at high risk of CaOx stones [41]. The abnormally high amount of fat in the colon of these individuals complexes calcium and leads to oxalate overabsorption. Compounding the picture, GI losses of fluids and alkali often produce lower urinary volume, pH, and citrate levels.

Hypocitraturia

Low levels of urinary citrate, an important inhibitor of crystallization, have been identified in 19–63% of patients with calcium urolithiasis [42]. Urinary citrate excretion is predominantly determined by the prevailing acid–base status within proximal tubular cells [43], which in the absence of systemic acidosis is most critically dependent on the net absorption of alkali from the diet [44]. Even though net alkali absorption and urinary citrate levels correlate, there is also residual scatter [44], suggesting that other factors are important co-determinants. Sex hormones may be one additional factor since urinary citrate excretion is higher in women [45]. In a single study that involved six families, individuals could be classified as low, intermediate or high citrate excretors, stone risk was associated with low citrate levels, and the pattern suggested co-dominant inheritance of alleles at a single genetic locus [46] The overall precise genetic determinants of citrate absorption and metabolism remain to be determined.

Hyperuricosuria

Approximately 5% of all stones are mixed CaOx and UA [47]. Excess excretion of UA in the urine is thought to be the pathological link, and this syndrome has been termed hyperuricosuric CaOx nephrolithiasis [48] to differentiate it from pure UA stones that have different pathogenic mechanisms. The pathways by which UA promotes CaOx stone formation could involve UA-induced spontaneous nucleation of CaOx by a "salting out" mechanism [49] or inactivation of urinary CaOx crystal growth inhibitors [50]. Hyperuricosuria has a clear dietary component [51] but a subgroup of CaOx stone formers demonstrate hyperuricosuria with a reduced fractional excretion of UA [52] Studies have found evidence for clustering of hyperuricosuria in certain stone-forming families [53]. The relationship of this phenotype to the anion exchanger *URAT1* (mutated in hyperuricosuric hyperuricemia [54]), or other genetic factors, is unknown.

Low urinary volume

Urinary excretion of key stone risk factors such as calcium, oxalate, or UA is not dependent on urinary flow. Therefore, it makes sense that drinking more fluid should decrease urinary concretion of these lithogenic molecules and benefit stone risk. Indeed, observational studies tie lower urine volume to the risk of first-time stone disease [55] as well as the risk of recurrent stones [56].

Stones without clear risk factors

Occasionally active stone formers are identified that have no clear urinary risk factors in a standard metabolic profile. It has been speculated that such individuals might harbor ineffective macromolecular inhibitors in their urine [57]. However, although many molecules have been identified in urine that can inhibit CaOx or CaP crystal growth, the key player(s) remain elusive.

Management algorithms

Diet

Nephrolithiasis has long been associated with affluence [58], hence dietary factors associated with higher socioeconomic status have been implicated [59]. More recently, two large prospective studies containing both men and women [60,61] have identified specific dietary components that correlated with subsequent stone events. Although there are subtle differences based upon gender and age, the following general patterns correlate with greater stone risk: higher animal protein intake, lower potassium intake, lower fluid intake, lower oxalate intake, and *lower* calcium intake [62]. Two prospective, randomized trials have demonstrated that counseling for increased fluid intake [63] and a normal-calcium (~1200 mg/day), low-salt (50 mEq), low-oxalate and low-protein (52 g) diet [64] both reduced the rate of calcium stone recurrence.

Based upon these observations, the standard diet recommendations for calcium stones contain five elements:

1 increased fluid intakes, with a target urine volume of 2000 mL or more per day
2 normal dietary calcium of ~1200 mg per day in the form of food or dairy products. Calcium pills, on the other hand, may slightly increase stone risk
3 lower sodium intake
4 moderate protein intake (0.8 g/kg/day)
5 avoid excessive intakes of high-oxalate foods.

Use of the Dietary Approaches to Stop Hypertension (DASH) diet plan may be one way to simplify overall compliance with this dietary pattern [65].

Patients with enteric hyperoxaluria benefit from extensive dietary counseling in a low-fat, low-oxalate diet replete with calcium [66]. This regimen can be supplemented with calcium pills to bind oxalate.

Medications

The pharmacological armamentarium for stone prevention is, unfortunately, not large. All are aimed at changing the urine composition and reducing crystallization potential. All are backed by clinical trials, albeit not particularly recent or with large numbers of patients.

Thiazide diuretics are well known to reduce urinary calcium excretion. It is now generally accepted that subtle volume depletion results in increased proximal tubular calcium reabsorption, and consequently less calcium in the urine. The utility of this approach using either hydrochlorothiazide [67] or chlorthalidone [68] is supported by several clinical trials. Indapamide is an alternative diuretic choice that also appears effective [69].

Oral administration of citrate salts increases urinary citrate excretion. Citrate is metabolized to bicarbonate in the liver; the alkali load inhibits proximal tubular citrate reabsorption. Potassium citrate is preferred, to limit sodium loads, but must be used in caution in patients with chronic kidney disease. The use of citrate salts in patients with calcium stones is supported by several trials [70,71]. Lemonade has been proposed as a natural source of citrate. However, the quantities needed (~2 L per day) are large, and studies are conflicting over whether or not lemonade can really increase urinary citrate levels.

There is at least theoretic concern regarding the undesired increase in urinary pH that occurs when citrate salts are used. In particular, the use of citrate must be monitored carefully in patients with CaP stones since potentially beneficial increases in urinary citrate, a crystallization inhibitor, may be outweighed by increases in urinary pH, the key driver of hydroxyapatite and brushite SS.

Neutral phosphate in the form of K-Phos neutral has also been used for the treatment of calcium stone disease [72]. Although no randomized trials have been completed, two effects of the medication should be helpful: increase of urinary pyrophosphate, a crystallization inhibitor, and lowering of urinary calcium, perhaps via inhibition of vitamin D hydroxylation. Diarrhea is a limiting side-effect at the doses needed to see an effect. Nevertheless, neutral phosphate remains a possibility in patients who have failed other approaches.

Since hyperuricosuria has been identified as a risk factor for CaOx stones, it makes sense to reduce urinary UA levels in this patient group. Indeed, a randomized trial supports the effectiveness of allopurinol to reduce recurrence rates in this subset of calcium stone formers [73].

In general, the choice of medications is driven by the results of 24-h urine collections. However, there is a school of thought that thiazides and/or citrate could be used in a stepped approach, much like we currently treat hypertension [74]. These approaches have never been compared head to head.

Key points

Major causes of calcium stones

CaOx

Hypercalciuria
Hyperoxaluria
Hypocitraturia
Hyperuricosuria
Low urine volume

CaP

High urine pH
Low urine citrate
Hypercalciuria

Components of a diet plan for calcium stones

High fluid intake (urine output >2 L/day)
Normal dietary calcium (1200 mg/day); no calcium pills
Moderate protein (0.8 g/kg)
Low sodium
Avoid excessive oxalate

Common drug treatments for calcium stones

Urine abnormality	*Drug*
Hypercalciuria	Thiazide diuretic
	Potassium citrate
	Neutral phosphate
Hypocitraturia	Potassium citrate
Hyperuricosuria	Allopurinol; febuxostat
	Potassium citrate

Grant funding

This work was supported by R01 DK077950, the Mayo Clinic O'Brien Urology Research Center P50 DK083007, and the Rare Kidney Stone Consortium (U54KD083908), a part of NIH Rare Diseases Clinical Research Network (RDCRN), funded by the NIDDK and the Office of Rare Diseases Research (ORDR), all funded by the National Institutes of Health. Its contents are solely the responsibility of the author and do not necessarily represent the official views of the NIH.

References

1. Unwin R, Wrong O, Cohen E, Tanner M, Thakker R. Unraveling of the molecular mechanisms of kidney stones. Lancet 1996; 348: 1561–5.
2. National Kidney and Urological Diseases Advisory Board. 1990 Long range plan: window on the 21st century. J Urol 1991; 145(3): 568–93.

3. Hesse A, Brändle E, Wilbert D, Köhrmann K-U, Alken P. Study on the prevalence and incidence of urolithiasis in Germany comparing the years 1979 vs. 2000. European Urol 2003; 44: 709–13.
4. Lieske JC, Pena de la Vega LS, Slezak JM, et al. Renal stone epidemiology in Rochester, Minnesota: an update. Kidney Int 2006; 69(4): 760–4.
5. Saigal CS, Joyce G, Timilsina AR. Direct and indirect costs of nephrolithiasis in an employed population: opportunity for disease management? Kidney Int 2005; 68(4): 1808–14.
6. Lingeman JE, Woods J, Toth PD, Evan AP, McAteer JA. Role of lithotripsy and its side effects. J Urol 1989; 141: 793–7.
7. Lemann JJ, Taylor AJ, Collier BD, Lipchick EO. Kidney hematoma due to extracorporeal shock wave lithotripsy causing transient renin-mediated hypertension. J Urol 1991; 145: 1238–41.
8. Lingeman JE, Woods JR, Toth PD. Blood pressure changes following extracorporeal shock wave lithotripsy and other forms of treatment for nephrolithiasis. JAMA 1990; 263: 1789–94.
9. Parks JH, Coward M, Coe FL. Correspondence between stone composition and urine supersaturation in nephrolithiasis. Kidney Int 1997; 51(3): 894–900.
10. Coe FL, Parks JH. *Nephrolithiasis: Pathogenesis and Treatment*, 2nd edn. Chicago: Year Book Medical Publishers, 1988.
11. Evan AP, Lingeman JE, Coe FL, et al. Randall's plaque of patients with nephrolithiasis begins in basement membranes of thin loops of Henle. J Clin Invest 2003; 111(5): 602–5.
12. Matlaga BR, Williams JC Jr, Kim SC, et al. Endoscopic evidence of calculus attachment to Randall's plaque. J Urol 2006; 175(5): 1720–4.
13. Kim SC, Coe FL, Tinmouth WW, et al. Stone formation is proportional to papillary surface coverage by Randall's plaque. J Urol 2005; 173(1): 117–19.
14. Evan AP, Bledsoe S, Worcester EM, Coe FL, Lingeman JE, Bergsland KJ. Renal inter-alpha-trypsin inhibitor heavy chain 3 increases in calcium oxalate stone-forming patients. Kidney Int 2007; 72(12): 1503–11.
15. Evan AP, Coe FL, Lingeman JE, et al. Mechanism of formation of human calcium oxalate renal stones on Randall's plaque. Anat Rec (Hoboken) 2007; 290(10): 1315–23.
16. Evan AP, Lingeman JE, Worcester EM, et al. Renal histopathology and crystal deposits in patients with small bowel resection and calcium oxalate stone disease. Kidney Int 2010; 78(3): 310–17.
17. Evan AP, Lingeman JE, Coe FL, et al. Histopathology and surgical anatomy of patients with primary hyperparathyroidism and calcium phosphate stones. Kidney Int 2008; 74(2): 223–9.
18. Evan AP, Lingeman J, Coe F, et al. Renal histopathology of stone-forming patients with distal renal tubular acidosis. Kidney Int 2007; 71(8): 795–801.
19. Evan AP, Lingeman JE, Coe FL, et al. Crystal-associated nephropathy in patients with brushite nephrolithiasis. Kidney Int 2005; 67(2): 576–91.
20. Linnes MP, Krambeck AE, Cornell L, et al. Phenotypic characterization of kidney stone formers via endoscopic and histological quantification of intrarenal calcifications. Kidney Int 2013; May 22 (epub ahead of print).
21. Arampatzis S, Ropke-Rieben B, Lippuner K, Hess B. Prevalence and densitometric characteristics of incomplete distal renal tubular acidosis in men with recurrent calcium nephrolithiasis. Urol Res 2012; 40(1): 53–9.
22. Coe FL, Parks JH, Asplin JR. The pathogenesis and treatment of kidney stones – medical progress. N Engl J Med 1992; 327: 1141–52.

23. Coe FL, Favus MJ, Crockett T, et al. Effects of low-calcium diet on urine calcium excretion, parathyroid function and serum 1,25(OH)2D3 levels in patients with idiopathic hypercalciuria and in normal subjects. Am J Med 1982; 72: 25–32.
24. Lemann J Jr, Worcester EM, Gray RW. Hypercalciuria and stones. Am J Kidney Dis 1991; 17: 386–91.
25. Xiao QL, Tembe V, Horwitz GM, Bushinsky D, Favus MJ. Increased intestinal vitamin D receptor in genetic hypercalciuric rats: a cause of intestinal calcium absorption. J Clin Invest 1993; 91: 661–7.
26. Sutton RAL, Walker VR. Responses to hydrochlorothiazide and acetazolamide in patients with calcium stones. N Engl J Med 1980; 13: 709–13.
27. Hou SH, Bushinsky DA, Wish JB, Cohen JJ, Harrington JT. Hospital-acquired renal insufficiency: a prospective study. Am J Med 1983; 74: 243–8.
28. Bianchi G, Vezzoli G, Cusi D, et al. Abnormal red-cell calcium pump in patients with idiopathic hypercalciuria. N Engl J Med 1988; 319: 897–901.
29. Moe OW, Bonny O. Genetic hypercalciuria. J Am Soc Nephrol 2005; 16(3): 729–45.
30. Smith LH. Hyperoxaluric states. In: Coe FL, Favus MJ, eds. *Disorders of Bone and Mineral Metabolism*. New York: Raven Press; 1992, pp. 707–28.
31. Robertson WG, Hughes H. Importance of mild hyperoxaluria in the pathogenesis of urolithiasis – new evidence from studies in the Arabian peninsula. Scanning Microsc 1993; 7(1): 391–401.
32. Chlebeck PT, Milliner DS, Smith LH. Long-term prognosis in primary hyperoxaluria type II (L-glyceric aciduria). Am J Kidney Dis 1994; 23(2): 255–9.
33. Krishnamurthy MA, Hruska KA, Chandhoke PS. The urinary response to an oral load in recurrent calcium oxalate stone formers. J Urol 2003; 169: 2030–3.
34. Holmes RP, Goodman HO, Assimos DG. Contribution of dietary oxalate to urinary oxalate excretion. Kidney Int 2001; 59: 270–6.
35. Massey LK, Palmer RG, Horner HT. Oxalate content of soybean seeds (Glycine max: Leguminosae), soyfoods, and other edible legumes. JAgric Food Chem 2001; 49: 4262–6.
36. Giannini S, Nobile M, Sartori L, et al. Acute effects of moderate dietary protein restriction in patients with idiopathic hypercalciuria and calcium nephrolithiasis. Am J Clin Nutr 1999; 69: 267–71.
37. Monico CG, Rossetti S, Olson JB, Milliner DS. Pyridoxine effect in type I primary hyperoxaluria is associated with the most common mutant allele. Kidney Int 2005; 67(5): 1704–9.
38. Cramer SD, Ferree PM, Lin K, Milliner DS, Holmes RP. The gene encoding hydroxypyruvate reductase (GRHPR) is mutated in patients with primary hyperoxaluria type II [published erratum appears in Hum Mol Genet 1999; 8(13): 2574]. Hum Mol Genet 1999; 8(11): 2063–9.
39. Monico CG, Rossetti S, Belostotsky R, et al. Primary hyperoxaluria type III gene HOGA1 (formerly DHDPSL) as a possible risk factor for idiopathic calcium oxalate urolithiasis. Clin J Am Soc Nephrol 2011; 6(9): 2289–95.
40. Goodman HO, Brommage R, Assimos DG, Holmes RP. Genes in idiopathic calcium oxalate stone disease. World J Urol 1997; 15(3): 186–94.
41. Lieske JC, Kumar R, Collazo-Clavell ML. Nephrolithiasis after bariatric surgery for obesity. Semin Nephrol 2008; 28(2): 163–73.
42. Pak CYC. Citrate and renal calculi: an update. Miner Electrolyte Metab 1994; 20: 371–7.
43. Pak CY, Fuller C, Sakhaee K, Preminger GM, Britton F. Long-term treatment of calcium nephrolithiasis with potassium citrate. J Urol 1985; 134: 11–19.

44. Sakhaee K, Williams RH, Oh MS, et al. Alkali absorption and citrate excretion in calcium nephrolithiasis. J Bone Miner Res 1993; 8: 789–94.
45. Parks JH, Coe FL. Urine citrate and calcium in calcium nephrolithiasis. Adv Exp Med Biol 1986; 208: 445–9.
46. Shah O, Assimos DG, Holmes RP. Genetic and dietary factors in urinary citrate excretion. J Endourol 2005; 19(2): 177–82.
47. Herring LC. Observations on the analysis of ten thousand urinary calculus. J Urol 1962; 88: 545–55.
48. Coe FL. Hyperuricosuric calcium oxalate nephrolithiasis. Kidney Int 1978; 13: 418–26.
49. Grover PK, Ryall RL, Marshall VR. Dissolved urate promotes calcium oxalate crystallization: epitaxy is not the cause. Clin Sci (Colch) 1993; 85: 303–7.
50. Robertson WG, Knowles F, Peacock M. Urinary acid mucopolysaccharide inhibitors of calcium oxalate cyrstallisation. In: Fleisch H, Robertson WG, Smith LH, Vahlensieck W, eds. *Urolithiasis Research*. London: Plenum, 1976, pp. 331–40.
51. Coe FL, Moran E, Kavalich AG. The contribution of dietary purine over-consumption to hyperpuricosuria in calcium oxalate stone formers. J Chronic Dis 1976; 29: 793–800.
52. Sakhaee K, Adams-Huet B, Moe OW, Pak CY. Pathophysiologic basis for normouricosuric uric acid nephrolithiasis. Kidney Int 2002; 62(3): 971–9.
53. Trinchieri A, Mandressi A, Luongo P, Coppi F, Pisani E. Familial aggregation of renal calcium stone disease. J Urol 1988; 139(3): 478–81.
54. Enomoto A, Kimura H, Chairoungdua A, et al. Molecular identification of a renal urate anion exchanger that regulates blood urate levels. Nature 2002; 417(6887): 447–52.
55. Curhan GC, Willett WC, Rimm EB, Spiegelman D, Stampfer MJ. Prospective study of beverage use and the risk of kidney stones. Am J Epidemiol 1996; 143(3): 240–7.
56. Hosking DH, Erickson SB, van den Berg CJ, Wilson DM, Smith LH. The stone clinic effect in patients with idiopathic calcium urolithiasis. J Urol 1983; 130: 1115–18.
57. Asplin JR, Parks JH, Chen MS, et al. Reduced crystallization inhibition by urine from men with nephrolithiasis. Kidney Int 1999; 56: 1505–16.
58. Andersen DA, ed. Historical and geographical differences in the pattern of incidence of urinary renal stones considered in relation to possible aetiological factors. Proceedings of the Renal Stone Research Symposium, 1968. Edinburgh: Churchill Livingstone.
59. Robertson WG, Peacock M, Heyburn PJ, Hanes FA. Epidemiological risk factors in calcium stone disease. Scand J Urol Nephrol 1980; 53(suppl): 15–28.
60. Curhan GC, Willet WC, Speizer FE, Stampfer MJ. Intake of vitamins B6 and C and the risk of kidney stones in women. J Am Soc Nephrol 1999; 10: 840–5.
61. Curhan GC, Willet WC, Rimm EB, Stampfer MJ. A prospective study of the intake of vitamins C and B6, and the risk of kidney stones in men. J Urol 1996; 155: 1847–51.
62. Curhan GC, Willett WC, Rimm EB, Stampfer MJ. A prospective study of dietary calcium and other nutrients and the risk of symptomatic kidney stones [see comments]. N Engl J Med 1993; 328: 833–8.
63. Borghi L, Meschi T, Amato F, Briganti A, Novarini A, Giannini A. Urinary volume, water and recurrences in idiopathic calcium nephrolithiasis: a 5-year randomized prospective study. J Urol 1996; 155(3): 839–43.

64. Borghi L, Schianchi T, Meschi T, et al. Comparison of two diets for the prevention of recurrent stones in idiopathic hypercalciuria. N Engl J Med 2002; 346(2): 77–84.
65. Taylor EN, Fung TT, Curhan GC. DASH-style diet associates with reduced risk for kidney stones. J Am Soc Nephrol 2009; 20(10): 2253–9.
66. Pang R, Linnes MP, O'Connor HM, Li X, Bergstralh E, Lieske JC. Controlled metabolic diet reduces calcium oxalate supersaturation but not oxalate excretion after bariatric surgery. Urology 2012; 80(2): 250–4.
67. Laerum E, Larsen S. Thiazide prophylaxis of urolithiasis: a double-blind study in general practice. Acta Med Scand 1984; 215: 383–9.
68. Ettinger B, Citron JT, Livermore B, Dolman LI. Chlorthalidone reduces calcium oxalate calculous recurrence but magnesium hydroxide does not. J Urol 1988; 139: 679–84.
69. Borghi L, Meschi T, Guerra A, Novarini A. Randomized prospective study of a nonthiazide diuretic, indapamide, in preventing calcium stone recurrences. J Cardiovasc Pharmacol 1993; 22(suppl 6): S78–86.
70. Barcelo P, Wuhl O, Servitge E, Rousaud A, Pak CYC. Randomized double-blind study of potassium citrate in idiopathic hypocitraturic calcium nephrolithiasis. J Urol 1993; 150(6): 1761–4.
71. Pak CY, Fuller C. Idiopathic hypocitraturic calcium-oxalate nephrolithiasis successfully treated with potassium citrate. Ann Intern Med 1986; 104: 33–7.
72. Smith LH, Thomas WC Jr, Arnaud CD. Orthophosphate therapy in calcium renal lithiasis. In: Cifuentes Delatte L, Rapado A, Hodgkinson A, eds. *Urinary Calculi: Recent Advances in Aetiology, Stone Structure and Treatment*. Basel: S. Karger, 1973, pp. 188–97.
73. Ettinger B, Tang A, Citron JT, Livermore B, Williams T. Randomized trial of allopurinol in the prevention of calcium oxalate calculi. N Engl J Med 1986; 315: 1386–9.
74. Pak CY. Medical prevention of renal stone disease. Nephron 1999; 81(suppl 1): 60–5.

CHAPTER 5

Struvite Stones

Brian H. Eisner[1], Sameer M. Deshmukh[2], and Dirk Lange[3]
[1]Massachusetts General Hospital, Harvard Medical School, Boston, MA, USA
[2]Stone Centre at Vancouver General Hospital, Vancouver, BC, Canada
[3]University of British Columbia, Vancouver, BC, Canada

Introduction

Nephrolithiasis is a common cause of morbidity with a lifetime estimated prevalence of 5–10% worldwide which appears to be increasing [1]. A subset of these stones, struvite stones, form in the presence of infection of the urinary tract and are caused by urease-splitting organisms. Struvite stones are composed of magnesium ammonium phosphate, although many struvite stones will also contain calcium phosphate (carbonate apatite or hydroxyapatite) [2]. Struvite stones account for 5% of all renal stones, and because of their association with urinary tract infection, gender prevalence favors females by a ratio of 2:1 [2,3].

Patients with struvite stones may present clinically with acute pyelonephritis. Common signs and symptoms include fevers, chills, irritative voiding symptoms, cloudy urine, and flank pain [4]. In contrast, patients with chronic infection and renal stones may have more non-specific symptoms, including malaise and generalized weakness [4]. If renal infection and obstruction are prolonged, the end-result can be xanthogranulomatous pyelonephritis (XGP), in which failure of either a particular renal segment or the entire kidney may occur due to chronic obstruction by a struvite calculus [4].

In the majority of cases, struvite stones form when urease-producing pathogens reach the kidneys and cause pyelonephritis. This generally occurs when the bacteria are able to overcome the host's natural defenses or if these defenses are absent all together. Examples of conditions which may predispose patients to struvite calculi include vesicoureteral reflux and bladder dysfunction leading to incomplete emptying [5]. This is a particular problem in patients suffering from spinal cord injury, as a correlation between urinary tract infections, specifically with urease-positive bacteria, and stone formation exists in this patient population [6,7,8].

Interestingly, recent series have shown that among spinal cord-injured patients, the relative number of struvite stones has decreased and the prevalence of calcium stones has increased [4,9]. It has been postulated

Urinary Stones: Medical and Surgical Management, First Edition. Edited by
Michael Grasso and David S. Goldfarb.

that this change in the stone composition of spinal cord-injured patients over time may be the result of reduced risk of urinary tract infection in this group due to the introduction of clean intermittent catheterization (CIC) and dedicated spinal cord injury rehabilitation units [4,10]. Voiding dysfunction may result in the retention of urine within the bladder, forming a stagnant reservoir for bacterial growth, while vesicoureteral reflux results in abnormal retrograde flow of urine from the bladder into the kidney. Foreign bodies in the urinary tract, including suture material or retained ureteral stents or catheters, can also result in bacterial colonization of the urine and a propensity to form struvite stones [4].

Microbiology

Struvite stone formation is associated with infections by urease-positive bacteria and other pathogens, of which more than 200 different species exist. While many pathogens may be associated with struvite calculi, the following is a list of the most common [11].

- Usually present (>90% of isolates):
  - gram-negative: *Proteus (rettgeri, vulgaris, mirabilis, morganii), Providencia stuartii, Haemophilus influenzae, Bordatella pertussis, Bacteroides corrodens, Yersinia enterocolitica, Brucella* species
  - gram-positive: *Flavobacterium* species, *Staphylococcus aureus, Micrococcus, Corynebacterium* (*ulcerans, renale, ovis, hofmanni*)
  - *Mycoplasma*: t-strain *Mycoplasma, Ureaplasma urealyticum*
  - yeasts: *Cryptococcus, Rhodotorula, Sporobolomyces, Candida humicola, Trichosporon cutaneum*
- Occasionally present (5–30% of isolates):
  - gram-negative: *Klebsiella* (*pneumoniae, oxytoca*), *Serratia marcescens, Haemophilus parainfluenzae, Bordatella bronchiseptica, Aeromonas hydrophila, Pseudomonas aeruginosa, Pasteurella* species
  - gram-positive: *Staphylococcus epidermidis, Bacillus* species, *Corynebacterium* (*murium, equi*), *Peptococcus asaccharolyticus, Clostridium tetani, Mycobacterium rhodochrous* group.

In humans *Proteus mirabilis* is the most common cause of struvite stones, accounting for more than half of all urease-positive infections [12]. *Pseudomonas, Klebsiella, Staphylococcus, Corynebacterium,* and *Providencia* species cause the remaining cases. Despite the fact that *Escherichia coli* (*E. coli*) is the most common cause of urinary tract infections, it does not play a prominent role in struvite stone formation due to the fact that only very few *E. coli* strains produce urease.

Urea is the major nitrogen-containing waste product in most animals. Produced in the liver by the urea cycle, it is carried to the kidneys via the blood where it is excreted in the urine. Along with low pH and the presence of various salts, the presence of urea is one of the main factors that reduces bacterial growth and survival in the urinary tract. The presence of urease is considered an important virulence factor that facilitates bacterial survival and promotes the pathogenicity of certain uropathogens.

Diagnosis and features

A definitive diagnosis of struvite calculus is made by urine microscopy or with stone composition – either by evaluating a stone which was spontaneously passed by the patient or one which was extracted during endourological or surgical procedures. It is important to note that a stone in the presence of cystitis or pyelonephritis may or may not represent a struvite calculus – a patient may have either a struvite calculus or a non-struvite calculus (i.e. calcium or uric acid) which is associated with bacteriuria. Light-microscopic analysis of the urine yields coffin-lid shaped crystals [13]. While efforts have been made to determine stone subtype based on radiographic findings, to date there are no studies which have reported the accurate differentiation of struvite calculi from calcareous stones using plain radiography, computed tomography (CT), or ultrasound. Recent *ex vivo* data using state-of-the-art dual-energy CT have shown promising results, but these findings have not been replicated in patients [14]. Urine pH is almost always elevated (i.e. >7.2) in patients with struvite calculi, due to urease-producing organisms generating high concentrations of ammonium ions in the urine. This elevated pH, in turn, may also drive precipitation of calcium phosphate (carbonate apatite) crystals whose presence depends on high urinary pH, leading to mixed struvite and carbonate apatite stones (also known as triple phosphate stones) [15,16].

Pathogenicity and pathophysiology

Conditions which promote the retention of uropathogens within the urinary system or their entry into the kidneys provide a mechanism for micro-organisms to adhere to the urothelium using specific outer membrane proteins called adhesins. These specialized outer membrane proteins recognize and tightly bind to target molecules on the surface of urothelial cells, resulting in bacterial retention within the kidneys. Once attached to the urothelial cells, the bacteria produce and secrete a thick capsular polysaccharide layer that connects neighboring bacteria, resulting in irreversible adhesion and the formation of a coherent bacterial biofilm on the urothelial surface [17]. This thick polysaccharide layer forms a physical barrier preventing antibiotics from reaching the underlying bacteria, rendering the bacterial biofilms highly resistant to antibiotic therapy, thus making the eradication of biofilms very difficult.

As a result of urease activity, the pH within the polysaccharide layer increases, resulting in the crystallization of struvite and apatite in the immediate vicinity of the biofilm and leading to the formation of nidi for subsequent stone formation [18,19,20]. However, urease activity, although responsible for struvite crystal formation, is not enough to trigger the formation of clinically relevant stones as this process involves additional factors that hold these crystals together to form a mature stone. Early studies suggested a role for the bacteria themselves, as the amount of urinary mucopolysaccharides and mucoproteins was increased in the presence of urease-positive bacteria [21,22,23]. Direct morphological studies on struvite stones surgically removed from patients further support this hypothesis, as these stones were found to contain bacteria as a part of the stone matrix, encased in a bacterial-induced anionic layer [24,25].

The anionic groups of the bacterial capsular polysaccharide are believed to significantly influence struvite and carbonate apatite formation, as they promote the binding of cations, affecting their supersaturation and the formation of stones [26,27]. Similarly, the endotoxic lipopolysaccharide (LPS) present on the surface of all gram-negative bacteria was also shown to affect struvite stone formation, as it consists of a lipophilic lipid A that anchors the LPS into the outer membrane, a core region, as well as a long polysaccharide chain termed the O-Antigen. The heterogeneous nature of this O-Antigen has been shown to promote or inhibit struvite crystal formation, depending on the composition of the O-Antigen and its ability to bind cations [28]. O-Antigen compositions that bound calcium and magnesium weakly were associated with increased crystallization rates (due to increased supersaturation), while those that bound large amounts of these cations inhibited crystallization [27,28]. These observations illustrate a significant role for bacterial polysaccharides in struvite and apatite crystallization. As the pH of the surrounding urine increases due to the actions of urease, the forming stone provides a surface for further bacterial attachment and subsequent biofilm formation. The subsequent incorporation of urinary components into the capsular polysaccharide layer results in the formation of further nidi, leading to the growth of the stone in concentric layers [24,25,29].

Of note, a murine model of struvite urolithiasis was recently reported – the authors created cutaneous vesicostomies in megabladder mice and a majority of experimental animals (>85%) formed struvite calculi. This model holds promise for future studies of struvite stone pathophysiology [30].

Effects on renal function

The potential deleterious effects of struvite calculi on renal function are well known. Large struvite stones will often grow in a staghorn configuration and studies have shown both an association with renal insufficiency as well as renal-related mortality in patients with untreated staghorn calculi [31]. Furthermore, recurrent cystitis is an independent risk factor for chronic kidney disease in patients with nephrolithiasis [32]. Also, as mentioned above, xanthogranulomatous pyelonephritis (XGP) is a chronic destructive granulomatous disease of the kidneys that arises from an atypical incomplete immune response to subacute bacterial infection with concomitant urinary tract obstruction by struvite and other calculi. Renal deterioration, infection, and abscess formation are common in XGP and patients are often treated with curative nephrectomy [33].

Metabolic evaluation and pharmacotherapy

Initial reports suggested that all patients with struvite (infection) stones should undergo metabolic evaluation, but more recent reports suggest that patients with struvite stones with or without calcium phosphate (carbonate apatite) typically do not merit complete metabolic stone evaluation due to the low likelihood of finding a non-infectious cause for their stone disease [3,34]. While surgical removal remains the mainstay of treatment for symptomatic struvite calculi, medications such as urease inhibitors and chronic suppressive antibiotics are used as well.

Acetohydroxamic acid (AHA), an inhibitor of urease production, has been evaluated in several randomized controlled trials including patients with spinal cord injury and struvite calculi. A significant decrease in recurrence of struvite calculi was shown, but significant side-effects were also noted, including headache, deep venous thrombosis, tremulousness, and pulmonary embolism [35,36,37]. The rate of side-effects has ranged from 22% to 62% [35,36]. Based on these side-effect profiles, urease inhibition is typically reserved for patients in whom endourological treatment and/or complete removal of stones is not possible or for struvite stones with high recurrence rates after endourological management. Hydroxyurea is another urease inhibitor which has not been studied in a randomized trial [35].

Chronic antibiotic suppression has also been suggested in patients with struvite calculi. It has been studied retrospectively, but there are no randomized studies to support this practice [35,38]. Despite the lack of data, many physicians will consider suppressive antibiotics even after complete removal of a struvite calculus (i.e. 3–6-month course) in an attempt to optimally sterilize the urinary tract and prevent the recurrence of both stones and infection. An alternative approach is to treat the patient with a course of perioperative antibiotics for 1–2 weeks after struvite stone removal, but to reserve the decision on chronic suppression for patients who have recurrent infection after stone removal. Certainly in patients in whom complete stone removal is not possible because of co-morbidities or stone complexity, chronic antibiotic therapy may be useful in slowing the rate of struvite stone growth [15].

Irrigation chemolysis

In select patients, typically those unfit for endourological treatment and/or those who have had significant side-effects of pharmacotherapy, irrigation chemolysis has been used effectively to treat struvite calculi [39,40]. Various techiques have been described which include the use of nephrostomy tubes with or without ureteral stents or catheters. The most common solutions used for chemolysis of struvite calculi are Suby's solution G (citric acid, magnesium oxide, sodium carbonate) and hemiacidrin (similar to Suby's solution, also contains d-gluconic acid). These acidic solutions provide hydrogen ions and citrate which may form soluble complexes with calcium and phosphate contained within the struvite calculus, as well as lowering the pH of the urine which further solubilizes struvite calculi [41]. While used successfully in several studies, percutaneous chemolysis is associated with long treatment duration (days to weeks), as well as a significant side-effect profile which includes sepsis, perirenal abscesses, pyelonephritis, epididymitis, and hypermagnesemia [39,40,42,43].

Surgical management

With the increasing popularity and practice of minimally invasive and endourological techniques (shock wave lithotripsy (SWL), ureteroscopy, percutaneous nephrolithotomy), the treatment of stone disease has radically changed over the past three decades. With specific reference to struvite calculi, an emphasis is placed on complete stone removal, as residual fragments can serve as nidi for recurrent stone formation. As described above, the thick exopolysaccharide layer formed on the stone by bacteria and the stone matrix itself make these stones difficult to treat with antibiotics and urease inhibitors alone. Even small residual stone fragments will harbor bacteria which may then break free, multiply, and lead to the formation of additional struvite calculi.

All three endourological techniques have been used successfully for treatment of struvite calculi, and treatment selection is based on a combination of stone-related and patient factors, including stone location and size and patient co-morbidities, body habitus, and genitourinary anatomy. The success and continued improvement of endourological techniques combined with the high side-effect profiles of the urease inhibitors are the two main reasons why pharmacotherapy is reserved for the highest risk patients with struvite calculi [35,44,45]. With the goal of complete stone removal, ureteroscopy and percutaneous extraction are often first-line treatments with the possible addition of SWL as an adjunct treatment, whereas SWL is rarely used as monotherapy. Nephrectomy is reserved for those whose stone-bearing kidneys have minimal function (typically <15% on nuclear functional studies) such as those with XGP or large chronic staghorn calculi which have resulted in severe renal cortical atrophy.

It is common practice to treat patients with struvite calculi with a course of antibiotics prior to endourological treatment. While patients with struvite calculi have not been studied specifically in this practice, two studies have noted a significant reduction in systemic inflammatory response (SIRS) or sepsis after percutaneous nephrolithotomy in patients receiving either ciprofloxacin or nitrofurantoin for 1 week prior to surgery. Whether this practice is appropriate for all patients undergoing percutaneous stone surgery is unclear, but it is a reasonable and common approach for patients with struvite calculi [46,47]. Postoperative, culture-specific antibiotics after removal of struvite calculi are often given for 5–7 days in the absence of infectious complications, though there are no randomized trials which have evaluated this practice.

When performing endourological procedures, it is important to obtain both renal pelvic and stone culture in patients with known or suspected struvite calculi. As the majority of urease-positive bacteria are harbored within the biofilm coating the stone or the stone matrix itself, stone culture is of particular importance. Both renal pelvis and stone culture have been shown to be more accurate predictors of organisms causing postoperative sepsis than bladder urine in patients undergoing percutaneous stone surgery for struvite stones [48,49]. In addition, patients with a positive renal pelvic urine or stone culture were found to have a four-fold greater relative risk of urosepsis [49].

Summary

Struvite stones, associated with recurrent infection of the urinary tract, present a treatment challenge due to the unique microbiological characteristics (i.e. biofilm formation) associated with these calculi. Endourological management, focused on complete stone removal, is the standard of care in patients who are fit for treatment, and other management strategies (pharmacotherapy, dissolution) have also been used successfully.

References

1. Scales CD Jr, Smith AC, Hanley JM, Saigal CS. Urologic Diseases in America Project. Prevalence of kidney stones in the United States. Eur Urol 2012; 62(1): 160–5.
2. Pearle MS, Lotan Y. Urinary lithiasis: etiology, epidemiology, and pathogenesis. In: *Campbell-Walsh Urology*, 10th edn. Philadelphia: Saunders-Elsevier, 2010.
3. Resnick MI. Evaluation and management of infection stones. Urol Clin North Am 1981; 8(2): 265–76.
4. Ferrandino MN, Pietrow PK, Preminger GM. Evaluation and medical management of urinary lithiasis. In: *Campbell-Walsh Urology*, 10th edn. Philadelphia: Saunders-Elsevier, 2010.
5. Bichler KH, Eipper E, Naber K, Braun V, Zimmermann R, Lahme S. Urinary infection stones. Int J Antimicrob Agents 2002; 19(6): 488–98.

6. DeVivo MJ, Fine PR. Predicting renal calculus occurrence in spinal cord injury patients. Arch Phys Med Rehab 1986; 67(10): 722–5.
7. DeVivo MJ, Fine PR, Cutter GR, Maetz HM. The risk of renal calculi in spinal cord injury patients. J Urol 1984; 131(5): 857–60.
8. Welk B, Fuller A, Razvi H, Denstedt J. Renal stone disease in spinal-cord-injured patients. J Endourol 2012; 26(8): 954–9.
9. Matlaga BR, Kim SC, Watkins SL, et al. Changing composition of renal calculi in patients with neurogenic bladder. J Urol 2006; 175: 1716–19.
10. Welk B, Fuller A, Razvi H, Denstedt J. Renal stone disease in spinal-cord-injured patients. J Endourol 2012; 26(8): 954–9.
11. Gleeson MJ, Griffith DP. Infection stones. In: Resnick MI, Pak CYC, eds. *Urolithiasis: A Medical and Surgical Reference*. Philadelphia: WB Saunders, 1990, p.115.
12. Kramer G, Klingler HC, Steiner GE. Role of bacteria in the development of kidney stones. Curr Opin Urol 2000; 10(1): 35–8.
13. Wasserstein AG. Nephrolithiasis: acute management and prevention. Dis Mon 1998; 44(5): 196–213.
14. Kulkarni NM, Eisner BH, Pinho DF, Joshi MC, Kambadakone AR, Sahani DV. Determination of renal stone composition in phantom and patients using single-source dual-energy computed tomography. J Comput Assist Tomogr 2013; 37(1): 37–45.
15. Rodman JS. Struvite stones. Nephron 1999; 81(suppl 1): 50–9.
16. Bichler KH, Eipper E, Naber K, Braun V, Zimmermann R, Lahme S. Urinary infection stones. Int J Antimicrob Agents 2002; 19(6): 488–98.
17. Costerton JW. Introduction to biofilm. Int J Antimicrob Agents 1999; 11(3–4): 217–21; discussion 37–9.
18. Choong S, Whitfield H. Biofilms and their role in infections in urology. BJU Int 2000; 86(8): 935–41.
19. Nickel JC, Olson M, McLean RJ, Grant SK, Costerton JW. An ecological study of infected urinary stone genesis in an animal model. Br J Urol 1987; 59(1): 21–30.
20. McLean RJ, Nickel JC, Noakes VC, Costerton JW. An in vitro ultrastructural study of infectious kidney stone genesis. Infect Immun 1985; 49(3): 805–11.
21. Finlayson B, Vermeulen CW, Stewart EJ. Stone matrix and mucoprotein from urine. J Urol 1961; 86: 355–63.
22. Griffith DP, Bragin S, Musher DM. Dissolution of struvite urinary stones. Experimental studies in vitro. Invest Urol 1976; 13(5): 351–3.
23. Wickham JE. Matrix and the infective renal calculus. Br J Urol 1975; 47(7): 727–32.
24. Nickel JC, Emtage J, Costerton JW. Ultrastructural microbial ecology of infection-induced urinary stones. J Urol 1985; 133(4): 622–7.
25. Nickel JC, Reid G, Bruce AW, Costerton JW. Ultrastructural microbiology of infected urinary stone. Urology 1986; 28(6): 512–15.
26. Clapham L, McLean RJC, Nickel JC, Downey J, Costerton JW. The influence of bacteria on struvite crystal habit and its importance in urinary stone formation. J Crystal Growth 1990; 104: 475–84.
27. Dumanski AJ, Hedelin H, Edin-Liljegren A, Beauchemin D, McLean RJ. Unique ability of the Proteus mirabilis capsule to enhance mineral growth in infectious urinary calculi. Infect Immun 1994; 62(7): 2998–3003.
28. Torzewska A, Staczek P, Rozalski A. Crystallization of urine mineral components may depend on the chemical nature of Proteus endotoxin polysaccharides. J Med Microbiol 2003; 52(Pt 6): 471–7.

29. McLean RJ, Nickel JC, Beveridge TJ, Costerton JW. Observations of the ultrastructure of infected kidney stones. J Med Microbiol 1989; 29(1): 1–7.
30. Becknell B, Carpenter AR, Bolon B, et al. Struvite urolithiasis and chronic urinary tract infection in a murine model of urinary diversion. Urology 2013; 81(5): 943–8.
31. Teichman JM, Long RD, Hulbert JC. Long-term renal fate and prognosis after staghorn calculus management. J Urol 1995; 153(5): 1403–7.
32. Bemis GG. Repair of enterocele (posterior vaginal wall hernia). Clin Obstet Gynecol 1975; 18(3): 3–19.
33. Hammond NA, Nikolaidis P, Miller FH. Infectious and inflammatory diseases of the kidney. Radiol Clin North Am 2012; 50(2): 259–70.
34. Lingeman JE, Siegel YI, Steele B. Metabolic evaluation of infected renal lithiasis: clinical relevance. J Endourol 1995; 9(1): 51–4.
35. Eisner BH, Goldfarb DS, Pareek G. Pharmacologic treatment of kidney stone disease. Urol Clin North Am 2013; 40(1): 21–30.
36. Griffith DP, Khonsari F, Skurnick JH, James KE. A randomized trial of acetohydroxamic acid for the treatment and prevention of infection-induced urinary stones in spinal cord injury patients. J Urol 1988; 140: 318–24.
37. Griffith DP, Gleeson MJ, Lee H, Longuet R, Deman E, Earle N. Randomized, double-blind trial of Lithostat (acetohydroxamic acid) in the palliative treatment of infection-induced urinary calculi. Eur Urol 1991; 20(3): 243–7.
38. Borghi L, Meschi T, Schianchi T. Medical treatment of nephrolithiasis. Endocrinol Metab Clin North Am 2002; 31(4): 1051–64.
39. Suby HI. Dissolution of urinary calculi. Proc Roy Soc Med 1944; 37(10): 609–20.
40. Smith AD, Reinke DB, Miller RP, Lange PH. Percutaneous nephrostomy in the management of ureteral and renal calculi. Radiology 1979; 133(1): 49–54.
41. Healy KA, Ogan K. Pathophysiology and management of infectious staghorn calculi. Urol Clin North Am 2007; 34(3): 363–74.
42. Dretler SP, Pfister RC. Percutaneous dissolution of renal calculi. Annu Rev Med 1983; 34: 359–66.
43. Dretler SP, Pfister RC. Primary dissolution therapy of struvite calculi. J Urol 1984; 131(5): 861–3.
44. Healy KA, Ogan K. Pathophysiology and management of infectious staghorn calculi. Urol Clin North Am 2007; 34(3): 363–74.
45. Borghi L, Meschi T, Schianchi T, et al. Medical treatment of nephrolithiasis. Endocrinol Metab Clin North Am 2002; 31(4): 1051–64.
46. Bag S, Kumar S, Taneja N, Sharma V, Mandal AK, Singh SK. One week of nitrofurantoin before percutaneous nephrolithotomy significantly reduces upper tract infection and urosepsis: a prospective controlled study. Urology 2011; 77(1): 45–9.
47. Mariappan P, Smith G, Moussa SA, Tolley DA. One week of ciprofloxacin before percutaneous nephrolithotomy significantly reduces upper tract infection and urosepsis: a prospective controlled study. BJU Int 2006; 98(5): 1075–9.
48. Korets R, Graversen JA, Kates M, Mues AC, Gupta M. Post-percutaneous nephrolithotomy systemic inflammatory response: a prospective analysis of preoperative urine, renal pelvic urine and stone cultures. J Urol 2011; 186(5): 1899–903.
49. Mariappan P, Smith G, Bariol SV, Moussa SA, Tolley DA. Stone and pelvic urine culture and sensitivity are better than bladder urine as predictors of urosepsis following percutaneous nephrolithotomy: a prospective clinical study. J Urol 2005; 173(5): 1610–14.

CHAPTER 6

Genetic Causes of Kidney Stones: Cystinuria, Primary Hyperoxaluria, Dent's Disease, and APRT Deficiency

Runolfur Palsson
Landspitali – The National University Hospital of Iceland *and* University of Iceland, Reykjavik, Iceland

Introduction

Nephrolithiasis encompasses a broad range of underlying disorders, many of which are directly caused or influenced by genetic factors. Idiopathic calcium nephrolithiasis, the most common form of stone disease, is a complex trait that results from interaction of multiple susceptibility genes and environmental factors [1]. Despite significant efforts, the search for major genetic variants contributing to this prevalent phenotype has largely been unsuccessful. In contrast, the characterization of several rare single gene defects associated with kidney stones and/or nephrocalcinosis has advanced our understanding of molecular pathways leading to stone formation, such as abnormalities in renal tubular transport and metabolic perturbations.

Collectively, monogenic disorders only account for approximately 2% of kidney stones in adults and 10% of childhood stones [2]. Nevertheless, these conditions are important in clinical practice due to their tendency to cause severe stone disease and progressive renal injury. The recognition of rare monogenic causes of kidney stones can be challenging for the clinician, owing to lack of awareness or absence of characteristic clinical features that distinguish these cases from the common type of nephrolithiasis. This frequently results in unacceptable delays in diagnosis and treatment, with identification of some patients after the onset of kidney failure. A genetic disorder should always be considered during evaluation of kidney stones in children and in unusual adult cases. Once a diagnosis of a single gene disorder has been made, screeing for genetic defect should be carried out in family members and genetic counseling provided.

Urinary Stones: Medical and Surgical Management, First Edition. Edited by Michael Grasso and David S. Goldfarb.

In this chapter, clues that should alert the clinician to a genetic cause of kidney stone disease will be reviewed along with several of the most common single gene disorders, cystinuria, primary hyperoxaluria (PH), Dent's disease and adenine phosphoribosyltransferase (APRT) deficiency. Other monogenic traits whose molecular defect has been characterized include familial hypomagnesemia with hypercalciuria and nephrocalcinosis, inherited forms of distal renal tubular acidosis, autosomal dominant hypocalcemic hypercalciuria, Bartter's syndrome and hereditary hypophosphatemic rickets with hypercalciuria, all of which are associated with hypercalciuria and calcium nephrolithiasis. Also, Lesch–Nyhan syndrome which is associated with uric acid stones, and xanthinuria which results in formation of xanthine stones.

When to suspect a genetic cause of kidney stones

Some of the key clinical and laboratory features that should alert the clinician to a possible genetic disorder in a patient who presents with kidney stones are shown in Box 6.1. Onset during childhood is an important clue as inherited disorders are much more common among children than adults with kidney stones. A detailed family history should always be obtained.

Box 6.1 When to suspect a genetic cause of kidney stones

Clinical manifestations	• First kidney stone in childhood or recurrent stones • Family history of nephrolithiasis or nephrocalcinosis or unexplained kidney failure • Growth retardation or rickets • Extrarenal features, particularly neurological abnormalities, ocular abnormalities or hearing loss • Symptoms of hypocalcemia or hypomagnesemia, such as tetany, muscle spasms and weakness and paresthesias • Reddish-brown diaper stain

Laboratory testing	• Unusual urinary crystals
	  ◦ Cystine
	  ◦ 2,8-Dihydroxyadenine
	• Proteinuria
	• Elevated serum creatinine and/or reduced GFR
	• Hypomagnesemia
	• Hypercalciuria
	• Severe hyperoxaluria

Imaging	• Nephrocalcinosis • Radiolucent or low-density kidney stones • Multiple stones or bilateral stones

GFR, glomerular filtration rate.

However, many of the monogenic disorders causing kidney stones have an autosomal recessive pattern of inheritance which may not be readily apparent in the family history.

A severe disease course as evidenced by frequent hospital admissions and urological interventions may suggest a genetic cause, and nephrocalcinosis should always prompt a search for a genetic disorder. Progressive chronic kidney disease (CKD) is a common feature of many single gene causes of nephrolithiasis [3]. Being uncommon in stone formers in general, early-onset or advanced CKD should alert the clinician to a possible underlying genetic disorder. The same applies to manifestations of renal tubulopathy, including hypocalcemia, hypomagnesemia, hypophosphatemia or rickets, metabolic acidosis and low molecular weight (LMW) proteinuria [4]. Furthermore, extrarenal manifestations such as neurological abnormalities, ocular defects and hearing loss are highly suggestive of a genetic cause of kidney stone disease [4].

Detection of crystals by urine microscopy may be pivotal in the diagnostic process, particularly the pathognomonic cystine crystals (Figure 6.1a) found

(a)

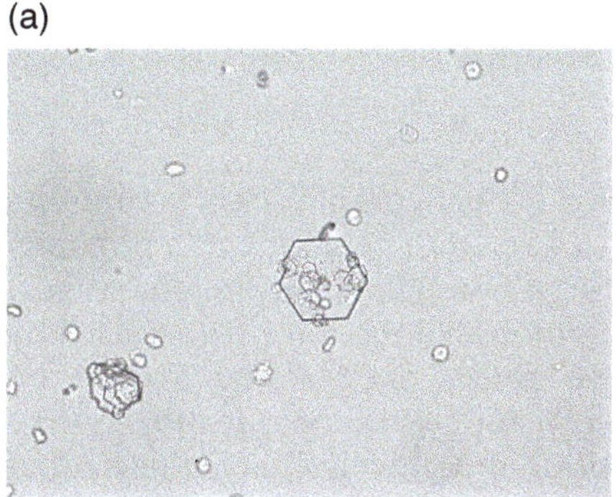

(b)

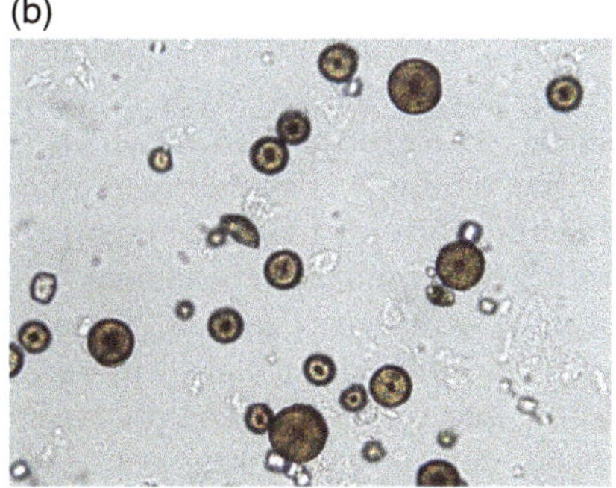

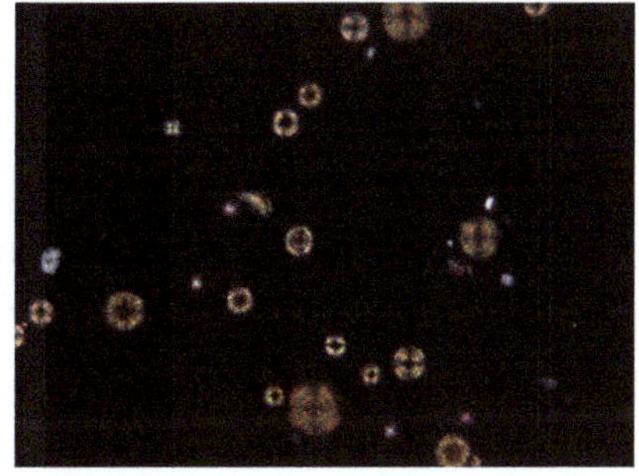

Figure 6.1 Characteristic urinary crystals. (a) Cystine crystals. The typical hexagonal crystals are diagnostic of cystinuria. (b) 2,8-Dihydroxyadenine crystals. Conventional light microscopy (*left panel*) shows brown crystals with dark outline and central spicules. When viewed by polarized light microscopy (*right panel*), the medium-sized cystals appear yellow in colour and produce a central Maltese cross pattern. Original magnification × 400.

in patients with cystinuria and the characteristic 2,8-dihydroxyadenine (DHA) crystals (Figure 6.1b) observed in patients with APRT deficiency [3]. Unfortunately, laboratory technicians may not recognize these crystals as skills in performing microscopic examination of the urine sediment have not been emphasized in many clinical laboratories. Stone analysis is an instrumental component of the evaluation of nephrolithiasis and may unravel an inherited cause such as cystinuria and APRT deficiency. It is important to use infra-red spectroscopy or X-ray diffraction techniques, while avoiding biochemical methods which are inaccurate and do not discriminate between uric acid stones and DHA or xanthine stones [3].

The results of imaging studies can also raise the suspicion of an underlying genetic disorder. While stones that are radiolucent on conventional radiographic studies or hypodense by computed tomography (CT) are usually composed of uric acid, it is important to consider DHA and xanthine stones in the differential diagnosis [4]. Radiographic findings consistent with nephrocalcinosis are also useful clues. However, it should be noted that increased medullary echogenicity by renal ultrasound is not specific for nephrocalcinosis as other deposits can give a similar picture, including crystalline DHA deposits [4].

Cystinuria

Cystinuria is the most common genetic cause of nephrolithiasis, accounting for about 1% of all cases. The disorder results from impairment in proximal tubular reabsorption of filtered cystine, a homodimer of the amino acid cysteine. Cystinuria is inherited as an autosomal recessive trait caused by inactivating mutations in one of two genes, *SLC7A9* and *SLC3A1* on chromosomes 19 and 2, respectively [3]. *SLC7A9* encodes for the cystine transporter $b^{0,+}$AT (amino acid transporter of positively charged or neutral amino acids), which forms a heterodimer with rBAT (related to $b^{0,+}$AT amino acid transporter), a product of *SLC3A1*, whose role is to target the transporting subunit to the apical membrane of proximal tubular epithelial cells. Patients who are homozygous for mutations of *SLC3A1* (type A genotype) or *SLC7A9* (type B genotype) will fail to reabsorb cystine which is excreted in excessive amounts in the urine where it is highly insoluble, predisposing to stone formation. Known mutations in these two genes do not explain all cases of cystinuria, suggesting additional genetic defects [5]. The cystinuria genotype does not appear to influence the rate of stone recurrence. The cystine transporter is also responsible for reabsorption of the dibasic amino acids ornithine, arginine, and lysine, but the increased urinary excretion of these compounds is not clinically relevant.

Clinical features

The clinical course is characterized by recurrent kidney stones. Most patients exhibit manifestations of kidney stones in childhood, with 50% forming a first stone in the first decade of life [3]. However, some patients have their first stone in late adulthood [6]. For unclear reasons, stones are more common in men than women with cystinuria. Cystine stones, which are less dense than calcium stones on CT images, frequently grow very large and can form staghorn calculi. Cystinuria can result in CKD due to recurrent stone episodes causing obstructive nephropathy and/or kidney damage resulting from repeated urological interventions [7]. The reduction in renal function is generally mild.

Diagnosis

Cystinuria should be suspected in patients presenting with their first kidney stone in childhood or adolescence. The diagnosis is often made by detection of the hexagonal cystine crystals on urine microscopy (see Figure 6.1a). The qualitative nitroprusside test is both sensitive and specific and is useful for screening [3]. Stone analysis will confirm the diagnosis and should always be performed when possible. Quantitative analysis of urinary cystine excretion is not required for diagnosis but is useful for guiding therapy. The normal range of cystine excretion is 30 mg/day (0.13 mmol/day) but patients with cystinuria excrete >400 mg per day (1.7 mmol/day) and in some cases up to 3600 mg per day (15 mmol/day). Genetic testing is not required for diagnosis of cystinuria.

Treatment

The treatment of cystinuria is centered on reducing the supersaturation of urinary cystine by targeting the cystine concentration and urine pH.

- Fluid intake of 1.5–4.5 L per day, depending on age, should be prescribed to maintain a dilute urine. The goal is to decrease the urine cystine concentration to <250 mg/L (approximately 1 mmol/L). In adults, this usually requires a urine output of at least 3 L per 24 h.
- The urinary cystine excretion can be reduced by dietary protein and sodium restriction. Modest limitation of animal protein (1.0 g/kg/day) and sodium (<100 mmol/day) intake is recommended.
- Urinary alkalinization reduces cystine supersaturation and requires raising the urine pH to above 7.5. The preferred alkalinizing agent is potassium citrate in a dose of 0.5–1.0 mmol/kg/day, administered 3–4 times daily. Maintaining an alkaline urine at all times is desirable for the most significantly affected individuals. Thus, the urine pH should be monitored by measurements at variable times and the alkali dose adjusted accordingly.
- The thiol drugs d-penicillamine and tiopronin may be useful when other measures prove ineffective [3]. Both drugs reduce stone formation by breaking the disulfide bonds linking the two cysteine molecules and forming more soluble drug–cysteine complexes. Unfortunately, many patients do not tolerate these agents due to severe adverse effects, including fever, rash, aplastic anemia, hepatotoxicity and rarely nephrotic syndrome caused by membranous nephropathy.

Several small, retrospective studies suggest a clear benefit of preventive therapies [8]. Nevertheless, many patients continue to form stones. Cystine stones are often not amenable to being fragmented by shock wave lithotripsy, but can be effectively broken up by laser treatment administered through ureteroscopy [9].

Primary hyperoxaluria

Primary hyperoxaluria (PH) is a rare autosomal recessive disorder of glyoxylate metabolism resulting in excessive production of oxalate which cannot be degraded in humans and is largely excreted by the kidneys. The high urinary oxalate concentration promotes the formation and aggregation of calcium oxalate crystals in renal tubules, leading to stone formation and nephrocalcinosis. Furthermore, attachment of crystals to the renal tubular epithelium causes cellular injury and appears to incite an inflammatory reaction in the renal interstitium, causing progressive renal damage and scarring [3]. A significant proportion of affected patients develop kidney failure [10]. When the glomerular filtration rate (GFR) has declined to below 30–35 mL/min/1.73 m^2, the renal excretion can no longer keep up with the oxalate production, resulting in rising plasma levels and deposition of calcium oxalate crystals in many organs, including the retina, myocardium, blood vessels, skin, bone and the central nervous system [10]. The incidence and prevalence of PH are unknown, though survey data from Europe suggest a prevalence of 1–3 per million population [11].

Three types of PH have been described, each involving a different enzyme of the oxalate metabolic pathways [3].

- Type 1 PH accounts for approximately 80% of cases and is caused by mutations of the *AGXT* gene on chromosome 2. The genetic defect results in reduced or abolished activity of the liver-specific enzyme alanine-glyoxylate aminotransferase (AGT), that catalyzes the conversion of glyoxylate to glycine, leading to accumulation of glyoxylate which is metabolized to oxalate and glycolate. Certain *AGXT* mutations cause mistargeting of AGT to mitochondria, resulting in hyperoxaluria despite detectable enzyme activity [12].
- Type 2 PH, which is observed in about 10% of patients, is caused by mutations in the *GRHPR* gene on chromosome 9, resulting in deficiency or absence of the hepatic cytosolic enzyme glyoxylate reductase/hydroxypyruvate reductase (GRHPR), that converts glyoxylate to glycolate. Increased levels of L-glyceric acid in the urine along with hyperoxaluria are indicative of type 2 PH.
- Type 3 PH is caused by mutations of the *HOGA1* gene (formerly *DHDPSL*) on chromosome 10. The metabolic defect is thought to be due to abnormalities of the enzyme 4-hydroxy-2-oxaloglutarate aldolase in hepatic mitochondria, which catalyzes the breakdown of 4-hydroxy-2-oxaloglutarate to pyruvate and glyoxalate [13].

Additional genes appear to be involved as patients with characteristic features of PH have been identified without demonstrable abnormalities of the genes responsible for types 1, 2, and 3 PH [3].

Clinical features

Most patients present with manifestations of nephrolithiasis and recurrent stone passage is characteristic of the disorder [2]. Nephrocalcinosis may also be observed without discrete stones. The median age of onset of symptoms is 5 years and >80% of patients present before 20 years of age. Progressive CKD develops over time and is most severe in patients with PH type 1, who frequently develop kidney failure in their early thirties [14]. Patients with PH types 2 and 3 appear to have better renal outcomes. Systemic oxalosis can result in refractory anemia, osteodystrophy, cardiac arrhythmias, oxalate cardiomyopathy, and painful ischemic ulcers, eventually leading to death [3].

Diagnosis

The diagnosis of PH should be suspected in any child or adolescent who presents with a calcium stone, especially if bilateral stones are present or if renal imaging studies demonstrate findings consistent with nephrocalcinosis. Stone analysis will generally reveal calcium oxalate monohydrate. A key component of the diagnostic evaluation is 24-h urine chemistries, while analysis of a random urine sample is an alternative option in young or developmentally delayed children. Patients with PH have a markedly increased urinary oxalate excretion, often >90 mg (1 mmol)/1.73 m^2 per day. Urinary oxalate levels in patients with dietary or enteric hyperoxaluria are generally lower than 63 mg (0.7 mmol)/1.73 m^2 per day. Urinary glycolate concentration >45 mg (0.5 mmol)/1.73 m^2 per day is strongly supportive of the diagnosis of type 1 PH, and patients with type 2 PH generally have urinary L-glyceric acid levels >5 µmol/L.

The diagnosis of PH can be confirmed by DNA testing. Identification of the genotype has potential therapeutic implications, as PH type 1 patients with mistargeting of AGT to mitochondria have been shown to respond to treatment with pyridoxine (vitamin B6), a co-enzyme of AGT [15].

Treatment

Early diagnosis is essential for successful management aimed at minimizing stone formation, delaying the progression of CKD and preventing systemic oxalosis. Conservative therapeutic strategies focus on decreasing urinary calcium oxalate crystal formation and oxalate production.

- Fluid intake >3 L/1.73 m^2 per day is generally recommended with a goal of maintaining the urinary oxalate concentration <40 mg/L (0.4 mmol/L).
- Orthophosphate 30–40 mg/kg daily [16] and potassium citrate 0.15 g/kg per day [17] reduce calcium oxalate crystal formation.
- All patients with PH type 1 should receive a trial of pyridoxine 7–9 mg/kg/day [3]. Pyridoxine promotes the conversion of glyoxylate to glycine

rather than to oxalate. The urinary oxalate excretion can correct into the normal range in patients homozygous for mutations causing mistargeting of AGT, while those heterozygous for these mutations demonstrate partial correction [15]. If a reduction in the urine oxalate excretion is demonstrated after 3 months, then the therapy should be continued. A pyridoxine dose of 5–7 mg/kg/day may be sufficient for long-term management [3].

Restriction of dietary oxalate is of limited benefit since the overwhelming majority of urinary oxalate in PH patients arises of from endogenous production.

In patients with advanced CKD, minimizing systemic oxalate accumulation is critically important for a favorable outcome of subsequent kidney transplantation [10]. Most patients with kidney failure require intensive dialysis for oxalate removal. However, removal by dialysis may be insufficient to keep up with the oxalate production and, therefore, kidney transplantation should be performed as soon as possible [3]. Combined liver-kidney transplantation is recommended for most patients with PH type 1. The liver allograft corrects the underlying metabolic defect. Kidney transplantation only is the current recommendation for PH type 2 patients who progress to end-stage renal disease (ESRD). Many PH patients require frequent urological intervention for stones.

Dent's disease

Dent's disease is a rare X-linked renal tubular disorder characterized by LMW proteinuria, hypercalciuria, nephrocalcinosis and/or nephrolithiasis and progressive CKD. Males are much more severely affected than females.

Approximately 60% of Dent's disease cases are caused by mutations in the *CLCN5* gene, whose protein product is a ClC-5 chloride channel, which is primarily expressed in the renal proximal tubule, cortical collecting duct, and the thick ascending limb of the loop of Henle [18]. In proximal tubular cells, this protein appears to be involved in the endocytic reabsorption of LMW proteins. Mutations in *OCRL1*, initially found to be associated with Lowe's (oculocerebral) syndrome, account for 15% of Dent's disease cases, now termed Dent's 2 disease [18]. *OCRL1* encodes a phosphatidylinositol 4,5-biphosphate 5-phosphatase located in the Golgi apparatus but the pathogenic mechanism of the molecular defect has not been elucidated. Mutations in *OCRL1* that are associated with Dent's 2 disease do not overlap with those causing Lowe's syndrome [3]. The phenotypic difference among patients with *CLCN5* or *OCRL1* mutations is unknown. Additional genes are assumed to be involved as there are patients with the characteristic phenotype of Dent's disease without detectable mutation in either of the two known genes [18].

Clinical features

The clinical presentation is variable but most commonly, the disease presents in childhood or early adult life with proteinuria, hypercalciuria and nephrolithiasis and/or nephrocalcinosis [3]. Proteinuria is a universal feature and is largely composed of LMW proteins. Many affected males (30–80%) will progress to ESRD in middle age. Nephrocalcinosis occurs in 75% of patients but only a minority of patients pass calcium oxalate or calcium phosphate kidney stones. Approximately 25% of affected males with Dent's disease have rickets or osteomalacia. Other manifestations of proximal tubular dysfunction, such as glycosuria, aminoaciduria and phosphaturia, are also common and hypophosphatemia occurs in about one-third of patients. Patients with Dent's 2 disease caused by *OCRL1* mutations exhibit none of the classic extrarenal manifestations of Lowe's syndrome such as mental retardation, bone disease, growth retardation, and congenital cataracts.

Diagnosis

Dent's disease should be suspected in children who present with proteinuria in conjunction with kidney stones and/or nephrocalcinosis, or in adult patients with unexplained CKD, proteinuria and nephrocalcinosis. A specific test for LMW proteins, such as retinol-binding protein and α1-microglobulin, must be carried out, as markedly increased levels are characteristic of the disease [3].

In patients with LMW proteinuria, the diagnosis of Dent's disease should be considered when at least one of the following features is present.

- Kidney stones or nephrocalcinosis.
- Hypercalciuria >4 mg (0.1 mmol)/kg in 24 h or >0.25 mg Ca^{2+}/mg Cr (0.57 mmol/mmol) in spot urine.
- Reduced GFR.
- Hypophosphatemia with or without rickets.
- Family history consistent with X-linked inheritance.

Genetic testing for *CLCN5* and *OCRL1* can be performed to confirm the diagnosis. Renal biopsy findings include nephrocalcinosis and interstitial fibrosis but these are not specific [3]. Stones, when present, are composed of calcium oxalate and/or calcium phosphate.

Treatment

The primary goal of therapy is delaying the progression of CKD, using an angiotensin-converting enzyme (ACE) inhibitor or an angiotensin receptor blocker (ARB) for controlling blood pressure and reducing proteinuria. However, the effect of this therapy is unclear. Additional therapeutic strategies are aimed at decreasing hypercalciuria and preventing kidney stones and nephrocalcinosis. Thiazide diuretics are often used for this purpose but may not be well tolerated in patients with Dent's disease, who frequently develop severe hypokalemia and/or volume depletion.

Adenine phosphoribosyltransferase deficiency (2,8-dihydroxyadeninuria)

Adenine phosphoribosyltransferase (APRT) deficiency is a rare autosomal recessive disorder of adenine metabolism, resulting in the generation and renal excretion of large amounts of poorly soluble DHA, which leads to kidney stone formation and CKD. Although the disorder has been described in all ethnic groups, the majority of reported cases have come from Japan, France, and Iceland [19]. The prevalence is unknown but has been estimated to be at least 1:50,000–100,000 based on a reported heterozygote frequency of 0.4–1.2% [20]. APRT deficiency appears to be seriously under-recognized and in a number of reported cases the disorder has not been diagnosed until after kidney transplantation [21].

The disease is caused by mutations that completely abolish the function of APRT, a cytoplasmic enzyme encoded by the *APRT* gene, located on chromosome 16 [22]. Absence of a functional APRT prevents the recycling of adenine and leads to the conversion of the 8-hydroxy intermediate metabolite by xanthine dehydrogenase (XDH) to DHA (Figure 6.2).

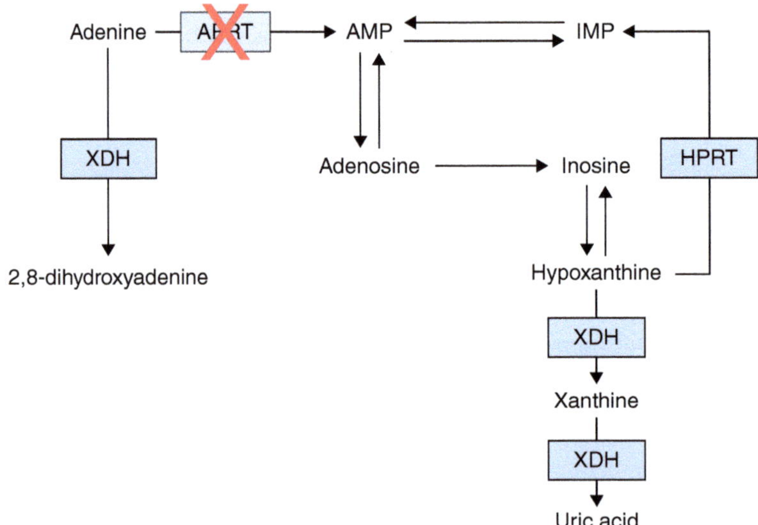

Figure 6.2 Schematic overview of adenine metabolism. In APRT deficiency, adenine cannot be converted to adenosine monophosphate and is instead converted by xanthine dehydrogenase to 2,8-dihydroxyadenine. AMP, adenosine monophosphate; APRT, adenine phosphoribosyltransferase; HPRT, hypoxanthine-guanine phosphoribosyltransferase; IMP, inosine monophosphate; XDH, xanthine dehydrogenase. Source: Edvardsson et al. 2013 [3]. Reproduced with kind permission from Springer Science and Business Media.

Clinical features

Symptoms related to kidney stones are by far the most common clinical manifestation of APRT deficiency [3]. CKD is a relatively common presenting feature in adult patients and progresses to ESRD in a significant proportion of untreated cases. Other common clinical features include lower urinary tract symptoms, hematuria, and reddish-brown diaper stains in infants [19,23]. However, many patients remain asymptomatic into adulthood. The kidney and urinary tract appear to be the only organ system affected in APRT deficiency.

Diagnosis

Early diagnosis of APRT deficiency is essential as timely institution of therapy prevents the development of kidney failure [19,23]. The disorder should be considered in all patients presenting with radiolucent kidney stones or unexplained CKD. The identification of kidney stones requires imaging techniques that are capable of detecting radiolucent stones, such as ultrasound or CT. The urine pH can provide a clue as uric acid stone formers generally have an acidic urine (pH <6), while DHA stones can form at any physiological pH [3]. Microscopic examination of the urine sediment usually reveals the characteristic round and brown DHA crystals which demonstrate a central Maltese cross pattern when viewed by polarized light (see Figure 6.1b). Analysis of DHA crystals and stone material using infra-red and ultraviolet spectrophotometry and/or X-ray crystallography easily differentiates DHA from uric acid.

The diagnosis of APRT deficiency should be confirmed by demonstrating the absence of APRT activity in red cell lysates. However, genetic testing is not required for diagnosis. In patients with CKD, renal biopsy will reveal DHA crystalline nephropathy [21]. It is important, however, not to confuse DHA nephropathy with other types of crystalline nephropathy, particularly those associated with oxalate and uric acid deposits.

Treatment

Treatment with the XDH inhibitor allopurinol, 5–10 mg/kg/day, administered as a single dose or divided into two doses, prevents stone formation and renal crystal deposition and thereby the progression of CKD [19,23]. Moreover, treatment with allopurinol can even result in a resolution of kidney stones and improvement of kidney function in patients with advanced renal failure [19,23]. The recently introduced XDH inhibitor febuxostat provides an alternative treatment option for patients allergic to or intolerant of allopurinol [3]. A low-purine diet and ample fluid intake provide adjunctive benefits to pharmacological therapy.

Acknowledgments

The support of the Rare Kidney Stone Consortium (U54KD083908), a part of the National Institutes of Health (NIH) Rare Diseases Clinical Research Network (RDCRN), funded by the NIDDK, and the NIH Office of Rare Diseases Research (ORDR) is gratefully acknowledged. The author thanks Gudridur Steinunn Oddsdottir of the Landspitali – The National University Hospital of Iceland Clinical Laboratory for the image of cystine crystals and Hrafnhildur L. Runolfsdottir, medical student at the University of Iceland, Reykjavik, for the images of urinary DHA crystals.

References

1. Vezzoli G, Terranegra A, Arcidiacono T, Soldati L. Genetics and calcium nephrolithiasis. Kidney Int 2011; 80(6): 587–93.
2. Monico CG, Milliner DS. Genetic determinants of urolithiasis. Nat Rev Nephrol 2012; 8(3): 151–62.
3. Edvardsson VO, Goldfarb DS, Lieske JC, et al. Hereditary causes of kidney stones and chronic kidney disease. Pediatr Nephrol 2013; 28(10): 1923–42.
4. Ferraro PM, d'Addessi A, Gambaro G. When to suspect a genetic disorder in a patient with renal stones, and why. Nephrol Dial Transplant 2013; 28(4): 811–20.
5. Bisceglia L, Fischetti L, Bonis PD, et al. Large rearrangements detected by MLPA, point mutations, and survey of the frequency of mutations within the SLC3A1 and SLC7A9 genes in a cohort of 172 cystinuric Italian patients. Mol Genet Metab 2010; 99(1): 42–52.
6. Thorleifsson G, Holm H, Edvardsson V, et al. Sequence variants in the CLDN14 gene associate with kidney stones and bone mineral density. Nat Genet 2009; 41(8): 926–30.
7. Worcester EM, Coe FL, Evan AP, Parks JH. Reduced renal function and benefits of treatment in cystinuria vs other forms of nephrolithiasis. BJU Int 2006; 97(6): 1285–90.
8. Pareek G, Steele TH, Nakada SY. Urological intervention in patients with cystinuria is decreased with medical compliance. J Urol 2005; 174(6): 2250–2.
9. Trinchieri A, Montanari E, Zanetti G, Lizzano R. The impact of new technology in the treatment of cystine stones. Urol Res 2007; 35(3): 129–32.
10. Hoppe B, Beck BB, Milliner DS. The primary hyperoxalurias. Kidney Int 2009; 75(12): 1264–71.
11. Cochat P, Liutkus A, Fargue S, Basmaison O, Ranchin B, Rolland MO. Primary hyperoxaluria type 1: still challenging! Pediatr Nephrol 2006; 21(8): 1075–81.
12. Danpure CJ. Molecular etiology of primary hyperoxaluria type 1: new directions for treatment. Am J Nephrol. 2005; 25(3): 303–10.
13. Belostotsky R, Seboun E, Idelson GH, et al. Mutations in DHDPSL are responsible for primary hyperoxaluria type III. Am J Hum Genet 2010; 87(3): 392–9.
14. Lieske JC, Monico CG, Holmes WS, et al. International registry for primary hyperoxaluria. Am J Nephrol 2005; 25(3): 290–6.
15. Monico CG, Olson JB, Milliner DS. Implications of genotype and enzyme phenotype in pyridoxine response of patients with type I primary hyperoxaluria. Am J Nephrol 2005; 25(2): 183–8.
16. Milliner D. Treatment of the primary hyperoxalurias: a new chapter. Kidney Int 2006; 70(7): 1198–200.
17. Leumann E, Hoppe B, Neuhaus T. Management of primary hyperoxaluria: efficacy of oral citrate administration. Pediatr Nephrol 1993; 7(2): 207–11.

18. Ludwig M, Utsch B, Monnens LA. Recent advances in understanding the clinical and genetic heterogeneity of Dent's disease. Nephrol Dial Transplant 2006; 21(10): 2708–17.
19. Edvardsson V, Palsson R, Olafsson I, Hjaltadottir G, Laxdal T. Clinical features and genotype of adenine phosphoribosyltransferase deficiency in Iceland. Am J Kidney Dis 2001; 38(3): 473–80.
20. Sahota AS, Tischfield JA, Kamatani N, Simmonds HA. Adenine phosphoribosyltransferase deficiency and 2,8-dihydroxyadenine lithiasis. In: Scriver CR, Beaudet AL, Sly WS, Valle D, Childs B, Kinzler K, Vogelstein B, editors. The Metabolic and Molecular Bases of Inherited Disease. 8th ed. New York, NY: McGraw-Hill; 2001. pp. 2571–84.
21. Nasr SH, Sethi S, Cornell LD, et al. Crystalline nephropathy due to 2,8-dihydroxyadeninuria: an under-recognized cause of irreversible renal failure. Nephrol Dial Transplant 2010; 25(6): 1909–15.
22. Edvardsson VO, Palsson R, Sahota A. Adenine phosphoribosyltransferase deficiency. In: Pagon RA, Bird TD, Dolan CR, et al., eds. GeneReviews™. Seattle, WA: University of Washington, 1993. Available from: www.ncbi.nlm.nih.gov/books/NBK100238/.
23. Bollee G, Dollinger C, Boutaud L, et al. Phenotype and genotype characterization of adenine phosphoribosyltransferase deficiency. J Am Soc Nephrol 2010; 21(4): 679–88.

CHAPTER 7

Evaluation and Management of Pediatric Stones

Vidar O. Edvardsson[1] *and Sherry S. Ross*[2]

[1]Landspitali – The National University Hospital of Iceland *and* University of Iceland, Reykjavik, Iceland

[2]Duke University Medical Center, Durham, NC, USA

Recent population-based studies suggest a significant increase in the frequency of kidney stone disease in children and adolescents younger than 18 years of age [1,2]. In a study by Sas et al., carried out in the state of South Carolina, the incidence of symptomatic kidney stones increased from 7.9 per 100,000 children in 1996 to 18.5 per 100,000 in 2007 [1]. Another study in the same age group, performed by Dwyer et al. in Rochester, Minnesota, showed an increase in incidence from 7.2 per 100,000 in the years 1984–1990 to 14.5 per 100,000 during the years 2003–2008 [2]. The greatest rise in incidence was seen in the oldest teenagers where it reached approximately 35 per 100,000 children in both of the above studies while only a limited increase was seen in children less than 10 years of age [1,2]. In the South Carolina study, children aged 14–18 years had an approximately 10 times greater risk of developing symptomatic kidney stones than children in the age group 0–3 years [1]. Stone disease has through the years been more frequently reported in males, both in children [3,4] and adults [5,6]. However, in recent pediatric studies, kidney stone disease has clearly been shown to be more common in females [1,7,8], particularly in the age group 10–17 years [1,9].

Children and adolescents predominantly form calcium-based stones. In the United States, 40–65% of urinary calculi in children are composed of calcium oxalate, 14–30% of calcium phosphate, 10–20% of struvite, 5–10% of cystine and 1–4% of uric acid [10,11]. Other stone types such as xanthine and 2,8-dihydroxyadenine (DHA) are seen more rarely [12]. These findings are supported by a recent pediatric study of the epidemiology of kidney stones based on the Rochester Epidemiology Project, in which 71% of the stones were composed of calcium oxalate, 25% calcium phosphate, 3% had infection-related stones, only 2% had stones composed of uric acid and none of the 84 incident stone formers had a cystine

Urinary Stones: Medical and Surgical Management, First Edition. Edited by Michael Grasso and David S. Goldfarb.

or other stone types [2]. Historically, a high proportion of kidney stones in younger boys was associated with uncorrected urinary tract anomalies and infections caused by *Proteus* or other urea-splitting organisms leading to the formation of magnesium ammonium phosphate, or struvite, stones [13]. The proportion of infection-related childhood stones has, however, decreased steadily during the last decades in association with the widespread use of antenatal screening for congenital anomalies of the urinary tract and prompt diagnosis and treatment of urinary tract infections [13].

Although the great majority of affected children have idiopathic calcium kidney stone disease, monogenic metabolic disorders such as adenine phosphoribosyltransferase (APRT) deficiency, cystinuria, Dent's disease, familial hypomagnesemia with hypercalciuria and nephrocalcinosis (FHHNC), primary hyperoxaluria (PH) and other inherited diseases should always be considered in the differential diagnosis of pediatric stone disease, particularly in prepubertal children and if stones are recurrent [12]. All of these inherited disorders with the exception of cystinuria frequently cause chronic kidney disease (CKD) that in a significant proportion of cases progresses to end-stage renal disease if left untreated. Unfortunately, the lack of recognition and knowledge of these disorders frequently results in unacceptable delay in diagnosis and treatment, often with serious consequences. Features suggestive of rare causes of kidney stones include first stone as a child or preadolescent, family history of stones or nephrocalcinosis or unexplained kidney failure, reddish-brown diaper stain (APRT deficiency), growth retardation or rickets.

Metabolic risk factors for stone formation have been reported in 40–95% of first-time pediatric stone formers [10,14] and up to 95% of adults with recurrent kidney stone disease [15]. Renal excretion of urinary constituents such as calcium, oxalate, phosphate and water determines the level of urinary supersaturation [16]; hypercalciuria, hyperoxaluria, hypocitraturia, and hyperuricosuria are important metabolic risk factors for idiopathic calcium nephrolithiasis [17,18]. Urinary pH is also an important risk factor for stone formation as acidic urine favors the formation of cystine (pH <7.5) and uric acid (pH <6.0) stones while calcium phosphate stones form more readily in alkaline urine (pH >6) [19]. Calcium oxalate crystal and stone formation does not appear to have a direct association with urinary pH in the physiological range. Tamm–Horsfall protein or uromodulin, albumin, RNA and DNA fragments, glycosaminoglycans, citrate, and magnesium are important inhibitors of calcium oxalate and calcium phosphate urinary crystallization and stone formation [16].

The clinical presentation of acute kidney stone events in childhood is highly variable. Colicky abdominal pain is the most common presenting symptom in older children, reported in approximately 50–80% of cases [7,20], while non-specific abdominal pain and irritability are more commonly seen in younger children and infants [4]. Gross hematuria is the presenting sign in 30–50% of cases and microhematuria is seen in most affected children [7,20]. Other frequently noted clinical features are urinary tract infection and/or lower urinary tract symptoms such as dysuria, frequency and voiding problems or even urinary retention when the stones are located in the distal ureter, bladder or urethra [4].

Clinical evaluation of children suspected of kidney stones includes a meticulous history and a complete physical examination followed by detailed laboratory evaluation and medical imaging. Medical history taking should focus on issues such as diet, medication use, specific disorders or conditions known to increase the risk of kidney stones and family history of nephrolithiasis [4,19]. Relevant dietary information includes special diets such as the ketogenic diet (acid urine pH, hyperuricosuria and hypocitraturia), vegetables (alkaline urine pH and hyperoxaluria), and the intake of fluids, salt, fruits, animal protein and of vitamin C (oxaluria) and vitamin D (hypercalciuria). Medication history should elicit the use of drugs known to increase the risk of kidney stones such as glucocorticoids and furosemide (hypercalciuria), acetazolamide (carbonic anhydrase inhibitor, calcium phosphate stones), anticonvulsants such as topiramate, felbamate and zonisamide (carbonic anhydrase inhibitors), protease inhibitors such as indinavir and antibiotics such as ceftriaxone (urinary crystallization of drugs) [4,19].

Specific disorders or conditions known to increase kidney stone risk include congenital malformations of the kidney and the urinary tract, either alone or in conjunction with abnormalities in urinary metabolic risk factor profile and/or urinary tract infections. Further, increased oxalate absorption associated with intestinal fat malabsorption in patients with disorders such as inflammatory bowel disease, short gut syndrome and cystic fibrosis increases the risk of kidney stone formation. Patients with severe neurological disorders are at particularly high risk of developing kidney stones due to their frequent anticonvulsant drug use, prolonged immobilization and inability to control fluid intake, which often is poor. Family history of kidney stones, kidney failure or specific metabolic diseases needs to be considered. Since most of these conditions follow an autosomal recessive inheritance pattern, there is a 25% chance of a sibling being affected while offsprings are unlikely to develop these disorders in the absence of consanguinity [4,12,19].

Physical examination should include the measurement of height, weight, blood pressure and the calculation of Body Mass Index percentile and/or z-score as overweight and obesity have been associated with kidney stones. Clinical features such as bony deformities, retarded growth (rickets) and tetany (FHHNC) associated with disorders of mineral and vitamin D metabolism should be carefully looked for [4,19].

All children with kidney stones need a thorough laboratory evaluation to search for modifiable risk factors for idiopathic kidney stone disease and to uncover rare causes of stones which may be associated with reduced kidney function and risk of kidney failure [12,19]. Urinalysis should be performed to look for hematuria and pyuria and changes consistent with tubular dysfunction such as hyposthenuria or isosthenuria, glycosuria and proteinuria, and urine should be cultured to rule out a bacterial infection. Further, urine microscopy should be performed at least once, screening for xanthine and the round reddish-brown 2,8-dihydroxyadenine (DHA) crystals and typical hexagonal cystine crystals. Stone analysis, a key part of kidney stone work-up, makes a definite diagnosis when the stones are composed of cystine, DHA, xanthine, and struvite (infection-related stones) [4,12,19]. The finding of calcium-based stones is helpful as it narrows the differential diagnosis while a uric acid stone should prompt an investigation for an inborn error of purine metabolism since this stone type is rare in healthy children. Urine should be strained for several days following a clinical stone event in an attempt to recover stone fragments for analysis of composition.

Metabolic evaluation in children with stone disease should include blood or serum studies and a complete assessment of urine metabolic risk factors [4,19]. Measurement of serum sodium, potassium, chloride, bicarbonate, calcium, phosphate, magnesium, creatinine, blood urea nitrogen, uric acid, and alkaline phosphatase should be performed in all these children to screen for tubular diseases, bone and mineral disorders, inborn errors of purine metabolism, and CKD. Parathyroid hormone levels should be evaluated in patients with raised serum calcium and/or reduced serum phosphate concentrations and a serum 25-hydroxyvitamin D level must be obtained when either hyper- or hypocalcemia is present. Patients with confirmed hyperoxaluria should have their plasma oxalate and vitamin B6 levels determined [4,12,19]. The urinary excretion of calcium, oxalate, citrate, uric acid, and sodium, and creatinine and urine pH should be measured in all children presenting with stones [4,19]. Cystinuria needs to be ruled out with a qualitative (nitroprusside test) or quantitative urinary cystine study [12]. Analysis of risk factors should preferably be carried out on 24 h samples while random urine specimens can be employed in children who are not toilet trained. Since intraindividual solute excretion varies significantly, several collections are frequently needed to confirm a normal or abnormal result. Urinary supersaturations of calcium oxalate, calcium phosphate, and uric acid can be calculated based on the results of urine collections [16]. Normal values for urinary solutes and other key variables associated with kidney stone formation are listed in Tables 7.1 and 7.2.

Hypomagnesemia and hypercalciuria in patients with kidney stones are strongly suggestive of FHHNC and in the absence of enteric hyperoxaluria, urine oxalate levels above 0.7 mmol/1.73 m^2 per 24 h are highly suggestive of PH [12]. Finally, all boys with stones of unknown etiology, nephrocalcinosis, and/or proteinuria should be screened for low molecular weight proteinuria (retinol binding protein, β2-microglobulin) to rule out the possibility of Dent's disease.

In adults, computed tomography (CT) scan is the gold standard for imaging in the diagnosis of stone disease, a fact that was used to justify the use of standard CT scan evaluation in children with suspected renal colic. In a recent US study by Routh et al., the use of CT scanning for the evaluation of renal colic in children increased from 26% to 45% over a 10-year period [21]. Radiation exposure from repeated CT scanning, a major concern in

Table 7.1 Random urine solute-to-creatinine ratio by age

Calcium/creatinine			Oxalate/creatinine			Cystine/creatinine			Uric acid/creatinine			Citrate/creatinine		
Solute-to-creatinine ratios (random urine samples)														
Age	mol/mol	mg/mg	Age	mol/mol	mg/mg	Age	mol/mol	mg/mg	Age	mol/mol	mg/mg	Age	mol/mol	mg/mg
0-1 y	2.29	0.81	<6 m	0.37	0.29	<1 m	<85	<180	<12 m	<1.5	<2.2	0-5 y	> 0.25	> 0.42
1-2 y	1.58	0.56	6 m – 2 y	0.26	0.20	1-6 m	<53	<112	1-3 y	<1.3	<1.9	>5 y	> 0.15	> 0.25
2-3 y	1.41	0.50	>2 y – 5 y	0.14	0.11	>6 m	<18	<38	3-5 y	<1.0	<1.5			
3-5 y	1.16	0.41	6 – 12 y	0.08	0.063				5-10 y	<0.6	<0.9			
5-7 y	0.85	0.30	>18 y	0.04	0.031				<10 y	<0.4	<0.6			
7-10 y	0.71	0.25												
10-17 y	0.68	0.24												

Sources: Adapted from Edvardsson 2013 [12] and Habbig 2011 [36].

Table 7.2 Normal values for the 24 h excretion of urinary solutes associated with kidney stone formation*

Calcium excretion		Oxalate excretion		Cystine excretion[†]		Uric acid excretion		Citrate excretion	
All age	<0.1 mmol/kg/day <4 mg/kg/day	All age	<0.5 mmol/1.73 m²/24 h <0.45 mg/1.73 m²/24 h	<10 y	<55 mmol/1.73 m²/24 h <13 mg/1.73 m²/24 h	<1 y 1-5 y	<70 μmol (1.29 mg)/kg/24 h <65 μmol (1.1 mg)/kg/24 h	All age (boys)	>1.9 mmol/1.73 m²/24 h >365 mg/1.73 m²/24 h
				>10 y	<200 mmol/1.73 m²/24 h <48 mg/1.73 m²/24 h	>5 y	<55 μmol (0.9 mg)/kg/24 h	All age (girls)	>1.6 mmol/1.73 m²/24 h >310 mg/1.73 m²/24 h

*Creatinine excretion should be measured to check for completeness of urine collection; normal range 15–25 mg/kg/day or 133–221 μmol/kg/day.

[†]A positive sodium-cyanide-nitroprusside test should be confirmed with 24 h urine collection. Sources: Adapted from Edvardsson 2013 [12] and Habbig 2011 [36].

Sources: Adapted from Edvardsson 2013 [12] and Habbig 2011 [36].

children, has led to the evaluation of alternative imaging modalities, specifically the combination of plain film (KUB) with ultrasound (US) for the evaluation of these children. In adults, studies have shown that the combination of KUB and US will adequately identify clinically significant stones with minimal loss of diagnostic accuracy [22,23]. Although CT is more sensitive for detecting kidney stones than ultrasound, the difference in usefulness between the two imaging modalities may not be clinically significant [24]. In 2009, Karmazyn et al. reported that a CT imaging technique using reduced radiation dose in children less than 50 kg did not change the sensitivity of detection of nephrolithiasis [25]. However, since low-dose CT scanning is not globally utilized in children, KUB and US remain the imaging modalities of choice in the diagnosis of suspected acute renal colic in children.

Acute symptomatic stone events in children should be managed much like in the adult population where careful attention must be paid to the control of pain, nausea and vomiting, and to hydration. Intravenous ketorolac has been found to be more effective than intravenous opioids to relieve pain caused by renal obstruction [26,27]. Sandhu et al. [28] compared ketorolac to meperidine in a prospective double-blind randomized study of adult patients with pain due to renal colic and found that 56% of patients receiving ketorolac required repeat analgesia within 24 h, compared to 80% of those receiving meperidine. In children, ketorolac has been shown to be a safe and effective pain medication [29,30,31]. In one study comparing 0.75, 1.0, and 1.5 mg/kg of intravenous (IV) ketorolac with 0.1 mg/kg of IV morphine given immediately prior to dental surgery [32], ketorolac at all doses was as effective an analgesic as morphine and was associated with a significant reduction in the incidence of postoperative vomiting. Therefore, ketorolac should be considered a first-line agent for pain management in children with renal colic while acetaminophen and opioids can be added if additional pain relief is needed.

Antiemetic treatment is often necessary, especially in the setting of an acute urinary obstruction. The most commonly used agents in pediatric patients are 5-HT_3 (serotonin) antagonists, specifically ondansetron, Antiemetic treatment is often necessary, especially in the setting of an acute urinary obstruction. The most commonly used agents in pediatric patients are 5-HT_3 (serotonin) antagonists, specifically ondansetron, promethazine, and metoclopramide [33]. Due to concerns regarding intravenous administration of promethazine, ondansetron is typically used in the acute setting while oral promethazine is frequently prescribed for outpatient management. Aggressive hydration in conjunction with adequate pain control is recommended only to replete extracellular volume lost to vomiting and not to facilitate stone passage [19].

Outpatient management of a child with symptomatic urolithiasis requires the patient's ability to tolerate oral intake with the hope that spontaneous stone passage will occur. Medical expulsion therapy has been evaluated in both adults and children. In adults, both calcium antagonists and α-adrenoceptor blockers appear to have beneficial effects when compared with placebo. A recent meta-analysis reported that treatment with tamsulosin after extracorporeal shock wave lithotripsy treatment appeared effective in assisting with stone clearance in adult patients with renal and ureteral calculi [34]. While studies in children are limited, some centers prescribe doxazosin or tamsulosin to older children. Historically, spontaneous stone passage rates in children are thought to be at least the same and perhaps better than in the adult population. In a report by Pietrow et al., the spontaneous passage rate for ureteral stones of all sizes in children aged 0–18 years was remarkably similar in all ages up to 4 mm in size but the passage rate was significantly lower for larger stones [35]. Based on these findings, it is reasonable to advocate attempted conservative therapy for pediatric ureteral stones less than 4–5 mm assuming there is no infection, severe pain, solitary system or renal dysfunction. In general, patients are typically given at least 2 weeks to allow for spontaneous stone passage before surgical intervention is considered.

Hospitalization followed by potential decompression is indicated for patients unable to tolerate oral hydration or have insufficient relief of pain with oral medical treatment. More aggressive management is also indicated in patients with a solitary kidney with renal colic or symptoms of renal obstruction. Patients with symptoms refractory to a trial of intravenous hydration and analgesics should be strongly considered for stent placement.

In the setting of urinary tract infection and urinary obstruction, emergency urinary decompression with either a ureteral stent or percutaneous nephrostomy tube is indicated, followed by hospitalization and aggressive antibiotic therapy.

A number of preventive therapeutic measures, including dietary modifications and drug therapy, can be taken to reduce the risk of new stone formation. High fluid intake is critically important for all patients with kidney stone disease and the minimum recommended intake is 1.5–2 L/m^2/day in children with idiopathic stone disease [19,36]. This fluid intake should be increased whenever insensible water loss is increased such as in warm weather conditions and during physical exercise. In patients with primary hyperoxaluria, cystinuria and other severe stone diseases, urine output as high as >750 mL/24 h in infants, >1000 mL/24 h in young children up to 5 years of age, >1500 mL/24 h up to 10 years of age, >2000 mL/24 h in older children and adolescents and >3000 mL/24 h in older adolescents and adults may be needed [12]. To achieve this goal, gastric tube placement may be needed in patients with the most severe disease manifestations. Children with calcium stone disease may benefit from drinking lemonade and orange juice as these are rich in citrate while grapefruit juice has been associated with an increased risk of calcium stones [19].

An inverse relationship has been described between dietary calcium intake and the risk of symptomatic kidney stones in several prospective observational studies [37]. Dietary calcium may decrease intestinal oxalate absorption, thereby preventing dietary hyperoxaluria and the resultant urinary calcium oxalate crystallization [36]. Indeed, a low-calcium diet has been shown to be a less effective treatment for calcium nephrolithiasis compared to a diet containing normal amounts of calcium and reduced amounts of animal protein and sodium [38]. Both diets reduced urine calcium to a similar amount but the low-sodium, low-protein diet also reduced urine oxalate excretion. The current recommendation for children with kidney stones is to avoid excess calcium intake but calcium restriction is contraindicated [19].

Animal protein ingestion induces an acid load which promotes skeletal calcium losses, leading to hypercalciuria and urinary acidification, reducing urinary citrate excretion [19]. Protein consumption in children with kidney stones should be aimed at approximately 100% of the recommended daily allowance and excessive animal protein consumption should be avoided [19]. In contrast to the effect of animal protein ingestion, fruits and vegetables generally deliver potassium and alkali load through citrate, the principal anion, which protects against kidney stone formation [39]. There is evidence suggesting that a reduction in the ingestion of sodium and an increase in potassium intake may benefit stone formers. Sodium may increase urinary calcium excretion so that a limitation of sodium intake to approximately 2–3 mEq/kg/day is recommended for pediatric stone formers [19,36].

Dietary oxalate makes a more significant contribution to urinary oxalate excretion than previously recognized and dietary oxalate may significantly contribute to calcium oxalate stone formation [40]. The current recommendation for children with calcium oxalate stone disease is to avoid certain oxalate-rich foods (different types of nuts, spinach, soy beans, rhubarb, tofu, beets, sweet potatoes, wheat bran, okra, parsley, chives, star fruit, green tea, and chocolate) and vitamin C supplementation should be discontinued in patients with documented hyperoxaluria [19,36].

Pharmacotherapy, guided by results of urine metabolic risk factor evaluation, is indicated for children with recurrent idiopathic calcium stone disease and immediately following diagnosis in treatable forms of genetic stone disease [19,36]. Oral potassium citrate (2–4 mEq/kg/day in children, adults 30–90 mEq/day) [19] is a safe and effective treatment that restores normal urinary citrate and has a significant preventive effect on recurrent calcium stone disease in children with hypocitraturia [41]. The goal of potassium citrate treatment is to normalize urinary citrate excretion but urinary alkalinization above pH 6.5 should be avoided as higher pH increases the risk of calcium phosphate stone formation [19]. In patients with cystinuria, potassium citrate should be prescribed in a dose sufficient to alkalinize the urine to a pH of 7.5. Thiazide diuretics are prescribed for children with stone disease and documented hypercalciuria [36]. Hydrochlorothiazide is the most frequently prescribed preparation, the recommended dose being 0.5–2 mg/kg/day in children, with twice-a-day use probably superior [19,36]. The longer acting chlorthalidone may lead to more satisfactory results. Amiloride can be added to thiazide treatment in the case of hypokalemia, hypocitraturia implying potassium depletion, or insufficient calciuric effect of thiazide treatment.

All patients with PH type 1 should be given a trial of pyridoxine therapy, at a dose of 7–9 mg/kg/day, for at least 3 months. Oxalate excretion should be evaluated with two or more timed urine collections before pyridoxine treatment is started and repeated after 3 months of therapy. Other types of PH do not respond to pyridoxine treatment [12]. The drugs d-penicillamine and tiopronin, that effectively break the disulfide bridge of cystine and form soluble drug–cysteine complexes, are prescribed to children with cystinuria when fluid intake and alkalinization fail to reduce stone formation [12]. Further, allopurinol in the dose of 5–10 mg/kg/day in children and 300–600 mg/day in adults has been shown to effectively prevent stone recurrence and improve kidney function in children and adults with APRT deficiency. The diagnosis and treatment of genetic forms of stone disease are discussed in depth in Chapter 6.

Summary

Ideally, all pediatric stone formers should be seen regularly in a stone prevention clinic where they are cared for by a medical team with special interest and training in childhood kidney stone disease. Correct and timely diagnosis of the underlying condition and adequate follow-up to assure compliance with prescribed therapies are essential to reduce stone recurrence and to optimize renal outcome in affected children.

References

1. Sas DJ, Hulsey TC, Shatat IF, Orak JK. Increasing incidence of kidney stones in children evaluated in the emergency department. J Pediatr 2010; 157(1): 132–7.
2. Dwyer ME, Krambeck AE, Bergstralh EJ, Milliner DS, Lieske JC, Rule AD. Temporal trends in incidence of kidney stones among children: a 25-year population based study. J Urol 2012; 188(1): 247–52.
3. VanDervoort K, Wiesen J, Frank R, et al. Urolithiasis in pediatric patients: a single center study of incidence, clinical presentation and outcome. J Urol 2007; 177(6): 2300–5.
4. Hoppe B, Kemper MJ. Diagnostic examination of the child with urolithiasis or nephrocalcinosis. Pediatr Nephrol 2010; 25(3): 403–13.
5. Edvardsson VO, Indridason OS, Haraldsson G, Kjartansson O, Palsson R. Temporal trends in the incidence of kidney stone disease. Kidney Int 2013; 83(1): 146–52.
6. Stamatelou KK, Francis ME, Jones CA, Nyberg LM, Curhan GC. Time trends in reported prevalence of kidney stones in the United States: 1976–1994. Kidney Int 2003; 63(5): 1817–23.

7. Edvardsson V, Elidottir H, Indridason OS, Palsson R. High incidence of kidney stones in Icelandic children. Pediatr Nephrol 2005; 20(7): 940–4.
8. Bush NC, Xu L, Brown BJ, et al. Hospitalizations for pediatric stone disease in United States, 2002–2007. J Urol 2010; 183(3): 1151–6.
9. Novak TE, Lakshmanan Y, Trock BJ, Gearhart JP, Matlaga BR. Sex prevalence of pediatric kidney stone disease in the United States: an epidemiologic investigation. Urology 2009; 74(1): 104–7.
10. Milliner DS, Murphy ME. Urolithiasis in pediatric patients. Mayo Clin Proc 1993; 68(3): 241–8.
11. Mckay CP. Renal stone disease. Pediatr Rev 2010; 31(5): 179–88.
12. Edvardsson VO, Goldfarb DS, Lieske JC, et al. Hereditary causes of kidney stones and chronic kidney disease. Pediatr Nephrol 2013; 28(10): 1923–42.
13. van't Hoff WG. Aetiological factors in paediatric urolithiasis. Nephron Clin Pract 2004; 98(2): C45–C8.
14. Coward RJM, Peters CJ, Duffy PG, et al. Epidemiology of paediatric renal stone disease in the UK. Arch Dis Child 2003; 88(11): 962–5.
15. Levy FL, Adams-Huet B, Pak CY. Ambulatory evaluation of nephrolithiasis: an update of a 1980 protocol. Am J Med 1995; 98(1): 50–9.
16. Coe FL, Evan A, Worcester E. Kidney stone disease. J Clin Invest 2005; 115(10): 2598–608.
17. Coe FL, Parks JH, Asplin JR. The pathogenesis and treatment of kidney stones. N Engl J Med 1992; 327(16): 1141–52.
18. Asplin JR, Lingeman J, Kahnoski R, Mardis H, Parks JH, Coe FL. Metabolic urinary correlates of calcium oxalate dihydrate in renal stones. J Urol 1998; 159(3): 664–8.
19. Copelovitch L. Urolithiasis in children: medical approach. Pediatr Clin North Am 2012; 59(4): 881–96.
20. Sas DJ. An update on the changing epidemiology and metabolic risk factors in pediatric kidney stone disease. Clin J Am Soc Nephrol 2011; 6(8): 2062–8.
21. Routh JC, Graham DA, Nelson CP. Trends in imaging and surgical management of pediatric urolithiasis at American pediatric hospitals. J Urol 2010; 184 (4 suppl): 1816–22.
22. Ripolles T, Agramunt M, Errando J, Martinez MJ, Coronel B, Morales M. Suspected ureteral colic: plain film and sonography vs unenhanced helical CT. A prospective study in 66 patients. Eur Radiol 2004; 14(1): 129–36.
23. Catalano O, Nunziata A, Altei F, Siani A. Suspected ureteral colic: primary helical CT versus selective helical CT after unenhanced radiography and sonography. Am J Roentgenol 2002; 178(2): 379–87.
24. Passerotti C, Chow JS, Silva A, et al. Ultrasound versus computerized tomography for evaluating urolithiasis. J Urol 2009; 182(4 suppl): 1829–34.
25. Karmazyn B, Frush DP, Applegate KE, Maxfield C, Cohen MD, Jones RP. CT with a computer-simulated dose reduction technique for detection of pediatric nephroureterolithiasis: comparison of standard and reduced radiation doses. Am J Roentgenol 2009; 192(1): 143–9.
26. Oosterlinck W, Philp NH, Charig C, Gillies G, Hetherington JW, Lloyd J. A double-blind single dose comparison of intramuscular ketorolac tromethamine and pethidine in the treatment of renal colic. J Clin Pharmacol 1990; 30(4): 336–41.
27. Bartfield JM, Kern AM, Raccio-Robak N, Snyder HS, Baevsky RH. Ketorolac tromethamine use in a university-based emergency department. Acad Emerg Med 1994; 1(6): 532–8.

28. Sandhu DP, Iacovou JW, Fletcher MS, Kaisary AV, Philip NH, Arkell DG. A comparison of intramuscular ketorolac and pethidine in the alleviation of renal colic. Br J Urol 1994; 74(6): 690–3.
29. Gonzalez A, Smith DP. Minimizing hospital length of stay in children undergoing ureteroneocystostomy. Urology 1998; 52(3): 501–4.
30. Eberson CP, Pacicca DM, Ehrlich MG. The role of ketorolac in decreasing length of stay and narcotic complications in the postoperative pediatric orthopaedic patient. J Pediatr Orthoped 1999; 19(5): 688–92.
31. Splinter WM, Reid CW, Roberts DJ, Bass J. Reducing pain after inguinal hernia repair in children: caudal anesthesia versus ketorolac tromethamine. Anesthesiology 1997; 87(3): 542–6.
32. Purday JP, Reichert CC, Merrick PM. Comparative effects of three doses of intravenous ketorolac or morphine on emesis and analgesia for restorative dental surgery in children. Can J Anaesth 1996; 43(3): 221–5.
33. Mee MJ, Egerton-Warburton D, Meek R. Treatment and assessment of emergency department nausea and vomiting in Australasia: a survey of anti-emetic management. Emerg Med Australasia 2011; 23(2): 162–8.
34. Zhu Y, Duijvesz D, Rovers MM, Lock TM. alpha-Blockers to assist stone clearance after extracorporeal shock wave lithotripsy: a meta-analysis. BJU Int 2010; 106(2): 256–61.
35. Pietrow PK, Pope JCI, Adams MC, Shyr Y, Brock JWI. Clinical outcome of pediatric stone disease. J Urol 2002; 167(2 Pt 1): 670–3.
36. Habbig S, Beck BB, Hoppe B. Nephrocalcinosis and urolithiasis in children. Kidney Int 2011; 80(12): 1278–91.
37. Taylor EN, Curhan GC. Role of nutrition in the formation of calcium-containing kidney stones. Nephron Physiol 2004; 98(2): 55–63.
38. Borghi L, Schianchi T, Meschi T, et al. Comparison of two diets for the prevention of recurrent stones in idiopathic hypercalciuria. N Engl J Med 2002; 346(2): 77–84.
39. Pak CY. Medical management of urinary stone disease. Nephron Clin Pract 2004; 98(2): c49–53.
40. Holmes RP, Goodman HO, Assimos DG. Contribution of dietary oxalate to urinary oxalate excretion. Kidney Int 2001; 59(1): 270–6.
41. Tekin A, Tekgul S, Atsu N, Bakkaloglu M, Kendi S. Oral potassium citrate treatment for idiopathic hypocitruria in children with calcium urolithiasis. J Urol 2002; 168(6): 2572–4.

CHAPTER 8

Primary Hyperparathyroidism and Stones

Marcella Donovan Walker and Shonni J. Silverberg
Columbia University College of Physicians and Surgeons, New York, NY, USA

Do's and don'ts box

Do:
- check serum intact PTH when hypercalcemia is present
- diagnose PHPT biochemically in the presence of elevated or inappropriately normal PTH levels in a hypercalcemic patient
- check 24-h urinary calcium excretion once in all patients with suspected PHPT in order to distinguish PHPT from FHH and secondary hyperparathyroidism
- refer patients with PHPT and nephrolithiasis for parathyroidectomy.

Don't:
- use parathyroid imaging to diagnose PHPT
- refer those with FHH or secondary hyperparathyroidism for parathyroidectomy.

Introduction

Primary hyperparathyroidism (PHPT) is a common disorder, with an estimated prevalence of 1 in 1000. PHPT is characterized by hypercalcemia and elevated or inappropriately normal serum parathyroid hormone (PTH) levels. PHPT results from excessive secretion of PTH from one or more of the four parathyroid glands. The disease is caused by a solitary parathyroid adenoma in 80% of cases. Less frequently, PHPT is due to four-gland hyperplasia (10–15%), multiple adenomas (5%), and rarely (<1%) parathyroid cancer.

Primary hyperparathyroidism has been dubbed a disease of "stones, bones, and groans," highlighting the manifestations of "classic PHPT" which included nephrolithiasis and the bone disease osteitis fibrosa cystica, as well as psychiatric and abdominal complaints. In the early part of the 20th century, nephrolithiasis occurred in over 50% of patients with PHPT [1].

Urinary Stones: Medical and Surgical Management, First Edition. Edited by Michael Grasso and David S. Goldfarb.

With the advent of routine biochemical testing of calcium in the 1970s, it became clear that PHPT was more common and less symptomatic than initially surmised. Today, the majority of PHPT patients in the United States have "asymptomatic PHPT" and are discovered incidentally when routine blood work is performed [2].

While nephrolithiasis has become less frequent, PHPT clearly remains a risk factor for urolithiasis. Today, approximately 15–20% of PHPT patients have symptomatic nephrolithiasis [2]. This figure is likely an underestimate of the true prevalence as a number of patients with asymptomatic PHPT have evidence of "subclinical" stone disease when imaging is performed [3,4]. In contrast, nephrocalcinosis is not commonly observed in PHPT today though the exact prevalence is unknown because patients are rarely formally evaluated for this manifestation [5]. About 2–8% of patients presenting with nephrolithiasis in the general population are found to have PHPT [6,7].

Urinary stones in PHPT may be composed of calcium phosphate or calcium oxalate or may be mixed in their composition [7]. Hypercalciuria is common in PHPT (35–40% of patients) and is thought to contribute to the pathogenesis of nephrolithiasis. Although PTH stimulates the distal tubular reabsorption of calcium, hypercalciuria occurs when the reabsorptive capacity of the kidney is overwhelmed by the hypercalcemia-induced increase in filtered calcium. Urinary calcium levels in PHPT patients are, however, influenced by other variables including vitamin D level, dietary calcium intake, glomerular filtration rate, and the extent of bone resorption, which may explain why not all patients are frankly hypercalciuric.

Urine calcium levels have not reliably been shown to predict the occurrence of nephrolithiasis in PHPT; younger age and male gender have more consistently been associated with nephrolithiasis in PHPT [4,8]. Marked hypercalciuria (>400 mg/day) was in the past an accepted indication for parathyroidectomy even in those without nephrolithiasis because of concerns about risk of stones and the effect on renal function. In the latest set (see p.000) of internationally accepted guidelines for the management of asymptomatic PHPT [8], hypercalciuria is no longer an indication for surgery because of poor correlation between urinary calcium excretion and stone formation, and poor reproducibility of findings on repeated 24-h collections.

The incidence of chronic kidney disease (CKD) in PHPT is not precisely known, with estimates varying between 17% and 40%. PHPT has the potential to cause CKD by a number of mechanisms, including hypercalcemia-induced diuresis, nephrocalcinosis, and nephrolithiasis. At this time, the contribution of PHPT to the pathogenesis of CKD in PHPT is unclear, but appears to be modest [9]. Most data suggest that renal function remains stable when PHPT is monitored over long-term follow-up [2,10], though one recent study suggests an increased risk of CKD in PHPT [11]. While data are limited, surgical cure of PHPT has not been shown to improve renal function. In fact, data in severe disease suggest CKD may worsen after parathyroidectomy, though one small study indicated that concentrating capacity improves [5,9].

Evaluation

Suspicion for PHPT as a cause of nephrolithiasis should be raised when stones occur in women or are multiple or recurrent. A metabolic panel (with serum calcium) is indicated in those with nephrolithiasis. The finding of hypercalcemia necessitates further evaluation to determine its cause. The first and most important test in evaluating hypercalcemia is serum PTH. The value of serum PTH distinguishes between the two most common causes of hypercalcemia: PHPT (PTH elevated or mid- to upper normal) and malignancy (PTH suppressed). PHPT is the most common cause of hypercalcemia in well-appearing outpatients while malignancy is most common in ill inpatients.

Differential diagnosis and laboratory evaluation

The diagnosis of PHPT is established biochemically. It can be confirmed by documenting hypercalcemia with a simultaneously elevated or inappropriately normal PTH level (PTH level typically >20 pg/mL). On repeat lab testing, it is important to note that not all serum calcium levels need be elevated. In PHPT, serum calcium may intermittently fall into the normal range. This finding is not inconsistent with the diagnosis as long as there is a "recurrent pattern" of hypercalcemia over time. In contrast, a single elevated calcium level must be repeated as spurious values can occur.

In contrast to PHPT, all non-parathyroid causes of hypercalcemia (malignancy, granulomatous disease such as sarcoidosis, etc.) are associated with a suppressed PTH level. In many malignancies, hypercalcemia is mediated by a PTH-like molecule, parathyroid hormone-related peptide. In granulomatous disease and some cancers, hypercalcemia is caused by elevated 1,25-dihydroxyvitamin D levels. In addition to PHPT, the differential diagnosis of elevated serum calcium and PTH includes:

- familial hypocalciuric hypercalcemia (FHH), an inherited disorder due to an inactivating mutation of the calcium sensing receptor (CaSR)
- drug-associated PHPT
- tertiary hyperparathyroidism
- and an ectopic PTH-secreting tumor (rare)

To distinguish PHPT from FHH, urine calcium excretion must be assessed by a 24-h urine collection. FHH has the same serum biochemical profile (elevated serum calcium and elevated or inappropriately normal PTH) as PHPT but the fractional excretion of calcium (FeCa) is typically <1% in FHH while it is generally >1–2% in PHPT. In practice, there is overlap of FeCa values between those with FHH and PHPT, particularly in patients with low vitamin D. The diagnosis of FHH rather than PHPT is supported by a history of hypercalcemia from an early age (presumably birth) and positive family history because FHH is an autosomal dominant condition with high penetrance. Family history of hypercalcemia does not entirely exclude PHPT, however, as there are inherited forms of PHPT (familial isolated PHPT, multiple endocrine neoplasia, hyperparathyroidism-jaw tumor syndrome). In contrast to PHPT, FHH is often accompanied by increased renal tubular reabsorption of magnesium and hypermagnesemia. Definitive diagnosis of FHH can be made with mutational analysis of the *CaSR* gene but current methods do not identify all *CaSR* mutations [12]. Differentiation of PHPT from FHH is important as parathyroidectomy is not indicated, curative or recommended in FHH.

Thiazide diuretics and lithium can lead to biochemical alterations mimicking PHPT. Thiazide diuretics reduce urine calcium excretion and increase serum calcium levels. While the majority of individuals treated with thiazides remain normocalcemic, a small percentage become hypercalcemic (estimated incidence 7.7/100,000 person-years) [13]. One study indicated that after thiazide discontinuation, the majority of hypercalcemic patients (64%) continued to have elevated calcium levels and most were ultimately diagnosed with PHPT [13]. Those with PHPT had higher serum calcium and PTH levels compared to the overall group with thiazide-associated hypercalcemia. The exact mechanism by which thiazides affect parathyroid gland function is debated. Some have suggested that thiazides may simply unmask "incipient" PHPT. In contrast, animal data indicate thiazides may stimulate parathyroid growth [14].

Treatment with lithium leads to elevations in serum calcium and PTH levels within the normal range in most patients, while hypercalcemia is estimated to occur in 3.6–10% [15,16]. Lithium leads to decreased parathyroid gland sensitivity, parathyroid growth, and a shift of the set-point of the calcium-PTH curve to the right, similar to what is observed in those with *CaSR* mutations [17]. Like patients with FHH, lithium decreases urinary calcium and magnesium excretion. Both adenomas and four-gland hyperplasia have been reported in lithium-induced hyperparathyroidism, with the latter being more common with longer treatment duration [18]. In cases of possible thiazide- or lithium-induced PHPT, we recommend withdrawal of the suspected medication for several (≥3) months, if medically safe, followed by retesting. In most instances, drug withdrawal does not change the biochemical findings and a reversible state of PHPT can be excluded. The medication can then be resumed if indicated.

Ectopic PTH secretion from a non-parathyroid tumor is extremely rare but has been described [19,20]. In most descriptions, such individuals were not asymptomatic. Rather, hypercalcemia was usually severe and a late-stage complication of their underlying malignancy.

Distinction from secondary and tertiary hyperparathyroidism

Primary hyperparathyroidism can be distinguished from secondary hyperparathyroidism by its different biochemical profile. Secondary hyperparathyroidism is associated with either a frankly low or normal serum calcium level and an appropriate secondary elevation in PTH in response to some hypocalcemic stimulus. Most commonly, secondary hyperparathyroidism is due to vitamin D deficiency, gastrointestinal malabsorption, chronic kidney disease or hypercalciuria. There is a subset of patients with secondary hyperparathyroidism who become hypercalcemic, and are ultimately found to have PHPT, when the underlying condition (for example, vitamin D deficiency) is corrected. In these cases, the hypercalcemia of PHPT is thought to have been "masked" by the co-existing hypocalcemic stimulus. Lastly, there is a subset of patients who have normal serum albumin-corrected calcium and ionized calcium values with an elevated PTH level in whom all known causes of secondary hyperparathyroidism have been excluded. These patients are said to have "normocalcemic primary hyperparathyroidism" which is thought to be an early form of PHPT. While data regarding the natural history of normocalcemic PHPT are limited, one study indicated that about 20% of patients became hypercalcemic within 3 years of follow-up [21]. Normocalcemic PHPT is not associated with elevated urinary calcium levels (by definition) and has not been reported to clearly increase risk of nephrolithiasis.

Tertiary hyperparathyroidism describes a condition in which prolonged severe secondary hyperparathyroidism (such as is seen in end-stage renal disease) evolves into a hypercalcemic state due to autonomous functioning of hyperplastic parathyroid glands. While this can be observed in patients on dialysis, it may also occur after renal transplant when calcitriol production and phosphate filtration normalize. After renal transplant, parathyroid hyperplasia often subsides, but some continue to have parathyroid hyperplasia and may remain hypercalcemic. Tertiary hyperparathyroidism is typically obvious from the history. A summary of biochemical profiles for various hypercalcemic and hyperparathyroid conditions can be found in Table 8.1.

Laboratory assays

When assessing for PHPT, PTH should be measured with an "intact" PTH assay. These assays detect both PTH (1-84), the entire 84-amino acid hormone, as well as PTH (7-84), an inactive fragment. Unless significant renal failure is present, the amount of circulating PTH (7-84) is low and its contribution to the measured PTH value is negligible. The intact assays do not cross-react with PTH-related peptide and can reliably distinguish PHPT from hypercalcemia of malignancy. Newer PTH assays (which detect only PTH (1-84)) do not clearly increase the diagnostic sensitivity over second-generation assays [12].

Serum calcium must be interpreted with respect to serum albumin. Because about 40% of calcium is protein bound, low albumin levels can make it appear that one is normocalcemic when hypercalcemia is present. Serum calcium should be corrected for low albumin: (4-albumin value)*(0.8) + serum calcium. Ionized calcium is typically elevated in PHPT, but does not add much to the evaluation except in individuals with acid–base disorders or when assessing for normocalcemic PHPT.

Imaging

Parathyroid imaging plays no role in the diagnosis of PHPT. Imaging studies, such as sestamibi scanning, ultrasound, computed tomography, magnetic resonance imaging or others, should only be obtained to assist the parathyroid

Table 8.1 Biochemical profile of hypercalcemic and hyperparathyroid conditions

	PHPT	Familial hypocalciuric hypercalcemia	Hypercalcemia of malignancy	Secondary hyperparathyroidism
Serum calcium	↑	↑	↑	↓ or normal
Serum PTH	↑ or inappropriately normal	↑ or inappropriately normal	↓	↑
Other features	Fractional excretion of calcium >1%; most often asymptomatic	Fractional excretion of calcium <1%; high or high normal serum magnesium; hypercalcemia present since birth/early age; positive family history	Constitutional symptoms and symptoms related to hypercalcemia typically present	Cause of secondary hyperparathyroidism such as low 25-hydroxyvitamin D, low glomerular filtration rate, malabsorption, hypercalciuria identifiable

surgeon in identifying the anatomical position of abnormal gland(s) when planning parathyroidectomy. While the accuracy of parathyroid imaging has improved, there is wide variation in the sensitivity and specificity for various imaging modalities, depending on where they are obtained. Negative imaging (more common among those with multiglandular PHPT) is not inconsistent with the diagnosis of PHPT and does not preclude surgical cure. Further, positive imaging is not needed to confirm the diagnosis and false-positive tests occur, particularly in those with concurrent nodular thyroid disease.

Clinical presentation

Primary hyperparathyroidism affects mainly women in middle age, with women outnumbering men by approximately 3:1 [2]. Hypercalcemia is typically within 1 mg/dL above the normal range. Elevations in PTH are generally within 1–2 times the upper limit of normal [2]. Serum phosphorus is typically in the lower half of the normal range and rarely frankly low. Vitamin D insufficiency or deficiency is common, while 1,25-dihydroxyvitamin D is elevated in close to half of patients, presumably due to increased PTH-induced transcription of α1-hydroxylase.

Because of the minimal elevation of serum calcium in the majority of patients, symptoms of hypercalcemia (nausea, vomiting, constipation, abdominal pain, polyuria, polydipsia, and altered mental status) are not typically observed in PHPT. Many patients with PHPT complain of non-specific symptoms such as weakness, memory impairment, and mild depression. Although some patients note improvement in these complaints after cure, a causal association with PHPT has not been established [22,23]. Patients reporting such symptoms are still described as "asymptomatic" if they lack the classic bone and renal manifestations of PHPT.

Osteitis fibrosa cystica, characterized by brown tumors of the long bones and periosteal bone resorption, was commonly seen in classic PHPT. Although these findings are not typically seen today, bone densitometry and bone biopsy studies document skeletal sequelae of PHPT. Low bone mineral density (BMD) is common in PHPT, particularly at the distal one-third radius, a site rich in cortical bone that is preferentially affected by PTH. Though fracture risk was increased in the classic form of PHPT, it is unclear if asymptomatic PHPT increases the risk of fracture.

The typical neuromuscular syndrome of classic PHPT, characterized by proximal muscle weakness and atrophy of type II muscle fibers [24], is not seen in modern PHPT. Pancreatitis and peptic ulcer disease were associated with classic PHPT. The former is virtually never seen as a consequence of the mild hypercalcemia in asymptomatic PHPT. Peptic ulcer disease is only causally associated with PHPT in patients with multiple endocrine neoplasia with gastrinoma.

Cardiovascular manifestations of severe PHPT include hypertension, cardiovascular calcifications, left ventricular hypertrophy, arrhythmia, and increased mortality. The increased cardiovascular morbidity and mortality in severe PHPT have not been definitively demonstrated in asymptomatic PHPT. There is, however, some evidence for subtle abnormalities, such as increased vascular stiffness, among others [25,26]. Results from observational studies assessing the effect of parathyroidectomy upon cardiovascular health have been conflicting. The single randomized controlled trial did not demonstrate that parathyroidectomy was beneficial [27].

Guidelines for surgery

All patients with symptomatic PHPT, which includes those with kidney stones, should be referred for parathyroidectomy. After successful surgery, the risk of nephrolithiasis declines, though some studies suggest that risk remains higher than that of the general population [4,28]. While 24-h urine calcium levels decline after parathyroidectomy (PTX) [23], some work indicates that stone formers have higher post-PTX urinary calcium excretion than non-stone formers [29]. Such findings suggest that at least some stone formers may have additional disorders of mineral metabolism such as a renal calcium leak [4]. Randomized studies of PTX versus medical observation in PHPT have not been designed or powered to compare nephrolithiasis risk reduction.

Controversy over the need to treat PHPT patients who are diagnosed in the absence of clear symptomatology has led to the development of guidelines for surgery [8]. A summary of the most recent guidelines follows.

1 **Serum calcium ≥1 mg/dL above upper limit of normal**: while there are no data to support a particular calcium threshold for requiring surgery, 1 mg/dL above the upper limit of normal is recommended because those above this threshold may be at greater risk for symptomatic disease and complications [8].
2 **Estimated glomerular filtration rate (eGFR) <60 mL/min**: parathyroidectomy is recommended in those with PHPT and concurrent stage 3 chronic kidney disease (eGFR < 60 mL/min/1.73 m^2). Data from the general population without PHPT indicate that serum PTH level typically increases at an eGFR <60 mL/min/1.73 m^2 [30]. Recent data found no difference in PTH or serum calcium in those with eGFR less than versus greater than 60 mL/min/1.73 m^2 [31], but on histomorphometric analysis of bone biopsies, those with reduced renal function did have greater bone resorption.
3 **T-score ≤ −2.5 or fragility fracture**: strong evidence from both observational studies and randomized trials of surgery versus observation demonstrates a salutary effect of surgical cure on BMD at all sites [2,22,32,33], particularly in those with low BMD [34]. Thus, parathyroidectomy is recommended in those with osteoporosis at any site, or with a history of fragility fracture.
4 **Age <50**: one study demonstrated that those under 50 years had a higher risk of developing a new surgical indication while under observation than those over the age of 50 years (60% versus 25%) [35].

Neither cardiovascular disease nor cognitive or psychiatric complaints are currently indications for surgery given conflicting data regarding their improvement after parathyroidectomy [8]. Some experts feel all patients with PHPT should be treated surgically. Implementation of these guidelines has always depended on conversations between the patient and physician. Given the benefits of surgery, cure of PHPT is never an incorrect approach, if the diagnosis is secure and there are no medical contraindications.

Non-surgical patients

The implication underlying the guidelines for surgery in asymptomatic PHPT is that it is safe to observe those without indications for surgery. Randomized clinical trials do not demonstrate deleterious effects of observation in asymptomatic patients over 1–2 years of observation [22,23,33]. No longer-term randomized trial data are available but observational studies report that over one-third of patients develop new surgical indications if observed for up to 15 years [32]. Stated in another way, however, approximately 60% of subjects followed for up to 15 years did not develop indications for parathyroidectomy. BMD is stable initially, but begins to decline particularly at the hip and forearm sites after ~8 years of observation.

The Third International Conference on Asymptomatic PHPT issued guidelines for following patients who do not have surgery (Box 8.1). In addition, patients should avoid bedrest and maintain adequate hydration and a modest (1000 mg daily) calcium intake, preferably from dietary sources rather than supplementation. Restriction of dietary calcium and vitamin D is not recommended as it can lead to further elevations in serum PTH level.

While several studies indicate that bisphosphonates improve BMD in PHPT patients followed without surgery, no specific pharmacological therapies are available to reduce the risk of nephrolithiasis. Cinacalcet, a calcimimetic that inhibits parathyroid cell function, normalizes serum calcium in PHPT [36]. Cinacalcet is not associated with improved BMD [36] or reduced urinary calcium excretion [37] and has not been shown to reduce the risk of nephrolithiasis. Cinacalcet is approved for PHPT patients with severe hypercalcemia who are unable to undergo PTX, for parathyroid cancer, and for secondary hyperparathyroidism in patients with chronic kidney disease on dialysis.

Box 8.1 Guidelines for follow-up of asymptomatic PHPT patients not undergoing parathyroidectomy

Serum calcium	Measure annually
Serum creatinine	Measure annually
BMD	Measure annually or biannually

Management of nephrolithiais in primary hyperparathyroidism

As noted above, parathyroidectomy is indicated in PHPT with nephrolithiasis. Some patients, however, refuse PTX despite meeting guidelines for surgery while others may be poor surgical candidates. Unfortunately, there are no specific data to aid in the medical or surgical management of nephrolithiasis in PHPT patients who do not undergo PTX. In the absence of such data, urolithiasis should be managed according to recommendations for those without PHPT, keeping in mind the guidelines regarding calcium intake and hydration noted above. While thiazide diuretics are not absolutely contraindicated in PHPT, they have the potential to exacerbate preexisting hypercalcemia. There are no data regarding their risks or benefit in reducing hypercalciuria or nephrolithiasis in PHPT. Thiazides should not be withheld if deemed medically necessary, as their effect on serum calcium is likely to be modest. The preferred management of urolithiasis in PHPT, however, is parathyroidectomy given its efficacy in reducing recurrence.

Summary

Primary hyperparathyroidism is a common endocrine condition that carries an increased risk for nephrolithiasis. The diagnosis of PHPT can be ascertained by biochemical testing of serum calcium and PTH along with measurement of the fractional excretion of calcium. Parathyroidectomy reduces the risk of recurrent stone disease and is recommended in PHPT patients with nephrolithiasis.

References

1. Albright F, Aub J, Bauer W. Hyperparathyroidism: common and polymorphic condition as illustrated by seventeen proven cases in one clinic. JAMA 1934; 102: 1276.
2. Silverberg SJ, Shane E, Jacobs TP, Siris E, Bilezikian JP. A 10-year prospective study of primary hyperparathyroidism with or without parathyroid surgery. N Engl J Med 1999; 341(17): 1249–55.
3. Suh JM, Cronan JJ, Monchik JM. Primary hyperparathyroidism: is there an increased prevalence of renal stone disease? Am J Roentgenol 2008; 191(3): 908–11.
4. Rejnmark L, Vestergaard P, Mosekilde L. Nephrolithiasis and renal calcifications in primary hyperparathyroidism. J Clin Endocrinol Metab 2011; 96(8): 2377–85.
5. Peacock M. Primary hyperparathyroidism and the kidney: biochemical and clinical spectrum. J Bone Miner Res 2002; 17(suppl 2): N87–94.
6. Pak CY. Etiology and treatment of urolithiasis. Am J Kidney Dis 1991; 18(6): 624–37.

7. Parks J, Coe F, Favus M. Hyperparathyroidism in nephrolithiasis. Arch Intern Med 1980; 140(11): 1479–81.
8. Bilezikian JP, Khan AA, Potts JT Jr. Guidelines for the management of asymptomatic primary hyperparathyroidism: summary statement from the third international workshop. J Clin Endocrinol Metab 2009; 94(2): 335–9.
9. Kristoffersson A, Backman C, Granqvist K, Jarhult J. Pre- and postoperative evaluation of renal function with five different tests in patients with primary hyperparathyroidism. J Intern Med 1990; 227(5): 317–24.
10. Rao DS, Wilson RJ, Kleerekoper M, Parfitt AM. Lack of biochemical progression or continuation of accelerated bone loss in mild asymptomatic primary hyperparathyroidism: evidence for biphasic disease course. J Clin Endocrinol Metab 1988; 67(6): 1294–8.
11. Yu N, Donnan PT, Leese GP. A record linkage study of outcomes in patients with mild primary hyperparathyroidism: the Parathyroid Epidemiology and Audit Research Study (PEARS). Clin Endocrinol (Oxf) 2011; 75(2): 169–76.
12. Eastell R, Arnold A, Brandi ML, et al. Diagnosis of asymptomatic primary hyperparathyroidism: proceedings of the third international workshop. J Clin Endocrinol Metab 2009; 94(2): 340–50.
13. Wermers RA, Kearns AE, Jenkins GD, Melton LJ 3rd. Incidence and clinical spectrum of thiazide-associated hypercalcemia. Am J Med 2007; 120(10): 911.
14. Pickleman JR, Straus FH 2nd, Forland M, Paloyan E. Thiazide-induced parathyroid stimulation. Metabolism 1969; 18(10): 867–73.
15. Mallette LE, Eichhorn E. Effects of lithium carbonate on human calcium metabolism. Arch Intern Med 1986; 146(4): 770–6.
16. Bendz H, Sjodin I, Toss G, Berglund K. Hyperparathyroidism and long-term lithium therapy – a cross-sectional study and the effect of lithium withdrawal. J Intern Med 1996; 240(6): 357–65.
17. Haden ST, Stoll AL, McCormick S, Scott J, Fuleihan Ge-H. Alterations in parathyroid dynamics in lithium-treated subjects. J Clin Endocrinol Metab 1997; 82(9): 2844–8.
18. Jarhult J, Ander S, Asking B, et al. Long-term results of surgery for lithium-associated hyperparathyroidism. Br J Surg 2010; 97(11): 1680–5.
19. VanHouten JN, Yu N, Rimm D, et al. Hypercalcemia of malignancy due to ectopic transactivation of the parathyroid hormone gene. J Clin Endocrinol Metab 2006; 91(2): 580–3.
20. Strewler GJ, Budayr AA, Clark OH, Nissenson RA. Production of parathyroid hormone by a malignant nonparathyroid tumor in a hypercalcemic patient. J Clin Endocrinol Metab 1993; 76(5): 1373–5.
21. Lowe H, McMahon DJ, Rubin MR, Bilezikian JP, Silverberg SJ. Normocalcemic primary hyperparathyroidism: further characterization of a new clinical phenotype. J Clin Endocrinol Metab 2007; 92(8): 3001–5.
22. Bollerslev J, Jansson S, Mollerup CL, et al. Medical observation, compared with parathyroidectomy, for asymptomatic primary hyperparathyroidism: a prospective, randomized trial. J Clin Endocrinol Metab 2007; 92(5): 1687–92.
23. Rao DS, Phillips ER, Divine GW, Talpos GB. Randomized controlled clinical trial of surgery versus no surgery in patients with mild asymptomatic primary hyperparathyroidism. J Clin Endocrinol Metab 2004; 89(11): 5415–22.
24. Patten BM, Bilezikian JP, Mallette LE, Prince A, Engel WK, Aurbach GD. Neuromuscular disease in primary hyperparathyroidism. Ann Intern Med 1974; 80(2): 182–93.

25. Walker MD, Fleischer J, Rundek T, et al. Carotid vascular abnormalities in primary hyperparathyroidism. J Clin Endocrinol Metab 2009; 94(10): 3849–56.
26. Iwata S, Walker MD, di Tullio MR, et al. Aortic valve calcification in mild primary hyperparathyroidism. J Clin Endocrinol Metab 2012; 97(1): 132–7.
27. Bollerslev J, Rosen T, Mollerup CL, et al. Effect of surgery on cardiovascular risk factors in mild primary hyperparathyroidism. J Clin Endocrinol Metab 2009; 94(7): 2255–61.
28. Mollerup CL, Vestergaard P, Frokjaer VG, Mosekilde L, Christiansen P, Blichert-Toft M. Risk of renal stone events in primary hyperparathyroidism before and after parathyroid surgery: controlled retrospective follow up study. BMJ 2002; 325(7368): 807.
29. Frokjaer VG, Mollerup CL. Primary hyperparathyroidism: renal calcium excretion in patients with and without renal stone sisease before and after parathyroidectomy. World J Surg 2002; 26(5): 532–5.
30. Fajtova VT, Sayegh MH, Hickey N, Aliabadi P, Lazarus JM, LeBoff MS. Intact parathyroid hormone levels in renal insufficiency. Calcif Tissue Int 1995; 57(5): 329–35.
31. Walker MD, Dempster DW, McMahon DJ, et al. Effect of renal function on skeletal health in primary hyperparathyroidism. J Clin Endocrinol Metab 2012; 97(5): 1501–7.
32. Rubin MR, Bilezikian JP, McMahon DJ, et al. The natural history of primary hyperparathyroidism with or without parathyroid surgery after 15 years. J Clin Endocrinol Metab 2008; 93(9): 3462–70.
33. Ambrogini E, Cetani F, Cianferotti L, et al. Surgery or surveillance for mild asymptomatic primary hyperparathyroidism: a prospective, randomized clinical trial. J Clin Endocrinol Metab 2007; 92(8): 3114–21.
34. Silverberg SJ, Locker FG, Bilezikian JP. Vertebral osteopenia: a new indication for surgery in primary hyperparathyroidism. J Clin Endocrinol Metab 1996; 81(11): 4007–12.
35. Silverberg SJ, Brown I, Bilezikian JP. Age as a criterion for surgery in primary hyperparathyroidism. Am J Med 2002; 113(8): 681–4.
36. Peacock M, Bolognese MA, Borofsky M, et al. Cinacalcet treatment of primary hyperparathyroidism: biochemical and bone densitometric outcomes in a five-year study. J Clin Endocrinol Metab 2009; 94(12): 4860–7.
37. Shoback DM, Bilezikian JP, Turner SA, McCary LC, Guo MD, Peacock M. The calcimimetic cinacalcet normalizes serum calcium in subjects with primary hyperparathyroidism. J Clin Endocrinol Metab 2003; 88(12): 5644–9.

CHAPTER 9

Renal Tubular Acidosis, Stones, and Nephrocalcinosis

Robert J. Unwin, Stephen B. Walsh, and Oliver M. Wrong
UCL Centre for Nephrology, University College London Medical School, London, UK

Historical background

The term "renal tubular acidosis," often abbreviated as RTA, could be applied to any form of renal disease that causes systemic acidosis, since the renal tubule is the critical renal structure responsible for acid excretion. However, RTA is not usually applied to acidosis in patients with end-stage renal disease (ESRD), even though these patients are almost always acidotic. For those patients who are acidotic and suffering from predominantly tubular disease, which is now called RTA, Fuller Albright had originally proposed the description "renal acidosis resulting from tubular insufficiency without glomerular insufficiency" [1]. Over the more than 60 years since his description, a mixture of different diseases has been described that could be covered by RTA, of which the best defined and most recognizable form, and the one in which the underlying molecular mechanisms have been clarified more recently, is the syndrome known today as distal renal tubular acidosis (dRTA), "classic," "type 1" or "hypokalemic" RTA. Distal RTA is characterized functionally by a hyperchloremic normal anion gap acidosis and defective urinary acid excretion with a urine pH that cannot fall below 5.3, and clinically by the presence of rickets or osteomalacia, renal stones or nephrocalcinosis, and hypokalemia.

Underlying acid–base physiology

In humans, the resting urinary hydrogen ion (H^+) or proton concentration averages about 1 µmol/L, or pH 6.0, and under acidotic stress urine pH can fall to values in the range 4.5–5.3. The main factor in total tubular H^+ secretion in humans is the tubular reabsorption of 3500 mmol of bicarbonate, equivalent to negative or retained acid, filtered at the glomerulus each day; normal subjects on a typical Western diet excrete an additional 70 mmolsof acid in their daily

Urinary Stones: Medical and Surgical Management, First Edition. Edited by Michael Grasso and David S. Goldfarb.

urine, ~30 mmol of which is H^+ bound to urinary buffers, mainly phosphate, as titratable acid (TA; $H_2PO_4^-$), and ~40 mmol H^+ bound to urinary ammonia (NH_3) as ammonium ion (NH_4^+); the ammonia is synthesized in the proximal tubule by deamination of glutamine. Pitts established that urinary NH_4^+ excretion had a reserve capacity of up to 250 mmol per day in humans when subjected to acidotic stress for several days, but that TA had very little reserve as the urine pH fell to its minimum of 4.5 in systemic acidosis; TA excretion was limited mainly by the rate of buffer (largely phosphate) excretion, and therefore the filtered load of phosphate. Urinary bicarbonate is negligible in urine more acid than pH 6.5, but can increase following an alkali load with corresponding increases in urine pH into the range 7–8. By general agreement, total daily net urinary acid (NAE) excretion has since been defined as TA plus NH_4^+ minus bicarbonate in mmol/day.

The two main processes alluded to above of bicarbonate reabsorption (or reclamation) and net acid excretion occur in distinct parts of the nephron (Figure 9.1): reclamation of the 3500 mmol of filtered bicarbonate (which does not contribute to net acid elimination) in the proximal tubule, and net excretion of the (typically) metabolically generated 70 mmol H^+ per day in the distal tubule and collecting duct. The main mediator of H^+ secretion in the proximal tubule is the NHE3 isoform of the electroneutral Na^+-H^+

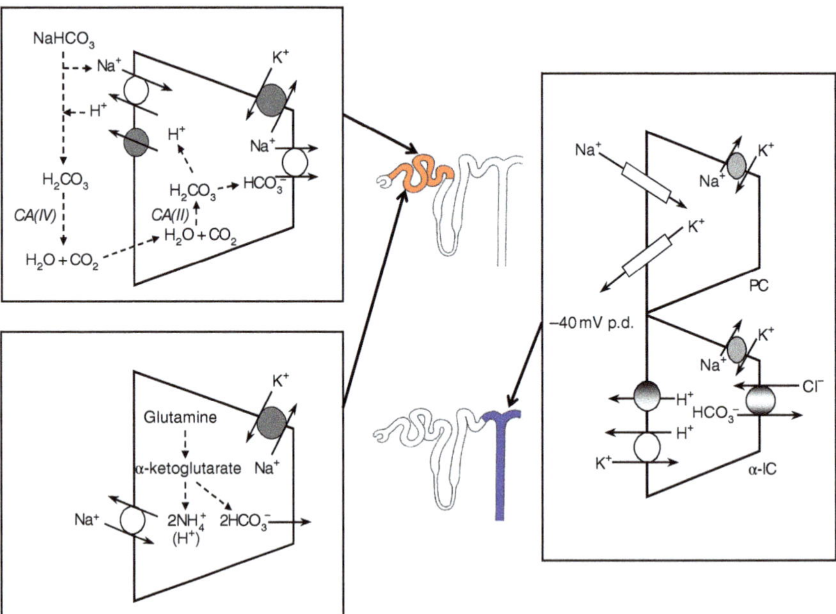

Figure 9.1 Simplified cell models of the mechanisms of H^+ secretion, bicarbonate absorption, and ammoniagenesis by the proximal tubular cell (orange part of the schematic nephron) and H^+ secretion by the α-intercalated cell of the distal tubule and collecting duct cells (blue part of the schematic nephron).

exchanger, and in the distal tubule and collecting duct the electrogenic H^+-ATPase of the α-intercalated cell. Hydrogen ion secretion is accompanied by bicarbonate reabsorption and the exit step for bicarbonate from cell to blood at each site depends on a basolateral membrane located electrogenic Na^+-coupled bicarbonate transporter in the proximal tubular cell and an electroneutral Cl^--bicarbonate exchanger in the distal tubular and collecting duct α-intercalated cell. NH_4^+ is generated in, and secreted by, proximal tubular cells, a process that also produces an additional bicarbonate ion. Thus, proximal RTA (pRTA) implies a defect in the process of bicarbonate reclamation, whereas distal RTA (dRTA) signifies a defect in distal tubular and collecting duct H^+ secretion, and net acid excretion. (When it occurs, defective ammoniagenesis is associated with a distal type of RTA – see p.000.)

In 1959 Wrong and Davies in Manchester published details of acid excretion in a large number of patients with various forms of renal disease, using as an oral acid load, a small dose (0.1 g/kg) of ammonium chloride (NH_4Cl) sufficient to lower plasma bicarbonate concentration by 3–4 mmol/L [2]. Normal subjects were able to lower their urine pH to <5.3 (5 µmol H^+/L), and most patients with chronic renal failure (CRF) were equally efficient in lowering their urine pH, but had a markedly reduced rate of NH_4^+ excretion that was roughly in proportion to their reduced glomerular filtration rate (GFR). Patients with dRTA had minimum urine pH values in the range 5.7–7.0, and urinary TA was reduced in keeping with their abnormally raised urine pH. Most strikingly, urinary NH_4^+ excretion rates in these dRTA patients were reduced in proportion to GFR, suggesting that a reduction in total renal mass (and therefore capacity for ammoniagenesis) was responsible for this defect (cf. CRF), rather than the tubular defect of dRTA *per se*. Support for this interpretation came from three patients with nephrocalcinosis, but no systemic acidosis, who were unable to lower their urine pH below 5.7–6.5, with matching reductions in urinary TA, but who had preserved GFRs and normal or even enhanced rates of urinary NH_4^+ excretion, which seemed to protect them from developing a systemic acidosis. This syndrome variant was described as "an incomplete form of renal tubular acidosis" (now known as incomplete dRTA), that is, a urinary acidification defect similar to that in "complete" dRTA, but not accompanied by acidosis. Such patients are almost certainly encountered clinically more commonly than those with complete dRTA, although they are more difficult to detect unless this diagnosis is considered.

Proximal renal tubular acidosis

Early work on RTA did not distinguish between the parts of the renal tubule where disease might cause acidosis, though it was clear from Albright's work that some patients had clinical features of proximal tubular disease, including the presence of glycosuria, phosphaturia, and amino-aciduria of so-called renal Fanconi's syndrome type, whereas others lacked these features and usually had nephrocalcinosis. These two groups were

Box 9.1 A clinical classification of renal tubular acidosis (RTA)

- **Proximal or type 2 RTA** is rarely an isolated defect and is usually part of a renal Fanconi's syndrome (with associated tubular proteinuria and variable glycosuria and phosphaturia)
- **Distal or type 1 RTA** with hypokalemia can be "complete" or "incomplete," depending on the presence of systemic acidosis (plasma bicarbonate concentration <20 mmol/L)
- **Mixed or type 3 RTA** was originally described in infants and children as transitory and due to an "immature tubule" but it is now used to describe a mixture of types 1 and 2, the best example being carbonic anhydrase deficiency or inhibition
- **Hyperkalemic or type 4 RTA** is "distal-like" and due to lack of aldosterone or resistance to its action, but unlike type 1 dRTA, patients are usually hyperkalemic rather than hypokalemic, and the main defect is reduced ammonia production

eventually described as "proximal" and "distal" forms of RTA, also designated as types 2 and 1, respectively (see Box 9.1). Later the label of type 3 was attached by Curtis Morris, and his group to rare pediatric cases that had features intermediate between types 1 and 2 [3], which is now considered to be a combination of proximal and distal forms of RTA, and the term type 4 was applied to patients with dRTA in whom mineralocorticoid deficiency or resistance results in hyperkalemia with acidosis due to reduced ammoniagenesis and NH_4^+ excretion (see p.000), and is better described as "hyperkalemic dRTA." The term "hypokalemic dRTA" is often used to refer to type 1 dRTA.

Although most patients with pRTA have features of a generalized proximal tubular defect (a renal Fanconi's syndrome), some patients do have an isolated defect of bicarbonate reabsorption along the proximal tubule, including a sporadic and transitory form occurring in infants and young children [3], and a rare recessive familial form caused by mutations in the above-mentioned electrogenic Na^+-bicarbonate co-transporter, which is also associated with various ocular defects [4]. Overall, proximal RTA in all its forms is much less common than dRTA and so has been less well studied.

Underlying mechanisms in distal RTA

Distal RTA is the form usually associated with both nephrocalcinosis and renal stone disease, and more causes of dRTA have been reported, including postrenal transplantation, hypercalcemic and obstructive renal damage, toluene/glue sniffing, chronic lithium administration, amiloride, use of the artificial sweetener cyclamate and the antifungal antibiotic amphotericin B, as well as in fetal alcohol syndrome. The number of reports in each of these categories has been small, many consisting of single case reports, so it has been difficult to establish the molecular basis of the underlying urinary acidification defect. However, two forms of dRTA have turned out to be relatively common: (i) the form associated with systemic autoimmune diseases, predominantly affecting adult females [5]; and (ii) various familial forms of dRTA, both autosomal dominant and recessive. The larger number of cases of these two forms of dRTA has encouraged an intensive study of their molecular basis, a summary of which is given below.

A large number of abnormal conditions might cause secondary clinical dRTA, including any cause of hypercalcemia or nephrocalcinosis, medullary sponge kidney (MSK), sickle cell disease, and various forms of chronic interstitial nephritis. However, secondary dRTA from these various causes is less common than dRTA in which no primary cause can be found. Among these cases were two distinct forms of primary dRTA: autoimmune and familial.

The familial forms of RTA, excluding the rare proximal form referred to earlier, cause dRTA and involve the two main molecular players involved in H^+ secretion along the distal tubule and collecting duct: the apical H^+-ATPase [6,7] and the basolateral bicarbonate secreting Cl^--bicarbonate exchanger, known also as AE1 (*SLC4A1*) [8]. The latter is a truncated form of the same anion exchanger present in red blood cells and is essential for normal CO_2 transport and transfer from tissues to lung. Mutations in these two transporters are responsible for all cases of familial dRTA described so far. Mutations of subunits of the H^+-ATPase cause a recessive and, more commonly, pediatric form of dRTA with early- (B1 subunit [*ATP6V1B1*] mutation) or late- (a4 subunit [*ATP6V04A*] mutation) onset deafness, because this pump is also present in the inner ear controlling the pH of endolymph. Mutations of the Cl^--bicarbonate exchanger cause a dominant form of dRTA that is usually detected later in life, particularly in patients who present with nephrocalcinosis and/or renal stones. While visible red cell abnormalities are not a feature of this form in Caucasians, this is not the case in tropical populations, where it can also be recessive when it occurs as a compound heterozygote of two different (usually recessive) mutations in the same patient or with the more common heterozygous form of South East Asian ovalocytosis (SAO) [9,10].

Familial and *de novo* autosomal dominant dRTA, as well as autoimmune dRTA, are more likely to be encountered and should be considered in any patient presenting with nephrocalcinosis and (calcium phosphate) renal stones. In autoimmune dRTA, hypokalemia is often striking and symptomatic, while nephrocalcinosis can be less prominent; MSK (a diagnosis that can still only be made confidently with an intravenous urogram) can also be inherited and confused with autosomal dominant dRTA, although both can occur in isolated cases without a family history. However, stone composition can sometimes provide a useful clue, since in dRTA it is almost invariably pure calcium phosphate, whereas in MSK it is more often mixed calcium oxalate and phosphate, as is true of most other forms of stone disease associated with nephrocalcinosis, although it is worth mentioning what is sometimes termed "secondary dRTA due to nephrocalcinosis" which seems more likely to occur when medullary nephrocalcinosis is heavy and extensive.

Diagnosis and management of RTA

A summary of how to diagnose RTA is set out in Box 9.2. Bearing in mind that the form of RTA most commonly encountered in a renal stone clinic is dRTA or type 1, the discussion will focus on the investigation and management of this form of RTA. It is worth remembering that in the context of renal stones or nephrocalcinosis, while an elevated random urine pH (especially if it is from a second void early morning sample), even if measured by urine dipstick, may raise the possibility of underlying dRTA, the urine pH (which is a measure of free H^+ concentration) can be increased for at least three reasons unrelated to an acidification defect: (i) urinary infection, especially with urea-splitting organisms (e.g. *Pseudomonas, Proteus*) that can generate ammonia/ammonium; (ii) a delayed measurement when a urine sample is left for several hours and not properly sealed or covered with oil, and CO_2 can volatize; (iii) high urinary content of ammonium (not due to infection), e.g. in hypokalemia.

Box 9.2 How to diagnose renal tubular acidosis (RTA)

- In the presence of a systemic acidosis when urine pH is >5.3
- A casual early morning (second void) urine pH >5.5* and a urine citrate:creatinine ratio that is low (in an alkaline urine) or undetectable, are highly suggestive

More active tests of urinary acidification

- The oral NH_4Cl (0.1 g/kg) test
- The oral furosemide (40 mg) plus fludrocortisone (1 mg) test (see text for details)
- Intravenous bicarbonate loading in suspected pRTA to raise plasma bicarbonate concentration and demonstrate a high fractional excretion of bicarbonate (>15%)

Less reliable or indirect tests of urinary acidification

- Urine-blood PCO_2 difference <30 mmHg (4 kPa)
- Urine anion gap or net charge (normally negative in acidosis) and osmolar gap (normally positive in acidosis) are surrogates for unmeasured ammonium (NH_4^+) excretion

*Urine pH should be measured with a glass pH electrode in the laboratory. Avoid delay in measuring after sample collection, since without collection under oil the urine pH can increase with time. Routine urine dipstick pH values can be a rough guide, but are less accurate and can be unreliable.

Most patients found to have dRTA will have been seen in a renal stone clinic and therefore they will have had a 24-h urine collection as part of their metabolic stone screen [11]. If not, this is something we do routinely, because it not only provides a valuable diagnostic clue, that is, a very low citrate excretion, but it may also identify other factors, such as high sodium excretion and hypercalciuria, contributing to stone risk that can be modified. However, in our UK experience, hypercalciuria is not a consistent finding in dRTA, even in those patients who have the complete form. We attribute this to the presence of an additional acid load from the diet, particularly in meat-eaters, which might explain why hypercalciuria in dRTA is reported more commonly in the US, where thiazides might be useful adjunctive therapy.

When the diagnosis of dRTA is suspected in a patient with recurrent stones, with or without nephrocalcinosis, a family history, rickets in children or osteomalacia in adults, an associated autoimmune disorder or a 100% calcium phosphate stone, it should be confirmed by carrying out a urinary acidification test (Figure 9.2). The urine minus blood (U-B) PCO_2, which has been proposed as a measure of normal H^+ secretion along the collecting duct, and ammonium excretion (particularly if estimated from the urine anion or osmolar gaps), even if seemingly more convenient, are too indirect and prone to error [12]. Although not yet as well validated as the short ammonium chloride test referred to earlier, an easier screening test is the recently described modification of the original furosemide test [13,14], now known as the "F+F test," which consists of the oral administration of single doses of furosemide 40 mg and fludrocortisone 1 mg, followed by immediate measurement of the pH (with a calibrated pH electrode) of each urine sample voided over at least 4 h (see Figure 9.2) [15]. Figure 9.3 is a graphical representation of the response to progressive acidosis in pRTA and dRTA compared with normal; note that the curve for pRTA is simply shifted to the left and that affected patients can acidify their urine when the serum or plasma bicarbonate concentration is low enough, whereas in dRTA the curve remains relatively flat and unresponsive.

While it may seem obvious that an acidotic (serum or plasma bicarbonate concentration <20 mmol/L) patient with a urine pH >6 and calcium phosphate stones and/or nephrocalcinosis is very likely to have dRTA, we still recommend an acidification test to confirm the diagnosis, and should not delay or prevent alkali treatment. However, is the diagnosis of the milder incomplete form of dRTA of any clinical value, apart from providing a diagnostic label (which many patients like to have)? While renal failure and death are unusual in patients with nephrocalcinosis and/or stones, and are usually the result of multiple stone-related surgical procedures with frequent complications such as infection or obstruction, making the diagnosis of dRTA ensures at least two things that are of potential benefit to the patient: (i) an effort to establish the actual cause of RTA, for example, a hitherto unrecognized family history and gene mutation, with its implications for relatives and children, or as

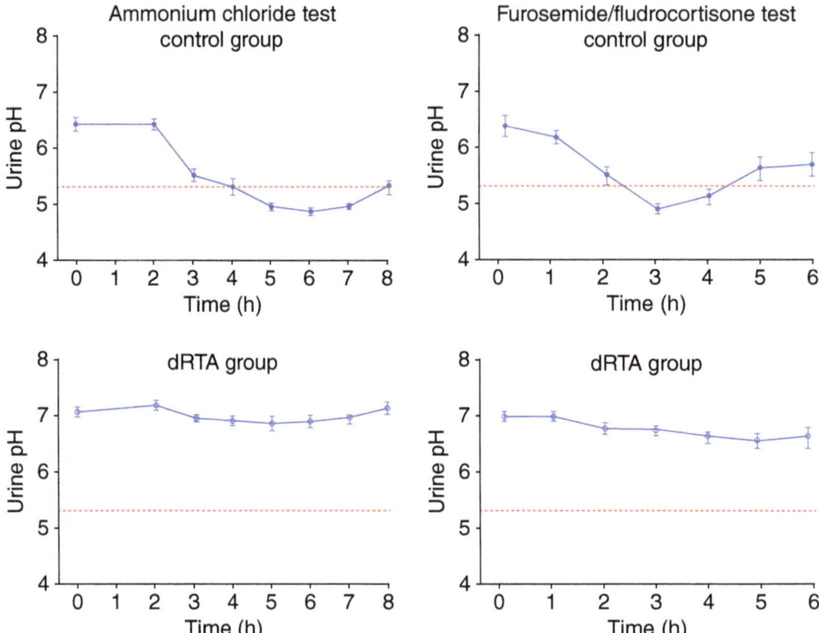

Figure 9.2 Responses to the short oral ammonium chloride and furosemide plus fludrocortisone tests of urinary acidification are compared in normal subjects and patients with known dRTA. Source: Walsh 2007 [12]. Reproduced with permission of John Wiley & Sons Ltd.

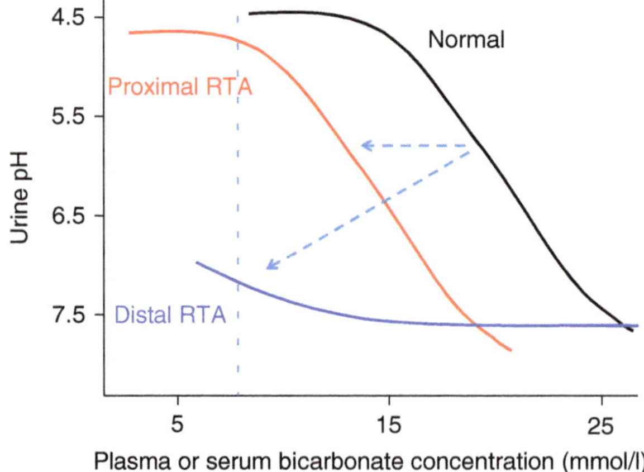

Figure 9.3 The pattern of change in the relationship between plasma or serum bicarbonate concentration and urine pH in normal subjects (*in black*), patients with proximal RTA (*pRTA in red*) and distal RTA (*dRTA in blue*); see text for details. Source: Rodriguez-Soriano 1969 [16]. Reproduced with permission of Annual Review Inc.

a manifestation of an unrecognized autoimmune disease; (ii) regular follow-up of a patient who is more likely to have episodes of stone recurrence in the long term. Reduced bone mineral density may be less of a problem in incomplete dRTA [17].

Whatever the underlying cause, the mainstay of treatment is alkali therapy, which probably benefits, and helps protect, the bones (Figure 9.4) more than reducing the risk of renal stones (at least in complete dRTA) [18,19], because it is difficult to boost urinary citrate excretion, even with large doses (typical recommendation is 1–2 mmol/kg). Alkali therapy can be given as bicarbonate or citrate, either one promoting citrate excretion by converting it from the readily reabsorbed divalent form to the less easily reabsorbed trivalent form. However, the potassium salt is more effective than the sodium salt in increasing citrate excretion (to offset any increase

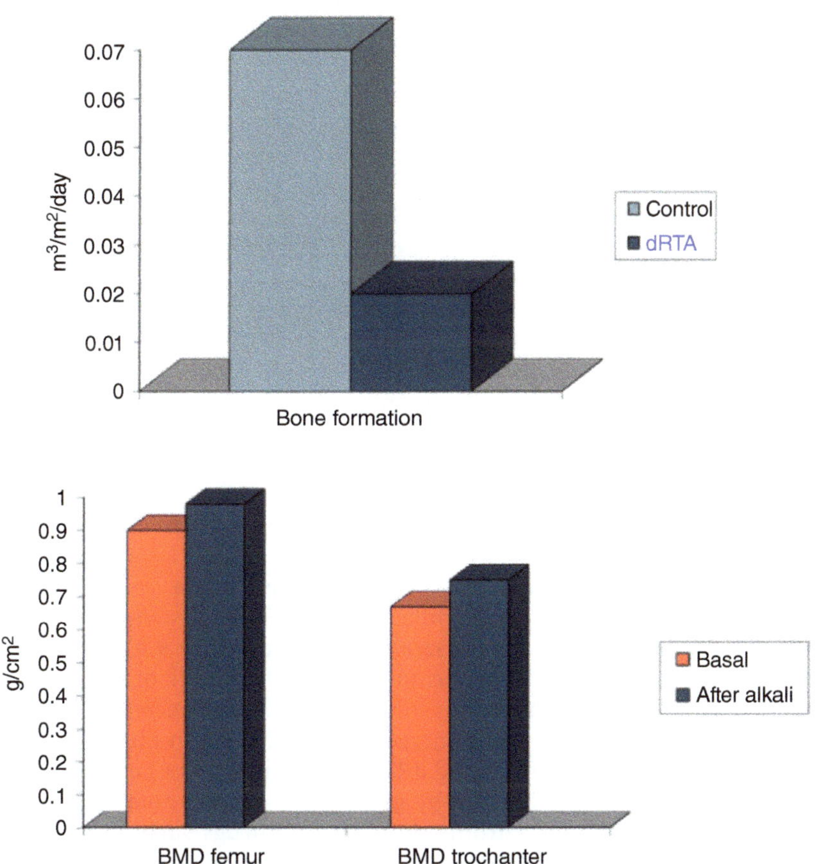

Figure 9.4 Bone formation in dRTA and the response to alkali therapy. Source: Adapted from Domrongkitchaiporn 2002 [18] and Domrongkitchaiporn 2001 [19].

in urine pH) and minimizing calcium excretion, and so correcting hypokalemia is also important in RTA treatment. Moreover, the balance between further increases in urinary pH with aggressive alkali therapy (and the attendant risk of more calcium phosphate stone formation) and increased citrate excretion is a potentially difficult one to manage. For this reason, as a first step we favor measures that we currently use in almost all stone formers, irrespective of the underlying cause, which includes boosting fluid intake to at least 2 L a day, mainly as water, which can be flavored with citrate-rich fresh lemon or lime juice, and encouraging a diet rich in fruit and vegetables (and to provide information on oxalate-rich foods as a simple precaution), and low in animal protein (red meat, white meat, and fish), recommending the Mediterranean-like Dietary Approaches to Stop Hypertension (DASH) diet [11].

If an autoimmune cause has not been suspected, it should be considered, especially in women. Almost all forms of autoimmune disease have been described in association with dRTA but dRTA is particularly common in patients with Sjögren's syndrome, with up to 40–70% affected in some series [20,21]. This form of dRTA can be difficult to manage and it should be done in conjunction with specialist rheumatologists, where efforts are directed at reducing elevated γ-globulin levels (with hydroxychloroquine) and may even require immunosuppression, especially if there is any evidence of active renal involvement with tubulointerstitial disease. Moreover, those cases with more pronounced tubulointerstitial inflammation (seen on renal biopsy) often have features of type 3 (mixed proximal and distal) RTA, which can be diagnosed clinically by the presence of tubular (e.g. retinol binding protein) proteinuria.

Figure 9.5 demonstrates the radiology of dRTA and an example of rickets. Although nephrocalcinosis is not always visible in autoimmune dRTA, when it is seen radiologically in the setting of renal stone disease, it should always raise the possibility of underlying dRTA, particularly if the stone composition is predominantly calcium phosphate. Around 20% of cases of nephrocalcinosis are due to dRTA, the most common cause still being primary hyperparathyroidism, and much less commonly MSK [22].

Again, alkali therapy (already in use in ancient India for "calculi") is given for all forms of RTA, and while it can normalize growth in children and preserve or restore bone mineralization (see Figure 9.4), it may not alter the progression of nephrocalcinosis or reduce the risk of renal stones, since, as already mentioned, any increase in citrate excretion may be offset by a rise in urine pH and increased risk of calcium phosphate precipitation. Patients with pRTA and dRTA (excluding type 4) are also often hypokalemic and correcting this by giving alkali as the potassium salt is recommended. Although chronic therapy with drugs such as oral acetazolamide, or those with carbonic anhydrase-inhibiting activity such as the antiepileptic topiramate, can cause calcium phosphate stones to form [23], in pRTA nephrocalcinosis and stones are less common (perhaps because citrate excretion is usually increased) than in dRTA, but giving alkali as

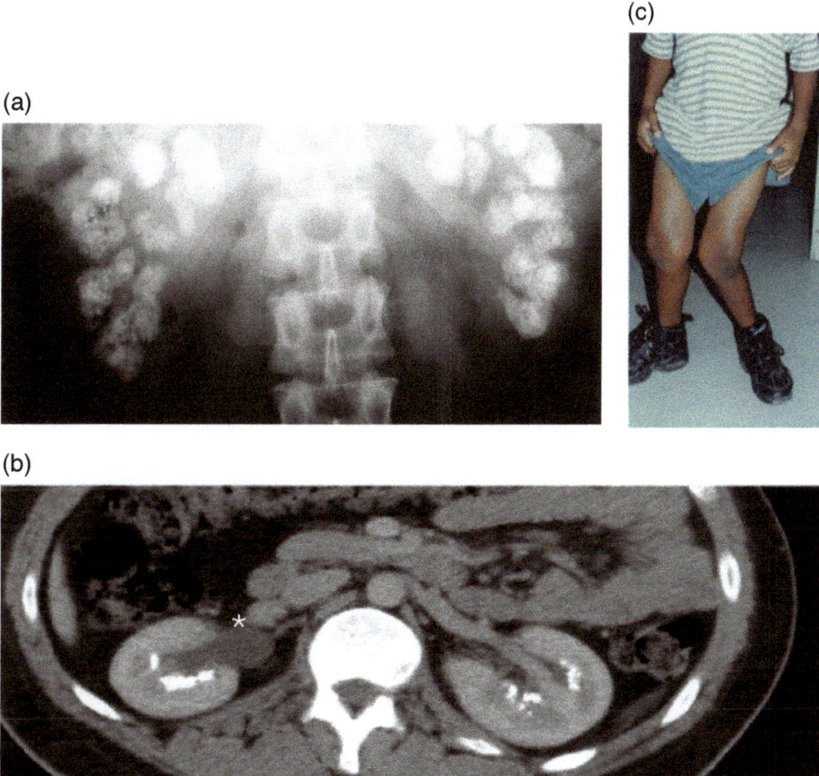

Figure 9.5 (a) Plain X-ray of a male with a reduced eGFR and autosomal dominant (complete) dRTA showing typical bilateral medullary nephrocalcinosis. (b) Non-contrast CT scan of a young male with autosomal recessive (complete) dRTA with late-onset deafness showing nephrocalcinosis (and dilated ureter – *asterisk*). Both patients had recurrent calcium phosphate (high urine pH) stones. (c) Young boy with inherited tropical (complete) dRTA and rickets which is rarely seen in the Western form. Source: (c) Khositseth 2012 [10]. Reproduced with permission of Oxford University Press.

sodium bicarbonate can still increase urinary potassium losses and worsen hypokalemia, because of its effect on distal tubule and collecting duct potassium secretion as a non-reabsorbable anion [24].

Summary

The distal form of renal tubular acidosis (dRTA) is encountered more commonly and should be suspected in a patient with nephrocalcinosis or calcium phosphate stones, especially with a family history or an associated autoimmune disease such as Sjögren's syndrome. While the X-linked familial Dent's disease presents typically with nephrocalcinosis and renal stones, an acidification defect is thought to be unusual in this genetic disorder, its hallmark being features of the renal Fanconi's syndrome, particularly tubular proteinuria (see p.000), often with significant renal impairment [25,26]. Alkali treatment for dRTA is aimed more at protecting the bones than preventing recurrent stones, which should be managed surgically and pre-emptively, if necessary, in those with a propensity to form recurrent stones. Alkali therapy should be given as the potassium rather than the sodium salt, and affected patients will require regular and long-term follow-up, although loss of renal function is rare. When it does occur, it is often the result of episodes of obstruction complicated by infection and the need for more invasive, repeated and urgent surgical interventions.

References

1. Albright F, Burnett CH, Parson W, Reifenstein Jr EC, Roos A. The various etiologies met in the United States with emphasis on that resulting from a specific form of renal acidosis, the therapeutic indications for each etiological sub-group, and the relationship between osteomalacia and milkman's syndrome. Medicine (Baltimore) 1946; 25: 399–479.
2. Wrong O, Davies H. The excretion of acid in renal disease. Q J Med 1959; 28: 259–313.
3. McSherry E, Sebastian A, Morris RC. Renal tubular acidosis in infants: the several kinds, including bicarbonate-wasting, classic renal tubular acidosis. J Clin Invest 1972; 51: 499–514.
4. Igarashi T, Sekine T, Inatomi J, Seki G. Unraveling the molecular pathogenesis of isolated proximal renal tubular acidosis. J Am Soc Nephrol 2002; 13: 2171–7.
5. Walsh S, Turner CM, Toye A, et al. Immunohistochemical comparison of a case of inherited distal renal tubular acidosis (with a unique AE1 mutation) with an acquired case secondary to autoimmune disease. Nephrol Dial Transplant 2007a; 22: 807–12.
6. Karet FE, Finberg KE, Nelson RD, et al. Mutations in the gene encoding B1 subunit of H^+-ATPase cause renal tubular acidosis with sensorineural deafness. Nature Genet 1999; 21: 84–90.
7. Smith AN, Skaug J, Choate KA, et al. Mutations in ATP6N1B, encoding a new kidney vacuolar proton pump 116-kD subunit, cause recessive distal renal tubular acidosis with preserved hearing. Nature Genet 2000; 26: 71–5.
8. Bruce LJ, Cope DL, Jones GK, et al. Familial distal renal tubular acidosis is associated with mutations in the red cell anion exchanger (Band 3, AE1) gene. J Clin Invest 1997; 100: 1693–707.
9. Wrong O, Bruce LJ, Unwin RJ, Toye AM, Tanner MJA. Band 3 mutations, distal renal tubular acidosis, and Southeast Asian ovalocytosis. Kidney Int 2002; 62: 10–19.
10. Khositseth S, Bruce LJ, Walsh SB, et al. Tropical distal renal tubular acidosis: clinical and epidemiological studies in 78 patients. Q J Med 2012; 105: 861–77.
11. Johri N, Cooper B, Robertson WG, Choong S, Unwin RJ. An update and practical guide to renal stone management. Nephron Clin Pract 2010; 116: c159–c171.

12. Wrong O. Distal renal tubular acidosis: the value of urinary pH, PCO_2 and NH_4^+ measurements. Pediatr Nephrol 1991; 5: 249–55.
13. Rastogi SP, Crawford C, Wheeler R, Flanigan W, Arruda JA. Effect of furosemide on urinary acidification in distal renal tubular acidosis. J Lab Clin Med 1984; 104: 271–82.
14. Batlle DC. Segmental characterization of defects in collecting tubule acidification. Kidney Int 1986; 30: 546–54.
15. Walsh SB, Shirley DG, Wrong OM, Unwin RJ. Urinary acidification assessed by simultaneous furosemide and fludrocortisone treatment: an alternative to ammonium chloride. Kidney Int 2007; 71: 1310–16.
16. Rodriguez-Soriano J, Edelmann CM. Renal tubular acidosis. Annu Rev Med 1969; 20: 363–82.
17. Arampatzis S, Ropke-Rieben B, Lippuner K, Hess B. Prevalence and densitometric characteristics of incomplete distal renal tubular acidosis in men with recurrent calcium nephrolithiasis. Urol Res 2012; 40: 53–9.
18. Domrongkitchaiporn S, Pongskul C, Sirikulchayanonta V, et al. Bone histology and bone mineral density after correction of acidosis in distal renal tubular acidosis. Kidney Int 2002; 62: 2160–6.
19. Domrongkitchaiporn S, Pongsakul C, Stitchantrakul W, et al. Bone mineral density and histology in distal renal tubular acidosis. Kidney Int 2001; 59: 1086–93.
20. Ren H, Wang W-M, Chen X-N, et al. Renal involvement and followup of 130 patients with primary Sjögren's syndrome. J Rheumatol 2008; 35: 278–84.
21. Ohtani H, Imai H, Kodama T, et al. Severe hypokalaemia and respiratory arrest due to renal tubular acidosis in a patient with Sjögren syndrome. Nephrol Dial Transplant 1999; 14: 2201–3.
22. Wrong O. The radiological significance of nephrocalcinosis. Hospital Update 1985; 11: 167–78.
23. Kuo RL, Moran ME, Kim DH, Abrahams HM, White MD, Lingeman JE. Topiramate-induced nephrolithiasis. J Endourol 2002; 16: 229–31.
24. Unwin RJ, Luft F, Shirley DG. Pathophysiology and management of hypokalemia: a clinical perspective. Nature Rev Nephrol 2010; 7: 75–84.
25. Wrong OM, Norden AG, Feest TG. Dent's disease; a familial proximal renal tubular syndrome with low-molecular-weight proteinuria, hypercalciuria, nephrocalcinosis, metabolic bone disease, progressive renal failure and a marked male predominance. Q J Med 1994; 87: 473–93.
26. Neild GH, Thakker RV, Unwin RJ, Wrong OM. Dent's disease. Nephrol Dial Transplant 2005; 20: 2284–5.

CHAPTER 10

Drug-Induced Stones

Michel Daudon[1] *and Paul Jungers*[2]
[1]Tenon Hospital, Paris, France
[2]Necker Hospital, Paris, France

Do's and don'ts box

Do:
- remember the possible formation of kidney stones in patients treated with protease inhibitors (especially atazanavir), sulfadiazine or carbonic anhydrase inhibitors (acetazolamide, topiramate or zonisamide), and in persons receiving calcium-vitamin D supplements or over-the-counter (OTC) compounds containing ephedrine and guaifenesin
- exercise clinical surveillance to detect drug-induced stones, remembering that they often are asymptomatic
- take into account the solubility characteristics of drugs used at high doses and/or for a long duration and try to optimally adapt urine pH, and maintain a high urine volume to prevent stone formation.

Do not:
- neglect immediate analysis of stones produced by subjects at risk, even in those with known history of urolithiasis
- systematically discontinue treatment in patients with severe diseases, but instead try to adapt the daily dose and solubility of the drug, and reinforce high fluid intake, when no equipotent alternative is available.

Introduction

Drug-induced kidney stones currently account for about 1% of cases of urolithiasis. Two different mechanisms are involved in the formation of such stones: (i) the drug or its metabolites is by itself the main component of calculi; (ii) the drug induces metabolic alterations leading to the formation of calcium or uric acid calculi [1]. Drug-induced stones are often undiagnosed or misdiagnosed, unless proper stone analysis (by means of X-ray diffraction or infra-red spectroscopy) and metabolic evaluation are performed, taking into account the co-morbidity and drug treatment of the patient.

Urinary Stones: Medical and Surgical Management, First Edition. Edited by Michael Grasso and David S. Goldfarb.

Table 10.1 Drug-related urolithiasis in our laboratory (1995–2012)

Drugs	Adults		Children	Components in stones
	Men	Women		
Total no of stones	n = 33,166	n = 14,557	n = 1761	
Drug-containing stones				
Protease inhibitors	*166*	*32*	*0*	
Indinavir (before 2005)	124	26	0	Indinavir monohydrate
Atazanavir (after 2005)	42	6	0	Atazanavir
Sulfonamides	*25*	*9*	*4*	
Sulfadiazine	17	8	4	N-acetylsulfadiazine ± sulfadiazine
Sulfamethoxazole	8	1	0	N-acetylsulfamethoxazole, HCl
Other antimicrobial agents	*1*	*3*	*12*	
Ceftriaxone	0	2	9	Ceftriaxone calcium salt
Ciprofloxacin	1	0	0	
Amoxicillin	0	1	3	Amoxicillin trihydrate
Antihypertensives: Triamterene	23	24	0	Triamterene and metabolites
Others	*12*	*5*	*4*	
Allopurinol	2	0	2	Oxypurinol + xanthine
Colloidal silica	0	0	2	Amorphous silica (opal)
Magnesium silicate	10	5	0	Amorphous silicia (opal)
Total	227	73	20	
Drug-induced stones				
Carbonic anhydrase inhibitors	*32*	*17*	*11*	
Acetazolamide	27	12	0	Carbapatite
Topiramate	5	5	11	Carbapatite
Vitamin D + calcium supplements	*27*	*34*	*7*	Calcium oxalate ± carbapatite
Laxative abuse		*2*	*0*	Ammonium hydrogen urate
Total	59	53	18	

Epidemiology

The epidemiology of drug-induced stones has markedly changed in the past two decades. Sulfonamides were the first drugs implicated in stone formation [1]. Since 1995, protease inhibitors, carbonic anhydrase inhibitors and calcium-vitamin D supplements have become increasingly frequent causes of drug-induced kidney stones.

Table 10.1 depicts the proportion and main causes of drug-induced calculi among 49,484 stones from adults and children analyzed by means of infra-red spectroscopy and morphology [2] since 1995 at our laboratory.

Drug-containing kidney stones

Triamterene

The potassium-sparing drug triamterene was commonly combined with thiazide diuretics in the long-term treatment of hypertension in order to minimize the risk of hypokalemia. Triamterene was identified in 0.4% of ~50,000 calculi in the USA [3] and a similar prevalence was observed in our experience [1]. Incidence of triamterene-induced stones has progressively declined in recent decades thanks to alternative use of drugs devoid of lithogenic potential, such as amiloride (see Table 10.1). Stones are made of triamterene and metabolites, which are poorly soluble especially in acidic urine (Figure 10.1a). Prevention of such stones is based on a daily dose not exceeding 100 mg of triamterene, urine pH no less than 6, and avoidance in patients with a history of calcium or uric acid stones [1].

Protease inhibitors

Protease inhibitors were introduced in the therapy of human immunodeficiency virus (HIV) infection in 1995 in combination with other antiretrovirals, mainly inhibitors of HIV reverse transcriptase [4].

Indinavir

Indinavir, initially the most widely prescribed protease inhibitor, was rapidly shown to induce the formation of calculi in 7–12% of patients. Indinavir calculi (Figure 10.1b) accounted for 0.74% of all calculi and for 61% of drug-containing calculi analyzed at our laboratory between 1996 and 2002 [1]. Infra-red spectroscopy identified indinavir monohydrate as the main component of these calculi [5].

The formation of stones is favored by the poor solubility of the drug at usual urine pH (35 mg/L at pH 6.0 compared to 300 mg/L at pH <5.5), while urine concentration achieved in the 3 h following an oral dose of 800 mg is 200–300 mg/L, and by the very large size of needle-shaped, plate-forming crystals (Figure 10.1c) [6]. As a result, crystalluria is a

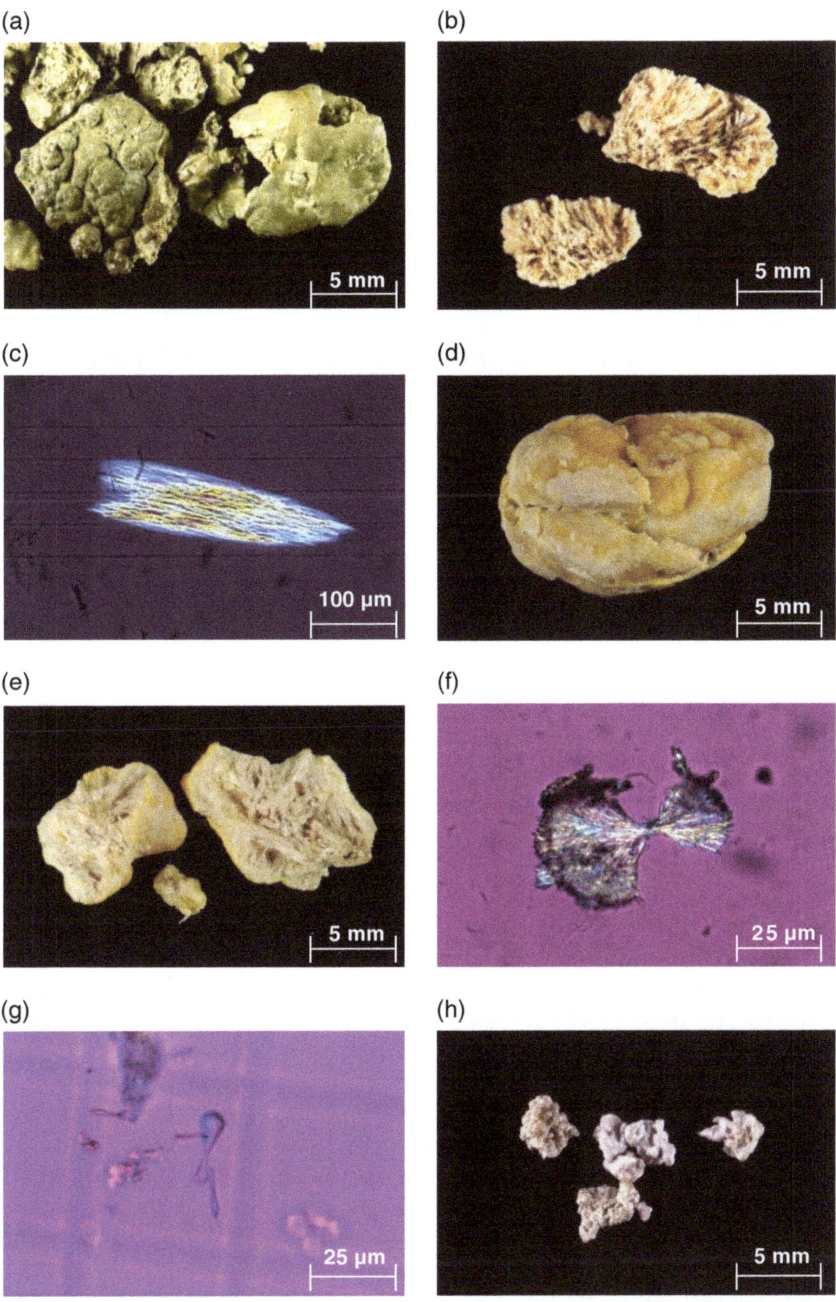

Figure 10.1 (a)Triamterene stones. (b) Cross-section of indinavir stone exhibiting a typical radial loose structure. (c) Indinavir plate-forming crystals in urine as seen by polarizing microscopy. (d) Atazanavir stone of pale yellow-orange color. (e) Atazanavir stone section. (f) Asymmetrical aggregate made of needle-shaped crystals of N-acetylsulfadiazine in urine (polarized light). (g) Small aggregates of crystals made of ceftriaxone calcium salt weakly birefringent in urine. (h) Calculi made of ceftriaxone calcium salt spontaneously passed in a child.

very frequent finding in indinavir-treated patients, with episodes of dehydration due to high temperature or diarrhea acting as triggering factors [7].

Indinavir renal complications may sometimes present with acute renal failure due to obstructive crystalluria with elevated serum creatinine [8]. Stones are totally radiolucent on X-ray and computed tomography (CT), but seen on echography [9]. They spontaneously pass in the majority of cases with conservative measures [6]. Urological intervention is only required in a minority of patients, preferably by ureteroscopy, as extracorporeal shock wave lithotripsy (ESWL) is usually ineffective due to the loose structure of calculi. The main preventive measure is to increase urine output by ingesting 150 mL fluids when taking the drug and during the following 2 h [5]. Cola soft drinks, which reduce urine pH, are useful in reducing the formation of crystals and stones [1].

In fact, the most effective measure was the development of new therapeutic protocols based on co-administration of protease inhibitors with ritonavir, acting as a "booster" which potentiates their action by increasing their plasma concentration. Indeed, ritonavir is a potent inhibitor of cytochrome P4503A4, the microsomal hepatic enzyme which metabolizes protease inhibitors [4]. However, despite generalized use of such protocols, some risk of crystalluria and stone formation still persists with certain anti-HIV agents.

Atazanavir

Atazanavir, an azapeptide inhibitor of HIV-1 protease first marketed in 2003, was soon reported as inducing urolithiasis [10] and sometimes acute interstitial nephritis [11]. Even in ritonavir-boosted protocols (ATZ/r), atazanavir was associated with a significantly higher risk of urolithiasis than other antiretroviral agents. Renal stone incidence was 7.3 cases/1000 patient-years in 1206 ATZ/r-treated patients, versus only 1.9/1000 patient-years among 4449 patients treated with other ritonavir-boosted protocols at a large HIV department in the UK [12]. An even more marked difference was reported in a recent study in Japan [13].

Atazanavir crystals present as thin needles which form smaller aggregates than do indinavir crystals. They form stones of yellow-orange color, resembling uric acid stones (Figure 10.1d), inasmuch as they also are radiolucent [14], and may induce crystalline acute kidney injury [15]. The sectioning of calculi reveals poorly organized aggregates of atazanavir needles (Figure 10.1e). As recommended for indinavir, increasing fluid intake when taking the drug is an effective measure to reduce urine concentration of the unchanged drug which is responsible for crystallization.

Nelfinavir and tenofovir

These protease inhibitors infrequently induce urolithiasis [16,17].

Sulfadiazine and other sulfonamides

Sulfadiazine

Sulfadiazine, which readily crosses the blood–brain barrier, is widely used for the treatment of cerebral toxoplasmosis, mainly ocular involvement. The high daily doses (4–8 g) needed in severe forms lead to intratubular crystallization of its poorly soluble metabolite N-acetylsulfadiazine, thus resulting in urolithiasis [18] or acute kidney injury due to bilateral obstruction by crystals [19]. Over the period 1987–1996, 16% of drug-containing calculi analyzed at our laboratory were made of sulfadiazine, with decreasing incidence over the following years.

Sulfadiazine stones are radiolucent but visible by echography. They give a very weak attenuation (<100 Hounsfield units, HU) with unenhanced helical CT. Examination of urinary sediment is of great diagnostic relevance, showing typical needle-shaped crystals forming large agglomerates (Figure 10.1f). Solubility of sulfadiazine and its metabolites markedly increases at alkaline pH. Thus, prevention relies on high fluid intake and alkalinization during the whole duration of sulfadiazine administration, unless the patient is simultaneously treated with a protease inhibitor. In such situations, active urine dilution is the only means of preventing precipitation of both drugs.

Other sulfonamides

Sulfasalazine, used in the treatment of ulcerative colitis, may induce bilateral stones [19]. Sulfamethoxazole, a component of co-trimoxazole, induces frequent crystalluria but stone formation [18] is infrequent relative to its wide use, likely due to the small size and smooth rhomboid shape of the crystals. Curative and preventive measures are the same as for sulfadiazine.

Other antibacterial or antiviral drugs

Quinolones and aminopenicillins are rarely involved in drug-induced nephrolithiasis (reviewed in [1]). Ciprofloxacin causes frequent asymptomatic crystalluria, especially in alkaline urine (in contrast with first-generation quinolones) but formation of stones is very infrequent [20].

Ceftriaxone is largely used for the treatment of bacterial meningitis, pneumonia or pyelonephritis, especially in children. The first cases of ceftriaxone-associated nephrolithiasis were reported in 1990 [21] and later in cohort studies with an incidence of 1.4–7.8% [22,23]. Stones are made of ceftriaxone calcium salt (Figure 10.1g), as ceftriaxone markedly increases urinary calcium excretion [24]. Ceftriaxone calcium salt may form small crystals (Figure 10.1g) and stones (Figure 10.1h) and, as shown in Table 10.1, accounts for a significant proportion of drug-induced calculi in children. Efavirenz, an antinucleosidase used in HIV+ patients, has induced several cases of urolithiasis [25].

Guaifenesin, ephedrine, and pseudoephedrine

A number of non-prescription oral cough suppressants, expectorants, and decongestants, often in the form of mixed preparations, are available OTC and freely available via the internet. This free access allows uncontrolled use of such preparations, leading in some cases to stone formation, besides other undesirable side-effects. In addition, these drugs may interfere with immunosuppression in solid-organ transplant patients [26].

Guaifenesin

Guaifenesin, an expectorant, was approved in 1989 by the FDA for OTC supply whereas prescription of ephedrine was limited in 1994. As a result, new OTC preparations were produced, combining guaifenesin and ephedrine in a 8:1 ratio, and subjects who previously took OTC ephedrine as a stimulant and switched to these new preparations were *ipso facto* consuming high doses of guaifenesin (some up to 24,000 mg/day). Thus, more than 30 cases of urolithiasis were reported in the following years [27,28].

Stones are radiolucent, but visualized on unenhanced helical CT scan, their weak density leading to frequent misdiagnosis as uric acid urolithiasis. Fourier-transform infra-red spectroscopy (FTIR) identifies a metabolite of guaifenesin in calculi, thus allowing differentiation from uric acid stones. Some stones contained in addition a minor amount of ephedrine or pseudoephedrine. Guaifenesin-induced calculi are often multiple, bilateral and recurrent, until diagnosis is made and the drug withdrawn. ESWL is variably effective, as well as alkalinization.

Ephedrine and pseudoephedrine

Ephedrine and pseudoephedrine are widely used as decongestants and bronchodilators. However, ephedrine is often used as a stimulant and ephedrine abuse has become popular due to its easy OTC availability (combined with guaifenesin) or as "herbal preparations." More than 200 kidney stones composed of ephedrine metabolites were identified in subjects who abused ephedrine, some taking more than 1000 mg/day [29].

Ephedrine stones are radiolucent but visible on CT, with a density of about 300 HU, i.e. similar to uric acid, these imaging characteristics leading to frequent diagnostic confusion with uric acid urolithiasis [30]. Stones are friable and easily fragmented by ESWL. Successful dissolution may be obtained by alkalinization with potassium citrate which enhances its tubular reabsorption [31]. Collectively, ephedrine- and guaifenesin-induced stones accounted for one-third of drug-induced stones recorded in the US [32].

Other drugs

Allopurinol used at high doses (≥600 mg/day) for the treatment of Lesch–Nyhan syndrome may induce the formation of stones made of its metabolite oxypurinol admixed with xanthine [33].

Silica-containing drugs, mainly as magnesium trisilicate, used as antacids over long periods, or as colloid silica, used as milk thickener for prevention of esophageal regurgitation in babies, may induce stones made of opaline silica [34].

Metabolically induced kidney stones

Carbonic anhydrase inhibitors and calcium-vitamin D supplements are now the leading drugs implicated in the formation of calculi resulting from metabolic induction.

Carbonic anhydrase inhibitors

Carbonic anhydrase inhibitors block the reabsorption of bicarbonate and sodium ions, and inhibit the excretion of H^+ ions, in the proximal tubule. This results in intracellular acidosis which enhances citrate reabsorption, thus inducing hypocitraturia, hypercalciuria and elevated urine pH. Such urine composition favors the precipitation of calcium phosphate crystals and formation of phosphate stones [35], mainly in the form of carbapatite [1].

Acetazolamide

Acetazolamide, used for a long time in the treatment of glaucoma and more recently epilepsy, provokes the frequent development of nephrolithiasis [35], as do its analogs methazolamide, dorzolamide, and dichlorphenamide (reviewed in [1]). Increased fluid intake is the safest preventive measure, associated with a thiazide diuretic to reduce hypercalciuria [36].

Topiramate

Topiramate, a novel neuromodulatory agent originally licensed as an antiepileptic medication and now increasingly prescribed in the treatment of a number of other neurological and psychiatric disorders, also induces the formation of calcium phosphate stones in a high proportion of long-term treated patients [37]. In 75 adult patients treated with a median daily dose of 300 mg for a median duration of 48 months, the incidence of symptomatic stones was 10.7% but CT scan detected asymptomatic stones in an additional 20% [38], whereas 13 of 23 (54%) neurologically impaired, institutionalized children on topiramate developed symptomatic stones after a mean duration of 3 years [39].

Zonisamide

Zonisamide, an antiepileptic drug used as adjunctive therapy for refractory partial seizures, is a weak inhibitor of carbonic anhydrase and accordingly induces a lower incidence of nephrolithiasis than the preceding drugs [40]. Symptomatic calculi developed in 1.4% of 1296 patients treated for up to 24 months, and CT imaging revealed an additional 2.6% asymptomatic stones [41].

Thus, the incidence of urolithiasis in adult and pediatric patients treated with topiramate or zonisamide is underappreciated when diagnosis is based only on clinical manifestations. As for acetazolamide, prevention essentially relies on high fluid intake and thiazides to reduce hypercalciuria, whereas the effectiveness of potassium citrate remains to be evaluated [36].

Of note, the ketogenic diet, prescribed for intractable epilepsy, either with or without topiramate or zonisamide, induced phosphate urolithiasis in 6.7% of treated children. Concomitant prescription of potassium citrate reduced the prevalence of stones and increased the duration free of symptomatic stones [42].

Calcium and vitamin D supplements

Calcium supplementation

Calcium supplements, especially when associated with vitamin D, may increase urinary calcium excretion and induce calcium nephrolithiasis, especially in subjects with underlying idiopathic hypercalciuria [43]. At variance with high dietary calcium, which reduces the risk of forming calcium stones, supplemental calcium increased the risk of calcium stone formation by 20% [44]. In the Women's Health Initiative (WHI) study involving 36,282 postmenopausal women randomly assigned to receive either a daily supplement with 1000 mg elemental calcium and 400 IU vitamin D3 or a placebo for 7 years, incidence of self-reported symptomatic renal calculi was 17% higher in the supplemented group, in parallel with a total calcium intake rising up to 2000 mg/day [45]. This finding suggests that dietary calcium sources are preferable to pharmacological formulations to achieve optimal calcium intake for the prevention of osteoporosis [46] and that urinary calcium output should be monitored in subjects receiving calcium-vitamin D supplements, particularly those having a history of nephrolithiasis or known hypercalciuria [1].

Vitamin D supplementation

Vitamin D supplements for the prevention or correction of vitamin D deficiency (serum concentration <30 ng/mL or <75 nmol/L) are increasingly prescribed, because a number of recent studies revealed a high prevalence of vitamin D deficiency in the general population [47]. They may induce the formation of calcium oxalate stones. However, prudent vitamin D repletion was not associated with increased urinary calcium excretion in healthy postmenopausal women [48], nor in institutionalized elderly [49] or even in patients with a history of calcium stones [50]. Therefore, the rising prevalence of papillary calcium oxalate calculi we observed over recent years in young adults and menopausal women [51] suggests the possible role of uncontrolled, excessive supplementation with vitamin D and/or calcium.

Other drugs

Furosemide therapy in preterm neonates may induce bilateral calcium calculi (and nephrocalcinosis) by rising urinary calcium concentration, unless combined with a thiazide diuretic [52]. Vitamin C overdosing (2 g/day or more) may increase oxaluria and the risk of formation of calcium oxalate stones [53]. Uricosurics and other drugs which inhibit net uric acid tubular reabsorption may induce uric acid nephrolithiasis [1]. Laxative abuse may induce the formation of radiolucent ammonium urate stones in weakly acidic urine [54].

Management of the patient with drug-induced nephrolithiasis

Diagnosis of drug-induced nephrolithiasis

Diagnosing the iatrogenic origin of kidney stones and identifying the offending drug are essential for an adequate therapeutic strategy. Diagnosis of drug-induced stones relies on clinical context, imaging characteristics, and stone analysis.

Carefully checking the medical history, co-morbidities, and current therapy is essential in every stone-forming patient and may immediately identify the diagnosis. For instance, infection with HIV implies the probable use of antiretroviral agents such as atazanavir and/or sulfadiazine. Recent or past bacterial infection, especially in children, suggests the possible implication of antibacterial agents such as ceftriaxone. Past or current treatment with acetazolamide or its analogs, topiramate or zonisamide, should be checked in patients suffering from glaucoma, epilepsy, migraines or neuropsychiatric diseases. Abuse of OTC guaifenesin and/or ephedrine preparations may be more difficult to recognize.

All drug-containing stones are radiolucent on conventional X-ray and need to be differentiated from uric acid, cystine, dihydroxyadenine or xanthine stones. Non-contrast helical CT is of major help as it visualizes all radiolucent stones, except those made of indinavir. In fact, analysis of stones by physical methods, such as X-ray diffraction or FTIR, which recognize all organic compounds, constitutes the most powerful, rapid, and cheap method allowing indisputable identification of drug-containing calculi based on the specific spectra of drugs and metabolites. Metabolically induced calculi do not differ in morphology and molecular composition from usual stones, so that the diagnosis is made by knowledge of the co-morbidities and nature of drugs taken by the patient, and also by the composition of stones, whether calcium phosphate, calcium oxalate or uric acid. When no stone is available for analysis or in patients presenting with acute kidney injury, a search for crystalluria and identification of crystals by morphology and FTIR may be highly contributory [1].

Therapeutic management

Medical management is often successful in patients with drug-induced nephrolithiasis. Solubilization of stones or obstructive crystalluria may be achieved by active urine dilution and/or adjustment of urine pH according to the specific pH dependence of the drug. Most drug-induced stones are easily fragmented by ESWL, with the exception of protease inhibitors. In cases of acute obstruction by heavy crystalluria, insertion of a ureteral stent is often efficient, whereas obstructive calculi will be extracted by ureteroscopy.

In any case, prevention of renal complications induced by drugs relies on adequate identification, taking into account the presence of risk factors, active hydration, and adaptation of urine pH whenever possible.

Key points

- Drug-induced kidney stones currently represent nearly 1% of all kidney stones.
- Atazanavir and sulfadiazine as prescription drugs and guaifenesin and ephedrine/pseudoephedrine OTC preparations are now the drugs most frequently involved in the formation of drug-containing stones, which are all radiolucent and variably visible on CT scan.
- Carbonic anhydrase inhibitors such as acetazolamide, topiramate and zonisamide, and calcium-vitamin D supplements, due to their metabolic effects, may induce respectively calcium phosphate and calcium oxalate stones, similar in composition to common stones, thus entailing the risk of misdiagnosis.
- Stone analysis by means of X-ray diffraction or infra-red spectroscopy reliably identifies drug-containing stones by their specific spectra. Etiological diagnosis of metabolically induced stones is oriented by medical history, co-morbidities, and composition of stones. Examination of urine for crystalluria is helpful in all cases.
- Close surveillance of patients on long-term treatment with potentially lithogenic drugs will allow early detection and management of drug-induced nephrolithiasis.

References

1. Daudon M, Jungers P. Drug-induced renal calculi: epidemiology, prevention and management. Drugs 2004; 64: 245–75.
2. Daudon M, Bader CA. Jungers P. Urinary calculi: review of classification methods and correlations with etiology. Scanning Microsc 1993; 7: 1081–106.
3. Ettinger B, Oldroyd NO, Sorgel F. Triamterene nephrolithiasis. JAMA 1980; 244: 2443–5.
4. Pokorná J, Machala L, Řezáčová P, Konvalinka J. Current and novel inhibitors of HIV protease. Viruses 2009; 1: 1209–39.
5. Daudon M, Estépa L, Viard JP, Joly D, Jungers P. Urinary stones in HIV-1-positive patients treated with indinavir. Lancet 1997; 349: 1294–5.
6. Kopp JB, Miller KD, Mican JA, et al. Crystalluria and urinary tract abnormalities associated with indinavir. Ann Intern Med 1997; 127: 119–25.
7. Martinez E, Leguizamon M, Mallolas J, et al. Influence of environmental temperature on incidence of indinavir-related nephrolithiasis. Clin infect Dis 1999; 29: 422–5.
8. Tashima KT, Horowitz J, Rosen S. Indinavir nephropathy. N Engl J Med 1997; 336: 138–40.

9. Schwartz BF, Schenkman N, Armenakas NA, et al. Imaging characteristics of indinavir calculi. J Urol 1999; 161: 1085–7.
10. Chang HR, Pella PM. Atazanavir urolithiasis. N Engl J Med 2006; 355: 2158–9.
11. Rho M, Perazella MA. Nephrotoxicity associated with antiretroviral therapy in HIV-infected patients. Curr Drug Saf 2007; 2: 147–54.
12. Rockwood N, Mandalia S, Bower M, Gazzard B, Nelson M. Ritonavir-boosted atazanavir exposure is associated with an increased rate of renal stones compared with efavirenz, ritonavir-boosted lopinavir and ritonavir-boosted darunavir. AIDS 2011; 25: 1671–3.
13. Hamada Y, Nishijima T, Watanabe K, et al. High incidence of renal stones in HIV-infected patients on ritonavir-boosted atazanavir than in those on other protease inhibitors-containing antiretroviral therapy Clin Infect Dis 2012; 55: 1262–9.
14. Couzigou C, Daudon M, Meynard JL, et al. Urolithiasis in HIV-positive patients treated with atazanavir. Clin Infect Dis 2007; 45: e105–8.
15. Izzedine H, M'Rad M B, Bardier A, Daudon M, Salmon D. Atazanavir crystal nephropathy. AIDS 2007; 21: 2357–8.
16. Engeler DS, John H, Rentsch KM, et al. Nelfinavir urinary stones. J Urol 2002; 167: 1384–5.
17. Cicconi P, Bongiovanni M, Melzi S, Tordato F, d'Arminio Monforte A, Bini T. Nephrolithiasis and hydronephrosis in an HIV-infected man receiving tenofovir. Int J Antimicrob Agents 2004; 24: 284–5.
18. Albala DM, Prien Jr EL, Galal HA. Urolithiasis as a hazard of sulfonamide therapy. J Endourol 1994; 8: 401–3.
19. Erturk E, Casemento JB, Guertin KR, et al. Bilateral acetyl-sulfapyridine nephrolithiasis associated with chronic sulfasalazine therapy. J Urol 1994; 151: 1605–6.
20. Chopra N, Fine PL, Price B, et al. Bilateral hydronephrosis from ciprofloxacin induced crystalluria and stone formation. J Urol 2000; 164: 438.
21. Cochat P, Cochat N, Jouvenet M, et al. Ceftriaxone-associated nephrolithiasis. Nephrol Dial Transplant 1990; 5: 974–6.
22. Mohkam M, Karimi A, Gharib A, et al. Ceftriaxone associated nephrolithiasis: a prospective study in 284 children. Pediatr Nephrol 2007; 22: 690–4.
23. Avci Z, Koktener A, Uras N, et al. Nephrolithiasis associated with ceftriaxone therapy: a prospective study in 51 children. Arch Dis Child 2004; 89: 1069–72.
24. Kimata T, Kaneko K, Takahashi M, Hirabayashi M, Shimo T, Kino M. Increased urinary calcium excretion caused by ceftriaxone: possible association with urolithiasis. Pediatr Nephrol 2012; 27: 605–9.
25. Izzedine H, Valantin MA, Daudon M, Ait Mohand H, Caby F, Katlama C. Efavirenz urolithiasis. AIDS 2007; 21: 1992.
26. Gabardi S, Carter D, Martin S, Roberts K. Recommendations for the proper use of nonprescription cough suppressants and expectorants in solid-organ transplant recipients. Prog Transplant 2011; 21: 6–13.
27. Pickens CL, Milliron AR, Fussner AL, et al. Abuse of guaifenesin-containing medications generates an excess of a carboxylate salt of beta- (2-methoxyphenoxy)-lactic acid, a guaifenesin metabolite, and results in urolithiasis. Urology 1999; 54: 23–7.
28. Assimos DG, Langenstroer P, Leinbach RF, et al. Guaifenesin- and ephedrine-induced stones. J Endourol 1999; 13: 665–7.
29. Powell T, Hsu FF, Turk J, et al. Ma-Huang strikes again: ephedrine nephrolithiasis. Am J Kidney Dis 1998; 32: 153–9.

30. Song GY, Lockhart ME, Smith JK, Burns JR, Kenney PJ. Pseudoephedrine and guaifenesin urolithiasis: widening the differential diagnosis of radiolucent calculi on abdominal radiograph. Abdom Imaging 2005; 30: 644–6.
31. Hoffman N, McGee SM, Hulbert JC. Resolution of ephedrine stones with dissolution therapy. Urology 2003; 61: 1035.
32. Bennett S, Hoffman N, Monga M. Ephedrine- and guaifenesin-induced nephrolithiasis. J Altern Complement Med 2004; 10: 967–9.
33. Kranen S, Keough D, Gordon RB, et al. Xanthine-containing calculi during allopurinol therapy. J Urol 1985; 133: 658–9.
34. Levison DA, Crocker PR, Banim S, et al. Silica urinary bladder. Lancet 1982; I (8274): 704–5.
35. Ahlstrand C, Tiselius HG. Urine composition and stone formation during treatment with acetazolamide. Scand J Urol Nephrol 1987; 21: 225–8.
36. Goldfarb DS. A woman with recurrent calcium phosphate kidney stones. Clin J Am Soc Nephrol 2012; 7: 1172–8.
37. Kuo RL, Moran ME, Kim DH, Abrahams HM, White MD, Lingeman JE. Topiramate-induced nephrolithiasis. J Endourol 2002; 16: 229–31.
38. Maalouf NM, Langston JP, van Ness PC, Moe OW, Sakhaee K. Nephrolithiasis in topiramate users. Urol Res 2011; 39: 303–7.
39. Goyal M, Grossberg RI, O'Riordan MA, Davis ID. Urolithiasis with topiramate in nonambulatory children and young adults. Pediatr Neurol 2009; 40: 289–94.
40. Zaccara G, Tramacere L, Cincotta M. Drug safety evaluation of zonisamide for the treatment of epilepsy. Expert Opin Drug Saf 2011; 10: 623–31.
41. Wroe S. Zonisamide and renal calculi in patients with epilepsy: how big an issue? Curr Med Res Opin 2007; 23: 1765–73.
42. Sampath A, Kossoff EH, Furth SL, Pyzik PL, Vining EP. Kidney stones and the ketogenic diet: risk factors and prevention. J Child Neurol 2007; 22: 375–8.
43. Pak CYC. Nephrolithiasis from calcium supplementation. J Urol 1987; 137: 1212–13.
44. Curhan GC, Willett WC, Speizer FE, Spiegelman D, Stampfer MJ. Comparison of dietary calcium with supplemental calcium and other nutrients as factors affecting the risk for kidney stones in women. Ann Intern Med 1997; 126: 497–504.
45. Wallace RB, Wactawski-Wende J, O'Sullivan MJ, et al. Urinary tract stone occurrence in the Women's Health Initiative (WHI) randomized clinical trial of calcium and vitamin D supplements. Am J Clin Nutr 2011; 94: 270–7.
46. Favus MJ. The risk of kidney stone formation: the form of calcium matters. Am J Clin Nutr 2011; 94: 5–6.
47. Visser M, Deeg DJ, Puts MT, Seidell JC, Lips P. Low serum concentrations of 25-hydroxyvitamin D in older persons and the risk of nursing home admission. Am J Clin Nutr 2006; 84: 616–22.
48. Penniston KL, Jones AN, Nakada SY, Hansen KE. Vitamin D repletion does not alter urinary calcium excretion in healthy postmenopausal women. BJU Int 2009; 104: 1512–16.
49. Demontiero O, Herrmann M, Duque G. Supplementation with vitamin D and calcium in long-term care residents. J Am Med Dir Assoc 2011; 12: 190–4.
50. Leaf DE, Korets R, Taylor EN, et al. Effect of vitamin D repletion on urinary calcium excretion among kidney stone formers. Clin J Am Soc Nephrol 2012; 7: 829–34.

51. Daudon M, Traxer O, Williams JC, Bazin DC. Randall's plaques. In: Rao PN, Preminger GM, Kavanagh JP, eds. *Urinary Tract Stone Disease*. London: Springer, 2011, pp.103–12.
52. Noe HN, Bryant JF, Roy III S, et al. Urolithiasis in pre-term neonates associated with furosemide therapy. J Urol 1984; 132: 93–4.
53. Traxer O, Huet B, Poindexter J, et al. Effect of ascorbic acid consumption on urinary stone risk factors. J Urol 2003; 170: 397–401.
54. Dick WH, Lingeman JE, Preminger GM, et al. Laxative abuse as a cause for ammonium urate renal calculi. J Urol 1990; 143: 244–7.

CHAPTER 11

Management of Renal Colic and Medical Expulsive Therapy

Michael S. Borofsky and Ojas Shah
New York University Langone Medical Center, New York, NY, USA

Do's and don'ts box

Do:

- consider low-dose CT, renal ultrasound and/or KUB for patients with history of nephrolithiasis
- use NSAIDs and opioids for symptomatic relief of renal colic
- prescribe α-blockers for use as medical expulsive therapy in the case of ureteral stone disease and to aid in pain management
- prescribe α-blockers for ureteral stent colic.

Don't:

- assume that all cases of renal colic arise from urinary stone disease
- always order CT scans for all patients with flank pain
- use NSAIDs for patients with history of chronic kidney disease or significant peptic ulcer disease
- treat ureteral obstruction with forced saline hydration.

Introduction

Patients suffering from renal colic can present in a variety of ways. While there is no formal medical definition of this term, it is generally used to describe an acute-onset, severe flank pain, often radiating to the ipsilateral groin and commonly associated with nausea and vomiting. Appropriately diagnosing and treating this painful condition can be challenging. In this chapter we will review the existing medical literature regarding renal colic and explore the most recent advances in diagnostic and medical treatment options for this disease.

A suggested management algorithm for patients with renal colic is shown in Figure 11.1.

Urinary Stones: Medical and Surgical Management, First Edition. Edited by Michael Grasso and David S. Goldfarb.

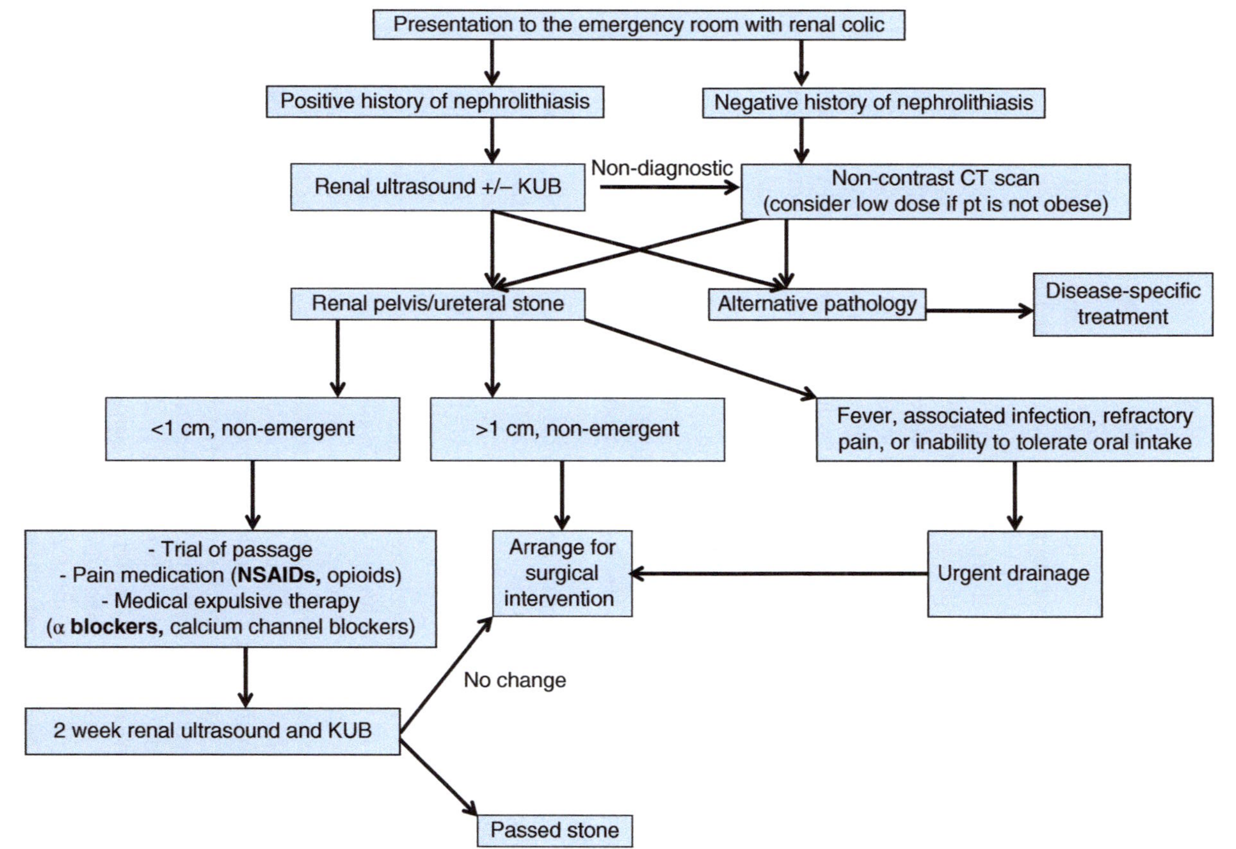

Figure 11.1 Suggested management algorithm for patient with renal colic.

Etiology

On a basic level, renal colic can be conceptualized as the end-result of ureteral obstruction causing stress on the kidney, ultimately leading to pain; however, the true pathophysiology of this disease is much more complex. The majority of the pain receptors in the upper urinary tract are located submucosally in the renal pelvis, calyces, capsule, and upper ureter [1]. Downstream obstruction causes back-up of urine and acute dilation of the collecting system, in turn leading to submucosal stretch and the activation of nociceptive nerve fibers. These nerve fibers then transmit afferent impulses to the T11–L1 spinal cord which are perceived as pain at that corresponding level [2].

Pain is propagated and exacerbated by a variety of mechanisms. The presence of ureteral obstruction causes ureteral hyperperistalsis and ultimately spasm which can lead to lactic acid build-up and initiation of an inflammatory cascade with subsequent irritation of slow type Aδ and fast type C sensory fibers [2,3]. A build-up in intrarenal pressure also mediates the release of prostaglandin E2 which in turn potentiates ureteral smooth muscle spasm [4]. Prostaglandin E2 also triggers vasodilation of the afferent arterioles, promoting a diuresis which further increases renal pelvic pressure and likely exacerbates the pain [5]. Finally, activation of pain receptors can occur in any organ that shares innervation with the kidney, including the organs of the gastrointestinal tract, thus explaining the frequent association of nausea and vomiting with renal colic [6].

The pathophysiology of ureteral obstruction can be broken down into several phases. In the case of unilateral ureteral obstruction, afferent arteriolar vasodilation leads to a progressive rise in renal blood flow and ureteral pressure for approximately 1–1.5 h. This time period is known as phase one. Phase two is marked by efferent arteriolar vasoconstriction that causes a decrease in renal blood flow. However, ureteral pressure continues to increase for up to 5 h. In phase three, the afferent arterioles begin to constrict, further decreasing renal blood flow and ureteral pressure as well [7,8,9]. Symptoms of renal colic appear to coincide with these physiological changes and classically are marked by three distinct phases as well. From the initiation of ureteral obstruction, pain waxes and wanes but progressively builds until reaching a maximum at 1–2 h. At this point the patient often enters the "constant phase" whereby pain is continuous and severe. This is frequently the point at which the patient is seen and treated in the emergency room, otherwise pain is likely to remit several hours later through physiological means of decreased ureteral/renal capsule distension or relief of obstruction [1]. On numerous occasions, episodes of renal colic may recur, likely owing to the fact that stones and other disease processes can be partially or intermittently obstructing, triggering episodes each time obstruction occurs.

While ureteral obstruction by stones is the most common cause of renal colic, other urological pathologies can present in a similar fashion

Table 11.1 Causes of renal colic

Renal	Ureteral	Extrinsic
Calculus	Calculi	Aneurysm
Staghorn calculus	Stricture	Retroperitoneal fibrosis
Tumor	Ureterocele	Pelvic lipomatosis
Cyst	Tumor	Adnexal mass
Infection	Fibroepithelial polyp	Endometriosis
Abscess	Retrocaval ureter	Pregnancy
Ureteropelvic junction obstruction	Foreign body (stent)	Lymphadenopathy
Calyceal diverticulum	Vesicoureteral reflux	Tumors
Papillary necrosis		
Renal vein thrombosis		
Infarction		

(Table 11.1). It should be noted that many of these pathologies occur gradually over time and as such may not lead to the acute rise in intrarenal pressure that triggers episodes of renal colic. While costovertebral angle tenderness and flank pain are hallmarks of these alternative conditions, the degree of pain is generally less than that seen for renal colic due to acute ureteral obstruction. Many of these patients will ultimately be diagnosed with non-obstructive intrarenal stones or papillary tip calcifications and rarely may be diagnosed with loin pain hematuria syndrome if noted to have hematuria associated with these episodes.

Epidemiology

Previous estimates show that nearly 1.2 million people suffer from episodes of renal colic each year and it is the primary diagnosis for approximately 1% of all hospital admissions [10]. Moreover, rates for urolithiasis are on the rise with recent studies estimating that the prevalence of the disease has nearly doubled over the past 15 years, with approximately 1 in 11 people reporting at least one previous episode [11].

Imaging

Diagnostic imaging is a critical step in the work-up of renal colic There are numerous imaging modalities available to the clinician, including plain abdominal X-ray of the kidneys, ureters, and bladder (KUB), intravenous urogram (IVU), renal ultrasound, computed tomography (CT) scans, and magnetic resonance imaging (MRI).

Non-contrast helical CT (NCCT) is the gold standard first-line imaging test for the patient with newly diagnosed, acute renal colic. NCCT has a sensitivity and specificity between 94% and 100% for identifying renal and ureteral stones and offers unique information regarding stone size, location, and composition that can be useful in guiding treatment recommendations [12,13]. Additionally, in the event that stones are not the source of pain, the NCCT offers detailed anatomical information that may lead to an alternative diagnosis. In a series of nearly 800 CT scans ordered for evaluation of renal colic, Nadeem et al. found a positive yield of 64% for urolithiasis, 15% for incidental/alternative findings, and 21% negative studies [14].

Unfortunately, the benefits of CT must be measured against the associated ionizing radiation and potential for carcinogenesis. While the overall risk of cancer is estimated to be low, patients with urolithiasis are at risk of undergoing numerous CT scans over their lifetime. Ferrandino et al. found that nearly 20% of patients received greater than 50 mSv of radiation, the recommended yearly dose limit, within 1 year following an acute stone-related episode [15]. One potential improvement in this regard is the introduction of low-dose CT that has comparable sensitivities and specificities to traditional CT with a 50–75% reduction in radiation exposure [16,17]. Performance parameters for this diagnostic tool may be lower among obese patients and those with small stones <4 mm in size [18].

Given growing concerns regarding the overuse of CT, numerous algorithms have been formulated to ideally utilize imaging modalities in the patient with acute renal colic. The majority of such recommendations involve more frequent use of KUB, renal ultrasound and occasionally both. Catalano et al. compared combination KUB and renal ultrasound to CT and demonstrated a 77% versus 93% sensitivity and 93% versus 96% specificity, each favoring CT [19]. Of note, 12.5% of the patients receiving KUB and renal ultrasound had false-negative results. MRI is another imaging test of potential utility, specifically the MR urogram (MRU). While this test eliminates the exposure to ionizing radiation, stones are not readily identifiable and must be inferred by the appearance of a filling defect and other secondary signs such as hydroureteronephrosis. One particular instance where this test may be useful is in the case of pregnancy, though White et al. found that the positive predictive value of renal ultrasound with MRU was 80% compared to 77% with renal ultrasound alone, bringing the usefulness of this test into question [20].

Pain management

Pain control is the critical first step in treating renal colic and the degree of pain relief is often the determining factor in deciding how to proceed. Historically, opioids and non-steroidal anti-inflammatory drugs (NSAIDs) have been recommended as first-line treatment options; however, several other classes of medications have been investigated as well [21].

Non-steroidal anti-inflammatory drugs versus narcotic analgesics

Non-steroidal anti-inflammatory drugs have a direct effect on pain from renal colic via inhibition of prostaglandin synthesis. Prostaglandin inhibition prevents renal arterial vasodilation which in turn prevents increased renal blood flow and a rise in collecting system pressure typically seen with obstruction. Furthermore, prostaglandin inhibition prevents ureteral smooth muscle spasm [22]. Prior to administration, the provider must first ensure that the patient does not have a significant history of peptic ulcer disease or baseline renal insufficiency, which could be exacerbated by the reduction in renal blood flow. Fifty mL/min has been suggested as the minimum creatinine clearance level, below which patients should avoid NSAIDs [23]. It remains unclear, however, whether these restrictions should be applied to patients with acute reductions in renal function secondary to obstruction compared to patients with baseline poor function.

Another scenario where NSAIDs should be avoided is in patients seeking shock wave lithotripsy for treatment of their stones as the platelet-inhibiting effect of NSAIDS may increase the risk of postprocedural bleeding. Opioids, on the other hand, do not have the potential to lower glomerular filtration rate like NSAIDs and do not increase the risk of bleeding and are thus preferred in the presence of renal insufficiency. Opioids work to treat pain via a complex array of interactions with neuronal pathways and other elements of the central nervous system. While they too have been shown to effectively relieve pain from renal colic, they carry the risk of numerous adverse effects not seen with NSAIDs, including constipation, urinary retention, respiratory depression, sedation, and potential for addiction [24].

Numerous studies have compared NSAIDs to narcotics for treatment of renal colic. A 2004 Cochrane review addressing this subject found that patients using narcotics were more likely to require additional analgesia at earlier times in greater doses [21]. These findings prompted the European Association of Urology to recommend NSAIDs as the first drug of choice for acute renal colic, with opioids generally recommended as an adjunct or alternative medication in the event of renal insufficiency [25]. NSAIDs have also been shown to reduce recurrent pain episodes in the event of ureteral stones expected to pass spontaneously [25]. Laerum et al. found that patients treated with diclofenac after being seen in the emergency room (ER) with renal colic had readmission rates of 10% compared to 67% when treated with placebo [26].

While previous studies have not found any significant efficacy differences between types of NSAIDs [25], general recommendations are to start with a dose of intravenous medication due to more rapid onset of pain relief. Currently ketorolac is the only parenteral NSAID available in North America [27].

Once the acute episode is resolved, treatment should continue with one of the less potent NSAIDs such as ibuprofen or diclofenac. Naproxen and ketorolac are more potent and thus may be reserved for patients with refractory pain. Indometacin is not recommended as a first-line agent given concern for central nervous system side-effects, especially in the elderly [27].

Desmopressin

Desmopressin has also been investigated for use in renal colic because of its ability to cause vasoconstriction of the afferent arteriole and potentially reduce renal pelvic pressure seen in obstruction [27]. The clinical benefit of desmopressin is its rapid onset of action via intranasal application; however, clinical results to date have been discordant. Published studies have mainly been small case series and some have demonstrated improved pain relief when administered along with NSAIDs [28] with others showing no difference at all [29].

α-Blockers and calcium channel blockers

α-Blockers and calcium channel blockers (CCBs) have been studied as pain relievers for renal colic given their ability to promote smooth muscle relaxation in the ureter. α-Adrenergic receptors are abundant in the ureter and when activated lead to a positive chronotropic and inotropic effect on the ureter. These mechanisms can be blocked by the administration of an α-blocker such as tamsulosin [30], which has been found to decrease both the overall degree and number of recurrent episodes of colic [31,32].

Calcium channel blockers such as nifedipine interfere with calcium signaling and cause a subsequent decrease in smooth muscle excitation, thereby diminishing ureteral smooth muscle spasm. They have also been associated with decreased analgesia requirements in patients passing ureteral stones [33].

Stent colic

Many of the same medications effective for renal colic are used for stent colic. The etiology of stent colic is proposed to be similar to that of a ureteral stone in the sense that a foreign body within the ureter leads to ureteral smooth muscle spasm [34]. Alternative theories that have been proposed include reflux of urine to the kidney leading to a rise in renal pelvic pressure [35] as well as bladder neck and trigone irritation from the distal curl [36].

α-Blockers have been studied as a potential treatment for stent-related symptoms given their ability to promote smooth muscle relaxation. Two recent meta-analyses reported favorable outcomes in terms of pain relief when α-blockers were used for patients with indwelling stents. Lamb et al. reviewed five studies with a total of 461 patients, all of which showed decreased pain scores with the use of α-blockers. The overall relative risk of pain when using an α-blockers compared to control was 0.6 [34]. A similar meta-analysis by Yakoubi et al. including 12 studies and 946 patients also found improvements in pain when α-blockers were used; however, there was no difference in terms of lost work-hours secondary to symptoms [37].

Several other novel therapies have been used to alleviate stent-related discomfort, including botox injections at the ureteral orifices [38] and intravesically administered medications such as oxybutynin, ketorolac, and lidocaine [39].

Medical expulsive therapy

The decision to observe versus intervene in the case of an obstructing ureteral stone is a commonly encountered clinical challenge. Observation avoids the need for anesthesia, trained subspecialists, and the associated risks and costs of the procedures itself. However, watchful waiting is not definitive and may be associated with recurrent pain, decreased quality of life, risks to renal function, and lost work productivity. Medical expulsive therapy (MET) bridges the gap between these two treatment options by using medications to expedite stone passage.

An understanding of ureteral physiology is necessary to comprehend how a pharmacological agent might be able to facilitate stone passage. Ureteral peristalsis, considered to be a promoter of stone passage, becomes disorganized and unco-ordinated in the case of acute obstruction. Furthermore, the stone induces ureteral spasm and edema, further inhibiting the ability of the stone to pass spontaneously [40]. Ideal therapy to facilitate stone passage would thus decrease ureteral spasm, allow for co-ordinated ureteral peristalsis and increase pressure proximal to the point of obstruction.

One commonly administered therapy for this purpose is the use of intense hydration and diuretics. The theoretical, though incorrect, premise for this treatment is that increased urine production increases pressure build-up proximal to the obstructing stone; however, in actuality the obstructed kidney has minimal to no GFR and is thus unable to contribute to increased urine production. As a result, there is little to no effect on the involved kidney. Prior comparisons between forced hydration and maintenance fluids found no differences with regard to pain perception, narcotic use, or stone passage rates [41] and a recent Cochrane review on the subject also failed to support this theory [42].

The two pharmacological agents most studied for this purpose are CCBs and α-blockers [40]. While both reduce the degree of ureteral contraction, it has been suggested that CCBs inhibit the force of ureteral peristalsis to a greater degree than α-blockers [43]. The use of CCBs and α-blockers for MET has been the subject of several randomized controlled trials. Three meta-analyses to date have investigated the efficacy of MET, all concluding that MET is associated with increased likelihood of stone passage. Use of CCBs led to a 1.5 times greater likelihood of spontaneous stone passage in all studies compared to α-blockers which were associated with a 1.5–1.6 times likelihood of spontaneous passage [44,45,46]. MET was also associated with decreased analgesia requirements and episodes of recurrent renal colic in a majority of studies [46].

Several studies have directly compared these medications to one another in terms of their ability to facilitate stone passage. Among 210 patients with ureteral stones greater than 4mm, Dellabella et al. found a higher spontaneous expulsion rate in those taking tamsulosin compared to those taking nifedipine (97% versus 77%). Furthermore, there was a shorter time to passage amongst the tamsulosin group (72 versus 120 hours). In a similar study by Porpiglia et al., tamsulosin was associated with an 85% success rate compared to 80% in the nifedipine group with a mean time to passage of 7.7 versus 9.3 days [47].

In 2007, a joint panel representing members from the American Urological Association and European Association of Urology developed a combined set of guidelines for urolithiasis based on a systemic review of available studies. Based on their review, the use of CCBs for MET was associated with a 9% increased likelihood of spontaneous stone passage, which was not statistically significant. Conversely, use of α-blockers was associated with a 29% increased likelihood of stone passage, which was significant. As a result, they concluded that α-blockers were the preferred agent for use in MET [48]. Despite their conclusions, the results of the aforementioned meta-analyses showed more comparable success rates, reinforcing the need for a large-scale, prospectively controlled study to determine the optimal choice of medication for MET [44,45,46].

Several other pharmacological agents have been investigated for the purpose of MET though they are far less studied than CCBs or α-blockers. Hamidi et al. investigated the use of nitrates (isosorbide-SR), given the smooth muscle-relaxing properties of this agent, and found no difference in likelihood of stone passage [49]. Corticosteroids have also been studied based on the premise that they might decrease ureteral edema and thus facilitate spontaneous passage. When used in combination with α-blockers, Dellabella et al. demonstrated a decreased time to stone passage but no overall difference in rate of expulsion [50]. Another study by Porpiglia et al. demonstrated that steroids only facilitated stone passage when used in combination with α-blockers [51].

Despite encouraging evidence supporting MET, studies have shown that it is vastly underutilized in clinical practice. National trends between the years 2000 and 2006 showed a steady increase in the utilization of MET; however, even during the peak year for usage, α-blockers or CCBs were only prescribed to 3.9% of patients visiting the emergency department with urinary stone disease [52]. Targeted educational efforts directed towards emergency room physicians are one successful way of improving utilization of MET. Brede et al. found a four-fold increase in the use of α-blockers after such educational efforts were made [53]. Another potentially useful tool would be establishing guidelines for how to treat patients with renal colic as previous studies estimate that nearly 90% of US emergency rooms lack them. Future efforts must ensure that urologists are not the only members of the medical community with a knowledgeable understanding of this common and treatable problem.

Key points

- Pain control and diagnostic imaging should be the first steps in the work-up of renal colic.
- Non-contrast CT is the gold standard in diagnostic imaging but alternative imaging modalities such as low-dose CT, renal ultrasound, and KUB can be diagnostic with less risk of ionizing radiation.
- NSAIDs and opioids are the most effective medications for pain relief secondary to renal colic.
- α-Blockers are effective at decreasing stent colic and may aid in pain management of ureteral stones.
- α-Blockers and calcium channel blockers both appear to increase the rate of spontaneous ureteral stone passage and should be considered for use as medical expulsive therapy

References

1. Smith AD. *Smith's Textbook of Endourology*, 3rd edn. Chichester: Wiley, 2012.
2. Shokeir AA. Renal colic: new concepts related to pathophysiology, diagnosis and treatment. Curr Opin Urol 2002; 12(4): 263–9.
3. Travaglini F, Bartoletti R, Gacci M, Rizzo M. Pathophysiology of reno-ureteral colic. Urol Int 2004; 72(Suppl 1): 20–3.
4. Morrison AR. Prostaglandins and the kidney. Am J Med 1980; 69(2): 171–3.
5. Moody TE, Vaughn ED Jr, Gillenwater JY. Relationship between renal blood flow and ureteral pressure during 18 hours of total unilateral uretheral occlusion. Implications for changing sites of increased renal resistance. Invest Urol 1975; 13(3): 246–51.
6. Shokeir AA. Renal colic: pathophysiology, diagnosis and treatment. Eur Urol 2001; 39(3): 241–9.
7. Vaughan ED Jr, Shenasky JH 2nd, Gillenwater JY. Mechanism of acute hemodynamic response to ureteral occlusion. Invest Urol 1971; 9(2): 109–18.
8. Vaughan ED Jr, Sorenson EJ, Gillenwater JY. The renal hemodynamic response to chronic unilateral complete ureteral occlusion. Invest Urol 1970; 8(1): 78–90.
9. Harris RH, Yarger WE. Renal function after release of unilateral ureteral obstruction in rats. Am J Physiol 1974; 227(4): 806–15.
10. Phillips E, Kieley S, Johnson EB, Monga M. Emergency room management of ureteral calculi: current practices. J Endourol 2009; 23(6): 1021–4.
11. Scales CD Jr, Smith AC, Hanley JM, Saigal CS. Prevalence of kidney stones in the United States. Eur Urol 2012; 62(1): 160–5.
12. Miller OF, Rineer SK, Reichard SR, et al. Prospective comparison of unenhanced spiral computed tomography and intravenous urogram in the evaluation of acute flank pain. Urology 1998; 52(6): 982–7.
13. Vieweg J, Teh C, Freed K, et al. Unenhanced helical computerized tomography for the evaluation of patients with acute flank pain. J Urol 1998; 160(3 Pt 1): 679–84.
14. Nadeem M, Ather MH, Jamshaid A, Zaigham S, Mirza R, Salam B. Rationale use of unenhanced multi-detector CT (CT KUB) in evaluation of suspected renal colic. Int J Surg 2012; 10(10): 634–7.

15. Ferrandino MN, Bagrodia A, Pierre SA, et al. Radiation exposure in the acute and short-term management of urolithiasis at 2 academic centers. J Urol 2009; 181(2): 668–72; discussion 673.
16. Kim BS, Hwang IK, Choi YW, et al. Low-dose and standard-dose unenhanced helical computed tomography for the assessment of acute renal colic: prospective comparative study. Acta Radiol 2005; 46(7): 756–63.
17. Ciaschini MW, Remer EM, Baker ME, Lieber M, Herts BR. Urinary calculi: radiation dose reduction of 50% and 75% at CT – effect on sensitivity. Radiology 2009; 251(1): 105–11.
18. Mancini JG, Ferrandino MN. The impact of new methods of imaging on radiation dosage delivered to patients. Curr Opin Urol 2010; 20(2): 163–8.
19. Catalano O, Nunziata A, Altei F, Siani A. Suspected ureteral colic: primary helical CT versus selective helical CT after unenhanced radiography and sonography. Am J Roentgenol 2002; 178(2): 379–87.
20. White WM, Johnson EB, Zite NB, et al. Predictive value of current imaging modalities for the detection of urolithiasis during pregnancy: a multi-center, longitudinal study. J Urol 2013; 189(3): 931–4.
21. Holdgate A, Pollock T. Systematic review of the relative efficacy of non-steroidal anti-inflammatory drugs and opioids in the treatment of acute renal colic. BMJ 2004; 328(7453): 1401.
22. Perlmutter A, Miller L, Trimble LA, Marion DN, Vaughan ED Jr, Felsen D. Toradol, an NSAID used for renal colic, decreases renal perfusion and ureteral pressure in a canine model of unilateral ureteral obstruction. J Urol 1993; 149(4): 926–30.
23. Barkin RL, Beckerman M, Blum SL, Clark FM, Koh EK, Wu DS. Should nonsteroidal anti-inflammatory drugs (NSAIDs) be prescribed to the older adult? Drugs Aging 2010; 27(10): 775–89.
24. Lasoye TA, Sedgwick PM, Patel N, Skinner C, Nayeem N. Management of acute renal colic in the UK: a questionnaire survey. BMC Emerg Med 2004; 4(1): 5.
25. Turk CKT, Petrik A, Sarica K, Straub M, Seitz C. Guidelines of urolithiasis. Uroweb 2013. Available at: www.uroweb.org/guidelines/online-guidelines/
26. Laerum E, Ommundsen OE, Gronseth JE, Christiansen A, Fagertun HE. Oral diclofenac in the prophylactic treatment of recurrent renal colic. A double-blind comparison with placebo. Eur Urol 1995; 28(2): 108–11.
27. Welk BK, Teichman JM. Pharmacological management of renal colic in the older patient. Drugs Aging 2007; 24(11): 891–900.
28. Roshani A, Falahatkar S, Khosropanah I, et al. Assessment of clinical efficacy of intranasal desmopressin spray and diclofenac sodium suppository in treatment of renal colic versus diclofenac sodium alone. Urology 2010; 75(3): 540–2.
29. Kumar S, Behera NC, Sarkar D, Prasad S, Mandal AK, Singh SK. A comparative assessment of the clinical efficacy of intranasal desmopressin spray and diclofenac in the treatment of renal colic. Urol Res 2011; 39(5): 397–400.
30. Richardson CD, Donatucci CF, Page SO, Wilson KH, Schwinn DA. Pharmacology of tamsulosin: saturation-binding isotherms and competition analysis using cloned alpha 1-adrenergic receptor subtypes. Prostate 1997; 33(1): 55–9.
31. Yencilek F, Erturhan S, Canguven O, Koyuncu H, Erol B, Sarica K. Does tamsulosin change the management of proximally located ureteral stones? Urol Res 2010; 38(3): 195–9.
32. Resim S, Ekerbicer H, Ciftci A. Effect of tamsulosin on the number and intensity of ureteral colic in patients with lower ureteral calculus. Int J Urol 2005; 12(7): 615–20.

33. Porpiglia F, Destefanis P, Fiori C, Fontana D. Effectiveness of nifedipine and deflazacort in the management of distal ureter stones. Urology 2000; 56(4): 579–82.
34. Lamb AD, Vowler SL, Johnston R, Dunn N, Wiseman OJ. Meta-analysis showing the beneficial effect of alpha-blockers on ureteric stent discomfort. BJU Int 2011; 108(11): 1894–902.
35. Ramsay JW, Payne SR, Gosling PT, Whitfield HN, Wickham JE, Levison DA. The effects of double J stenting on unobstructed ureters. An experimental and clinical study. Br J Urol 1985; 57(6): 630–4.
36. Rane A, Saleemi A, Cahill D, Sriprasad S, Shrotri N, Tiptaft R. Have stent-related symptoms anything to do with placement technique? J Endourol 2001; 15(7): 741–5.
37. Yakoubi R, Lemdani M, Monga M, Villers A, Koenig P. Is there a role for alpha-blockers in ureteral stent related symptoms? A systematic review and meta-analysis. J Urol 2011; 186(3): 928–34.
38. Gupta M, Patel T, Xavier K, et al. Prospective randomized evaluation of periureteral botulinum toxin type A injection for ureteral stent pain reduction. J Urol 2010; 183(2): 598–602.
39. Beiko DT, Watterson JD, Knudsen BE, et al. Double-blind randomized controlled trial assessing the safety and efficacy of intravesical agents for ureteral stent symptoms after extracorporeal shockwave lithotripsy. J Endourol 2004; 18(8): 723–30.
40. Tzortzis V, Mamoulakis C, Rioja J, Gravas S, Michel MC, de la Rosette JJ. Medical expulsive therapy for distal ureteral stones. Drugs 2009; 69(6): 677–92.
41. Springhart WP, Marguet CG, Sur RL, et al. Forced versus minimal intravenous hydration in the management of acute renal colic: a randomized trial. J Endourol 2006; 20(10): 713–16.
42. Worster AS, Bhanich Supapol W. Fluids and diuretics for acute ureteric colic. Cochrane Database Syst Rev 2012; 2: CD004926.
43. Troxel SA, Jones AW, Magliola L, Benson JS. Physiologic effect of nifedipine and tamsulosin on contractility of distal ureter. J Endourol 2006; 20(8): 565–8.
44. Hollingsworth JM, Rogers MA, Kaufman SR, et al. Medical therapy to facilitate urinary stone passage: a meta-analysis. Lancet 2006; 368(9542): 1171–9.
45. Singh A, Alter HJ, Littlepage A. A systematic review of medical therapy to facilitate passage of ureteral calculi. Ann Emerg Med 2007; 50(5): 552–63.
46. Seitz C, Liatsikos E, Porpiglia F, Tiselius HG, Zwergel U. Medical therapy to facilitate the passage of stones: what is the evidence? Eur Urol 2009; 56(3): 455–71.
47. Porpiglia F, Ghignone G, Fiori C, Fontana D, Scarpa RM. Nifedipine versus tamsulosin for the management of lower ureteral stones. J Urol 2004; 172(2): 568–71.
48. Preminger GMTH, Assimos DG, et al. 2007 guideline for the management of ureteral calculi. 2007. Available at: www.auanet.org/education/guidelines/ureteral-calculi.cfm
49. Hamidi Madani A, Kazemzadeh M, Pourreza F, et al. Randomized controlled trial of the efficacy of isosorbide-SR addition to current treatment in medical expulsive therapy for ureteral calculi. Urol Res 2011; 39(5): 361–5.
50. Dellabella M, Milanese G, Muzzonigro G. Medical-expulsive therapy for distal ureterolithiasis: randomized prospective study on role of corticosteroids used in combination with tamsulosin-simplified treatment regimen and health-related quality of life. Urology 2005; 66(4): 712–15.

51. Porpiglia F, Vaccino D, Billia M, et al. Corticosteroids and tamsulosin in the medical expulsive therapy for symptomatic distal ureter stones: single drug or association? Eur Urol 2006; 50(2): 339–44.
52. Hollingsworth JM, Davis MM, West BT, Wolf JS Jr, Hollenbeck BK. Trends in medical expulsive therapy use for urinary stone disease in U.S. emergency departments. Urology 2009; 74(6): 1206–9.
53. Brede C, Hollingsworth JM, Faerber GJ, Taylor JS, Wolf JS Jr. Medical expulsive therapy for ureteral calculi in the real world: targeted education increases use and improves patient outcome. J Urol 2010; 183(2): 585–9.

PART 2
Surgical Management of Urinary Stones

CHAPTER 12

Indications for Conservative and Surgical Management of Urinary Stone Disease

Brian D. Duty and Michael J. Conlin
Oregon Health & Science University/Portland VA Medical Center, Portland, OR, USA

Introduction

The lifetime risk of developing nephrolithiasis in the United States exceeds 10% in men and 5% in women [1]. Beyond patient morbidity, urinary stone disease also exacts a significant economic burden. Over $2.1 billion was spent in 2000 treating stone disease within the United States [2].

Following the introduction of percutaneous nephrolithotomy (PCNL) in the late 1970s and extracorporeal shock wave lithotripsy (ESWL) in the early 1980s, there was a rapid shift away from open stone surgery. With rare exceptions, patients are presently managed with medical expulsive therapy (MET), ureteroscopy (URS), ESWL, or PCNL. Each treatment has its own potential advantages and associated risks. It can be challenging to choose one treatment option over another because the indications for each modality are rarely mutually exclusive.

The purpose of this chapter is to help guide treatment decisions through a comprehensive literature review. Unfortunately, multiple methodological challenges exist in the literature making definitive, evidence-based recommendations impossible for many of the questions in stone disease. Most studies have been observational or non-randomized comparative series. Differences in equipment between series make direct comparisons difficult. The timing and means of assessing treatment outcomes frequently vary. The definition of success has not been standardized, with some studies including residual fragments under a certain size as a success. Lastly, the use of adjuvant therapies also frequently differs between series.

Urinary Stones: Medical and Surgical Management, First Edition. Edited by Michael Grasso and David S. Goldfarb.

Ureteral calculi

Indications for treatment

Ureteral stones are rarely diagnosed incidentally. The majority of patients present with acute renal colic (flank/abdominal pain), gross hematuria, or fever. Indications for urgent intervention include urinary tract infection (UTI), intractable pain or nausea, obstruction of a solitary unit, and renal insufficiency not responsive to hydration.

The initial goal of treatment for patients with an acute stone episode is often decompression of the collecting system. Lithotripsy is then deferred until the patient's infection has resolved or renal function has recovered. Upper urinary tract drainage may be accomplished by placement of either a retrograde ureteral stent or percutaneous nephrostomy tube. The optimal mode of decompression for infection has been debated. In 1998 Pearle and colleagues published a randomized study comparing percutaneous nephrostomy tube placement with retrograde ureteral catheterization in 42 consecutive patients presenting with obstructive ureteral stones and clinical evidence of infection [3]. The authors found no difference in time to decompression, time to defervescence, and length of hospital stay. Ureteral stent placement was twice as costly as percutaneous nephrostomy.

Expectant management

Observation may be considered in the absence of the above-mentioned indications for urgent treatment. Stone size and location are the two most important predictors of spontaneous stone passage. Hübner et al. performed a meta-analysis of six studies including a total of 2704 patients with ureteral calculi and found that 38% of stones 4 mm or less passed without the need for intervention compared to only 1.2% larger than 6 mm [4]. Stones within the distal ureter at presentation were more likely to pass (45%) compared to the mid (22%) and proximal ureter (12%). Of the stones that passed, two-thirds did so within 1 month of symptom onset.

A more recent retrospective study of 172 patients with ureteral stones diagnosed by non-contrast computed tomography (CT) reported more encouraging results [5]. The spontaneous passage rate was 87% for 1 mm, 76% for 2–4 mm, 60% for 7–9 mm, and 48% for stones larger than 9 mm. Once again, stones within the proximal ureter were less likely to pass than those within the distal ureter (48% compared to 75%).

Miller and colleagues published a prospective study of 75 patients with ureteral calculi [6]. Patients with stones 2–4 mm in size had a 95% chance of spontaneously passing their stone. Half of the patients in the study with stones 5 mm or larger required surgical intervention. Mean time to stone passage was 12.2 days, but the time to clearance was highly variable with one patient requiring 40 days to pass their stone.

Although evidence-based guidelines do not exist, many experts recommend periodic imaging to assess stone position and monitor for hydronephrosis. Failure of stone migration after 2 months of observation, even in the absence of symptoms, is a relative indication for surgical treatment. Roberts and colleagues found a 24% rate of ureteral stricture following endoscopic treatment of stones fixed in the same location for more than 2 months [7].

Medical expulsive therapy

A variety of pharmacological agents have been found to affect ureteral function. These include cyclo-oxygenase inhibitors, angiotensin-converting enzyme inhibitors, phosphodiesterase inhibitors, β-adrenergic agonists, calcium channel blockers, and α1-adrenergic antagonists. While cyclo-oxygenase inhibitors have been found to reduce renal colic, only calcium channel and α-blockers have been shown to improve stone passage rates [8].

Singh et al. performed a meta-analysis of all randomized or controlled trials involving calcium channel blockers and α-antagonists in patients with radiographically diagnosed ureteral stones [9]. Data from nine calcium channel blocker trials including 686 patients were analyzed. Compared to standard therapy calcium channel blockers were associated with improved expulsion rates (relative risk [RR] 1.50; 95% confidence interval [CI] 1.34–1.68) and a number needed to treat of 3.9. A total of 1235 patients from 16 trials were used to evaluate α-blocker therapy. α-Antagonists were associated with improved likelihood of spontaneous passage (RR 1.59; 95% CI 1.44–1.75) and a decreased time to expulsion ranging from 2 to 6 days. The number needed to treat was 3.3. It should be noted that additional medications (e.g. low-dose steroids) were prescribed along with the study drug in many of these trials despite not being utilized in the control group, resulting in pooled data heterogeneity.

The EAU/AUA Ureteral Calculi Clinical Guidelines Panel conducted a meta-analysis of medical expulsive therapy trials [10]. In contrast to the Singh review, calcium channel blockers were found to increase the stone passage rate by only 9%, which was not statistically significant. α-Blocker therapy was associated with a 29% improved passage rate, which was significant. As a result, until a large, multicenter, randomized placebo-controlled trial has been performed α-blocker should be considered the first-line agent for MET.

Surgical treatment overview

Lithotripsy procedures should be performed in patients without evidence of UTI who are poor candidates for or fail expectant management. The two primary treatment modalities utilized are shock wave lithotripsy and ureteroscopy. Percutaneous, laparoscopic, and open procedures are reserved for selected cases.

Three large meta-analyses have been published evaluating surgical treatment for ureteral stones [10,11,12]. The EAU/AUA Ureteral Calculi Clinical Guidelines Panel extracted data from 244 publications. The vast majority were single-center case series. A hierarchical model was used to combine the studies. The panel divided treatment outcomes by stone size

(≤10 mm versus >10 mm) and location (proximal, mid, versus distal ureter). The Cochrane Collaboration analyzed outcomes from seven randomized trials comparing ESWL to URS in 1205 patients. Case series were not included. Unlike the EAU/AUA Guidelines, the Cochrane Collaboration did not break down treatment outcomes by ureteral stone location. Neither meta-analysis attempted to account for the type of shock wave machine used (HM3 versus non-HM3) despite level 1 data showing superior results for the HM3 machine [13]. The latest meta-analysis included only randomized studies, but also evaluated treatment outcomes by stone location and type of shock wave machine used [12].

Proximal ureteral stones

The EAU/AUA meta-analysis included 6428 and 2242 patients with proximal ureteral stones treated by ESWL and URS, respectively [10]. The overall stone-free rate was equivalent between the two modalities (ESWL 82%; URS 81%). Shock wave lithotripsy was found to be more efficacious than URS for stones less than 10 mm (90% versus 80%). However, stone-free rates following ureteroscopy were better than ESWL for stones larger than 10 mm (79% versus 68%). These findings likely reflect the fact that shock wave lithotripsy results are more dependent on stone size than ureteroscopy.

A direct comparison of ESWL and URS complication rates was not possible due to a lack of variance data. Regardless, complications were low for both modalities. Postoperative sepsis occurred in 3% and 4% of ESWL and URS patients, respectively. Steinstrasse following ESWL developed 5% of the time. Ureteral injury was reported in 6% of URS cases compared to only 2% of ESWL procedures. However, the ureteral stricture rate was 2% for both groups. No quality of life data were reported.

Four randomized trials that included proximal ureteral stones were analyzed by Matlaga et al. [12]. These trials compared HM3 to non-HM3 ESWL, semi-rigid URS to HM3 ESWL, flexible URS to non-HM3 ESWL, and semi-rigid URS to PCNL. The authors found a 35% greater probability of being rendered stone free following semi-rigid URS compared to HM3 ESWL. Surprisingly, the superiority of URS was less pronounced compared to non-HM3 ESWL (15%). Differences in stone-free rates tended to decrease with longer follow-up.

The need for retreatment following semi-rigid ureteroscopy was less common compared to both HM3 (RR 0.14) and non-HM3 (RR 0.08) ESWL. Complication rates were low for all modalities, but HM3 ESWL patients experienced more complications than those treated with non-HM3 ESWL or URS. However, the authors ultimately concluded that "meaningful comparisons were not possible" between ureteroscopy and shock wave lithotripsy for proximal ureteral stones due to the great variability in the clinical characteristics of the four randomized studies.

Distal ureteral stones

The EAU/AUA meta-analysis compared 6981 patients treated by ESWL to 5952 individuals managed by URS for distal ureteral stones [10]. The overall stone-free rate was significantly better in the URS group compared to ESWL (94% versus 74%). Unlike proximal ureteral stones, these findings were consistent across stone size. Stone-free rates for calculi less than 10 mm and greater than 10 mm were 86% and 74% for ESWL compared to 97% and 93% for ureteroscopy, respectively.

As with proximal stones, a direct comparison of adjuvant procedure and complication rates between ESWL and URS was not possible. Postoperative sepsis remained low at 3% for ESWL and 2% for URS patients. Steinstrasse following ESWL occurred 4% of the time. Ureteral stricture formation did not occur after ESWL and was found in only 1% of URS patients.

Matlaga's meta-analysis of distal ureteral stones included five randomized studies [12]. Four compared semi-rigid URS to non-HM3 ESWL (443 total patients) and one study of semi-rigid URS versus HM3 ESWL (32 patients). The pooled analysis found a 55% greater probability of being rendered stone free following URS compared to non-HM3 ESWL. However, as with the proximal stone data, the stone-free rates following ESWL approached those of URS over time. No difference was found between URS and HM3 ESWL [14]. Ureteroscopy was associated with significantly more auxiliary procedures, likely related to stent removal, while non-HM3 ESWL patients had a seven-fold higher retreatment rate compared to URS. No difference was noted in the overall complication rate between URS and ESWL.

Role of antegrade ureteroscopy and ureterolithotomy

More invasive treatment options such as antegrade ureteroscopy and ureterolithotomy may be considered in selected cases. Antegrade ureteroscopy should be considered in patients with a large stone impacted in the upper ureter. Retrograde URS in this setting carries with it a high risk of ureteral injury. Other indications for antegrade URS include patients with a significant renal stone burden and individuals with urinary diversions making retrograde access challenging or impossible.

Indications for ureterolithotomy are fortunately quite rare. The procedure may be contemplated when intra-abdominal surgery for another purpose is being performed or when less invasive treatment modalities have already failed.

Renal calculi

Asymptomatic renal calculi

Renal calculi causing pain, obstruction, demonstrating growth, associated with infection, and staghorn calculi require treatment in the majority of cases. Other high-risk clinical situations when treatment of renal calculi is encouraged are patients with a solitary kidney, reconstructed urinary tract, immunodeficiency, high-risk occupations, poor medical access or compliance, and children [14]. The more challenging clinical scenario is in low-risk patients with truly asymptomatic renal calculi. Just as we are seeing increasing numbers of small renal masses identified due to the expanded use of diagnostic CT scans, urologists are now faced with increasing numbers of asymptomatic, incidentally identified renal calculi.

There are several options for management of these asymptomatic renal calculi: active surveillance or treatment options including shock wave lithotripsy, ureteroscopy, and percutaneous nephrolithotomy. In rare situations laparoscopic or open intervention may be indicated. There are multiple reasons to consider elective intervention for asymptomatic renal calculi. These include avoiding future potential complications such as pain, obstruction, infection, and acute kidney injury. Also, by treating asymptomatic renal stones early rather than later after the stones may have grown, we may be able to avoid more difficult and more invasive procedures required for the resulting larger stone burden. However, not all renal calculi need to be treated. Some will remain asymptomatic and not grow. We also see renal calculi in elderly patients and those with significant medical co-morbidities, when the risks of treatment might outweigh any potential benefit. Unfortunately, despite the increasing number of renal calculi identified and treated over many years worldwide, we do not yet have well-performed prospective studies to help guide our decision making.

Active surveillance for asymptomatic renal calculi

Many of these patients with asymptomatic renal calculi can be managed initially with active surveillance, but the risk of failure remains high. It was shown by Hübner et al. in renal calculi that are followed closely (62 patients with an average follow-up of 7.4 years), although 16% passed spontaneously without intervention, 45% increased in size, and only 11% remained symptom free after 10 years [15]. In a separate study, Glowacki et al. followed a cohort of 107 patients with asymptomatic urolithiasis for a mean follow-up period of 31.6 months [16]. They found that 73 patients (68.2%) remained asymptomatic during the follow-up period, and 34 (31.8%) developed a symptomatic event. Of those 34, about half (16) passed their stones spontaneously, and the other half (18) required some type of treatment (ESWL, ureteroscopy, or PCNL). They calculated a 5-year probability of developing a symptomatic event of 48.5%.

A more recent observational study was reported by Burgher et al. involving 300 men who were followed for a mean of 3.26 years for their asymptomatic renal calculi [17]; 77% had disease progression (stone growth, development of pain, or required surgical intervention). Factors that correlated with progression were stone size >4 mm, lower pole or renal pelvic location, and elevated urine and serum uric acid levels. All patients with stones larger than 15 mm demonstrated disease progression, 71% with growth, 57% pain, and 26% requiring intervention. Overall, using survival analysis, this study demonstrate a required intervention rate of 50% at just over 7 years follow-up for these asymptomatic renal calculi.

Koh et al. followed 50 patients with asymptomatic renal calculi [18]. This study differed from the previously reviewed studies in that the stones were on average smaller (average diameter 5.7 mm versus 10.8 mm in the Burgher study). This may more accurately represent a contemporary patient population given the increase in stones identified incidentally by CT. They found a lower 7.1% rate of required intervention in these patients with smaller stones. Likewise, a higher number of patients (20%) spontaneously passed their stones. A study with a similar average stone size (4.39 mm) was reported by Kang et al. [19] who reviewed the records of 347 patients with asymptomatic renal calculi. Rates of progression (53.6%) and required intervention (24.5%) were similar to previous reports; 29.1% of patients spontaneously passed their stones.

Active surveillance should consist of routinely scheduled visits every 6–12 months, with imaging (CT alternating with renal US for instance), urinalysis, and consideration for metabolic analysis. One could argue that any patient with renal calculi who is not surgically treated should undergo metabolic evaluation and treatment. It is likely that the condition in the urinary milieu that led to the formation of the stone is still present and may cause the growth of the existing and new stones.

In summary, when active surveillance is chosen for patients with asymptomatic renal calculi, we should expect a rate of progression of 45–77% and a need for intervention in 7–26%. These existing data (summarized in Table 12.1) are helpful, but there has not yet been a randomized prospective trial comparing active surveillance to ureteroscopic management for asymptomatic renal calculi.

Table 12.1 Results with untreated renal calculi

Author	Year	# Patients	Months follow-up	Mean stone diameter	Spontaneous passage	Progression %	Intervention %
Hübner [15]	1990	62	88.8		16		40
Glowacki [16]	1992	107	31.6		15	32	16.8
Keeley [21]	2001	99	26.4		17		21
Burgher [17]	2004	300	39	10.8		77	26
Inci [37]	2007	24	52.3	8.8	12.5	33.3	11.1
Koh [18]	2012	50	46	5.7	20	45.9	7.1
Kang [19]	2012	347	31	4.39	29.1	53.6	24.5

Choice of treatment for renal calculi

When renal calculi require treatment, the most common options are ESWL, URS or PCNL. Laparoscopic treatment may be utilized for stones in a calyceal diverticulum, or for stone removal at the time of laparoscopic pyeloplasty. Some surgeons may perform atrophic nephrolithotomy for those patients with full staghorn calculi who require reconstruction of stenotic infundibula, though these are increasingly rare [20]. The most common procedure performed to treat renal calculi is ESWL, although URS utilization is increasing because of wider availability and superior stone-free rates [2].

Stone size

Symptomatic renal stones less than 4 mm in diameter can be safely allowed to pass. A period of attempted passage with medical expulsive therapy is warranted given an acceptable rate of successful passage of what will soon become a small ureteral calculus. Shock wave lithotripsy is most effective for smaller, non-lower pole, renal calculi. Stones less than 1 cm in diameter that are located in the renal pelvis and non-lower pole calyces are ideal for ESWL. There has been one randomized trial comparing ESWL to active surveillance for asymptomatic calyceal stones less than 15 mm in diameter. The study consisted of 228 patients with a mean follow-up of 2.2 years. Stone-free rates between the ESWL group (28%) and the active surveillance group (17%) were not significantly different. There were also no differences in the rates of additional treatments and quality of life [21]. An additional trial comparing shock wave lithotripsy, observation, and percutaneous nephrolithotomy for the management of asymptomatic lower pole calculi found a stone-free rate in the ESWL group of only 54.8% [22].

Ureteroscopic laser lithotripsy can also be used to treat these smaller renal calculi. The use of the holmium laser, which will fragment any composition of calculus and has the ability to directly visualize the calculi and remove fragments, permits superior stone-free rates when compared to shock wave lithotripsy.

As the stone size increases beyond 1 cm, ureteroscopic treatment should be favored. One of the weaknesses of shock wave lithotripsy treatment for larger calculi is the limitation on total session shock wave energy permitted to prevent renal trauma. It may not be safely possible to fully fragment larger stone burdens with ESWL due to this limit. There is no limitation to the total amount of laser energy that may be utilized ureteroscopically. Laser lithotripsy does not expose the kidney to potentially harmful energy. This versatility of ureteroscopic laser lithotripsy enables greater success than shock wave lithotripsy for the treatment of larger kidney stones. Although there are no randomized controlled trials comparing URS to ESWL for treatment of renal calculi, there are URS series reported demonstrating excellent results. One of the earliest series by Fabrizio et al. reported an overall success rate of 89% for ureteroscopic treatment of intrarenal calculi [23].

Stones larger than 2 cm in diameter are generally treated with percutaneous nephrolithotomy. However, with greater ureteroscopy experience, more results are being reported of successful ureteroscopic treatment of these larger stones. One of the first of these reports by Grasso et al. demonstrated success (<2 mm fragments) in 76% of 45 patients with renal calculi after one ureteroscopic treatment [24]. Use of a second ureteroscopy when needed increased the success rate to 91% overall. A study by Breda et al. of 15 patients with large (mean diameter 22 mm) intrarenal stones treated ureteroscopically resulted in a stone-free rate of 93.3% after a mean number of 2.3 procedures [25]. A matched paired analysis was performed by Akman et al. comparing PCNL to URS for the management of 2–4 cm stones [26]. They demonstrated a stone-free rate of 73.5% after one URS session in 34 patients. This increased to 88.2% after a second ureteroscopy when needed. Overall, these encouraging results in selected patients with very large renal calculi support ureteroscopy as a viable alternative to the more invasive percutaneous treatment of these patients.

Staghorn calculi will generally require treatment because of the risk of kidney injury and life-threatening sepsis [27,28]. The most successful treatment for staghorn calculi remains PCNL, with stone-free rates of 78% reported from a systematic review of the literature performed by the AUA staghorn calculi clinical guidelines committee. Inferior stone-free rates (54%) were found for SWL [29].

Stone location

The location of intrarenal calculi affects the success rate of ESWL treatment. Renal calculi located in the renal pelvis treated with SWL will result in stone-free rates of 56–80%. Stones in the middle and upper calyces that are less than 2 cm can be treated with SWL with stone-free rates between 57.4% and 76.5% [30]. However, in a prospective randomized study, stones in the lower pole treated with SWL achieved a stone-free rate of only 21% for stones larger than 1 cm [31]. A similar randomized trial comparing URS to SWL for lower pole calculi demonstrated a higher stone-free rate for ureteroscopy (50%) than for shock wave lithotripsy (35%) though this difference was not statistically significant [32].

Another advantage of ureteroscopic holmium laser lithotripsy is the ability to reposition lower pole stones into the upper kidney to allow easier laser lithotripsy and more successful residual fragment passage. A review by Schuster et al. compared patients who had their lower pole stones repositioned using a nitinol stone basket during ureteroscopic treatment to patients whose lower pole stones were treated *in situ* [33]. The stone-free rates were better in those patients whose lower pole stones were repositioned, particularly for calculi larger than 1 cm (stone-free rates of 29% *in situ* versus 100% with repositioning).

Stone composition

Shock wave lithotripsy will be less successful for cystine, calcium oxalate monohydrate, and brushite stones because of their resistance to fragmentation.

This can be useful in selecting appropriate treatment methods for patients with prior stone analysis. However, many patients will not have a current stone analysis. Imaging with CT and measurement of Hounsfield units have been shown to be helpful in determining stone fragility and success with SWL. Gupta et al. found a Hounsfield unit value of 750 to be predictive of SWL success for renal calculi [34]. Above this level, 65% of stones were successfully treated versus 90% for those stones with attenuation less than 750 Hounsfield units. A similar study by Shah et al. examined 99 patients prospectively [35]. Using a Hounsfield unit value of 1200, they had better results with SWL for those stones with attenuation levels less than 1200 (efficiency quotient 80.4%) compared to stones with attenuation values

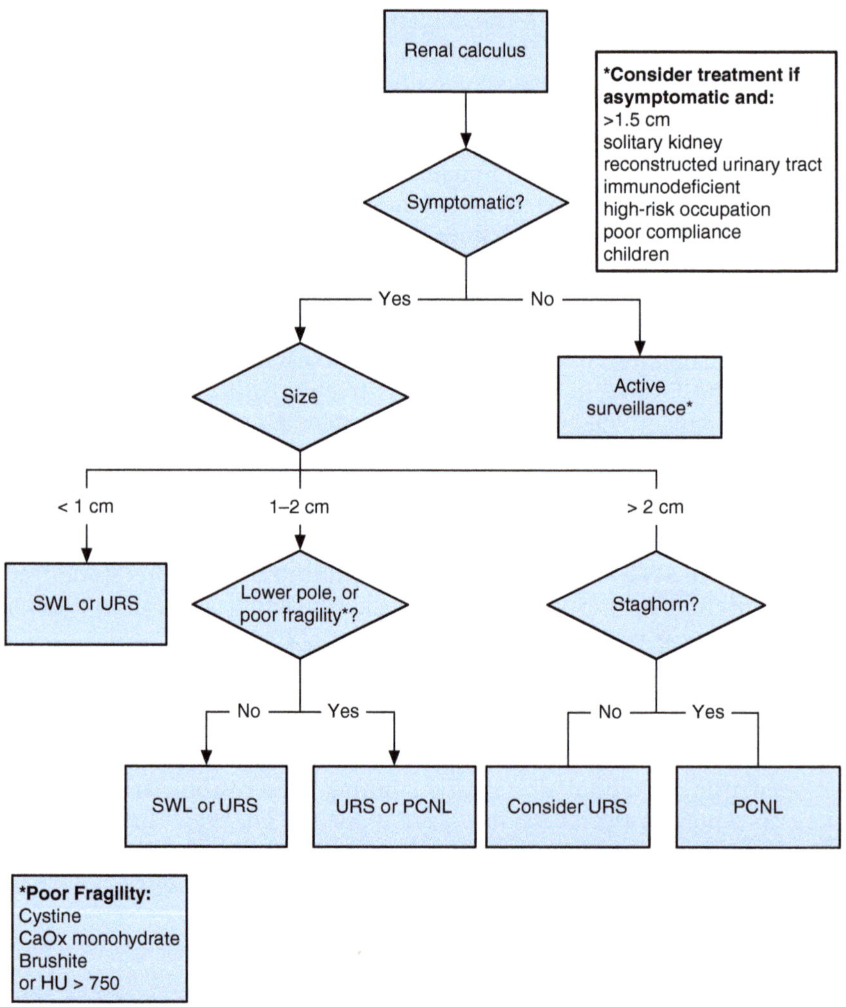

Figure 12.1 Treatment selection for renal calculi.

greater than 1200 (efficiency quotient 66.2%). Dual-energy multidetector CT imaging has been shown to improve our ability to predict stone composition [36]. These methods may prove to be more routinely helpful in correctly choosing patients in whom SWL may be ineffective due to stone density. Stone density will have less effect on ureteroscopic laser lithotripsy success, because of the ability of the holmium laser to fragment any composition of calculus.

Figure 12.1 proposes a treatment algorithm based on the data we presented.

Summary

Most stones will require treatment. There are multiple factors that affect the success of the available treatment techniques in different clinical settings. Although SWL revolutionized the treatment of urolithiasis and remains an excellent option for many patients, there is expanding use of and improving success with endoscopic treatments for ureteral and renal calculi. There remains a need for well-designed prospective studies to help guide our choice of appropriate treatment for patients with urolithiasis.

References

1. Curhan GC. Epidemiology of stone disease. Urol Clin North Am 2007; 34(3): 287–93.
2. Pearle MS, Calhoun EA, Curhan GC, Urologic Diseases of America Project. Urologic Diseases of America Project: Urolithiasis. J Urol 2005; 173(3): 848–57.
3. Pearle MS, Pierce HL, Miller GL, et al. Optimal method of urgent decompression of the collecting system for obstruction and infection due to ureteral calculi. J Urol 1998; 160(4): 1260–4.
4. Hübner WA, Irby P, Stoller ML. Natural history and current concepts for the treatment of small ureteral calculi. Eur Urol 1993; 24(2): 172–6.
5. Coll DM, Varanelli MJ, Smith RC. Relationship of spontaneous passage of ureteral calculi to stone size and location as revealed by unenhanced helical CT. Am J Roentgenol 2002; 178(1): 101–3.
6. Miller OF, Kane CJ. Time to stone passage for observed ureteral calculi: a guide for patient education. J Urol 1999; 162(3 Pt 1): 688–90; discussion 690–1.
7. Roberts WW, Cadeddu JA, Micali S, Kavoussi LR, Moore RG. Ureteral stricture formation after removal of impacted calculi. J Urol 1998; 159(3): 723–6.
8. Sterrett SP, Nakada SY. Medical expulsive therapy. Semin Nephrol 2008; 28(2): 192–9.
9. Singh A, Alter HJ, Littlepage A. A systematic review of medical therapy to facilitate passage of ureteral calculi. Ann Emerg Med 2007; 50(5): 552–63.
10. Preminger GM, Tiselius HG, Assimos DG, et al. 2007 guideline for the management of ureteral calculi. Eur Urol 2007; 52(6): 1610–31.
11. Aboumarzouk OM, Kata SG, Keeley FX, McClinton S, Nabi G. Extracorporeal shock wave lithotripsy (ESWL) versus ureteroscopic management for ureteric calculi. Cochrane Database Syst Rev 2012; 5: CD006029.

12. Matlaga BR, Jansen JP, Meckley LM, Byrne TW, Lingeman JE. Treatment of ureteral and renal stones: a systematic review and meta-analysis of randomized, controlled trials. J Urol 2012; 188(1): 130–7.
13. Zehnder P, Roth B, Birkhäuser F, et al. A prospective randomised trial comparing the modified HM3 with the MODULITH® SLX-F2 lithotripter. Eur Urol 2011; 59(4): 637–44.
14. Goldsmith ZG, Lipkin ME. When (and how) to surgically treat asymptomatic renal stones. Nat Rev Urol 2012; 9(6): 315–20.
15. Hübner W, Porpaczy P. Treatment of caliceal calculi. Br J Urol 1990; 66(1): 9–11.
16. Glowacki LS, Beecroft ML, Cook RJ, Pahl D, Churchill DN. The natural history of asymptomatic urolithiasis. J Urol 1992; 147(2): 319–21.
17. Burgher A, Beman M, Holtzman JL, Monga M. Progression of nephrolithiasis: long-term outcomes with observation of asymptomatic calculi. J Endourol 2004; 18(6): 534–9.
18. Koh LT, Ng FC, Ng KK. Outcomes of long-term follow-up of patients with conservative management of asymptomatic renal calculi. BJU Int 2012; 109(4): 622–5.
19. Kang HW, Lee SK, Kim WT, et al. Natural history of asymptomatic renal stones and prediction of stone related events. J Urol 2013; 189(5): 1740–6.
20. Galvin DJ, Pearle MS. The contemporary management of renal and ureteric calculi. BJU Int 2006; 98(6): 1283–8.
21. Keeley FX, Tilling K, Elves A, et al. Preliminary results of a randomized controlled trial of prophylactic shock wave lithotripsy for small asymptomatic renal calyceal stones. BJU Int 2001; 87(1): 1–8.
22. Yuruk E, Binbay M, Sari E, et al. A prospective, randomized trial of management for asymptomatic lower pole calculi. J Urol 2010; 183(4): 1424–8.
23. Fabrizio MD, Behari A, Bagley DH. Ureteroscopic management of intrarenal calculi. J Urol 1998; 159(4): 1139–43.
24. Grasso M, Conlin M, Bagley D. Retrograde ureteropyeloscopic treatment of 2 cm. or greater upper urinary tract and minor staghorn calculi. J Urol 1998; 160(2): 346–51.
25. Breda A, Ogunyemi O, Leppert JT, Lam JS, Schulam PG. Flexible ureteroscopy and laser lithotripsy for single intrarenal stones 2 cm or greater – is this the new frontier? J Urol 2008; 179(3): 981–4.
26. Akman T, Binbay M, Ozgor F, et al. Comparison of percutaneous nephrolithotomy and retrograde flexible nephrolithotripsy for the management of 2–4 cm stones: a matched-pair analysis. BJU Int 2012; 109(9): 1384–9.
27. Koga S, Arakaki Y, Matsuoka M, Ohyama C. Staghorn calculi – long-term results of management. Br J Urol 1991; 68(2): 122–4.
28. Rous SN, Turner WR. Retrospective study of 95 patients with staghorn calculus disease. J Urol 1977; 118(6): 902–4.
29. Preminger GM, Assimos DG, Lingeman JE, Nakada SY, Pearle MS, Wolf Jr JS. AUA guideline on management of staghorn calculi: diagnosis and treatment recommendations. J Urol 2005; 173(6): 1991.
30. Saw KC, Lingeman JE. Lesson 20: Management of calyceal stones. AUA Update Series 1999; 20: 154–9.
31. Albala DM, Assimos DG, Clayman RV, et al. Lower pole I: A prospective randomized trial of extracorporeal shock wave lithotripsy and percutaneous nephrostolithotomy for lower pole nephrolithiasis – initial results. J Urol 2001; 166(6): 2072–80.

32. Pearle MS, Lingeman JE, Leveillee R, et al. Prospective, randomized trial comparing shock wave lithotripsy and ureteroscopy for lower pole caliceal calculi 1 cm or less. J Urol 2005; 173(6): 2005–9.
33. Schuster TG, Hollenbeck BK, Faerber GJ, Wolf JS. Ureteroscopic treatment of lower pole calculi: comparison of lithotripsy in situ and after displacement. J Urol 2002; 168(1): 43–5.
34. Gupta NP, Ansari MS, Kesarvani P, Kapoor A, Mukhopadhyay S. Role of computed tomography with no contrast medium enhancement in predicting the outcome of extracorporeal shock wave lithotripsy for urinary calculi. BJU Int 2005; 95(9): 1285–8.
35. Shah K, Kurien A, Mishra S, et al. Predicting effectiveness of extracorporeal shockwave lithotripsy by stone attenuation value. J Endourol 2010; 24(7): 1169–73.
36. Boll DT, Patil NA, Paulson EK, et al. Renal stone assessment with dual-energy multidetector CT and advanced postprocessing techniques: improved characterization of renal stone composition – pilot study 1. Radiology 2009; 250(3): 813–20.
37. Inci K, Sahin A, Islamoglu E, Eren MT, Bakkaloglu M, Ozen H. Prospective long-term followup of patients with asymptomatic lower pole caliceal stones. J Urol 2007; 177(6): 2189–92.

CHAPTER 13

Perioperative Imaging: Plain Film, Sonography, Contrast-Based Fluoroscopic Imaging, Computed Tomography, and Magnetic Resonance Urography

Nicole Hindman
New York University Langone Medical Center, New York, NY, USA

Introduction

The diagnosis of urinary stones is rising, due in part to an increase in overall prevalence [1,2]. Imaging plays an important role in the diagnosis, therapeutic planning, and follow-up of patients with urolithiasis. Techniques utilized for imaging include conventional radiography (KUB), intravenous urography (IVU), ultrasound (US), magnetic resonance urography, and computed tomography (CT) scans; each of these modalities is associated with advantages and limitations. Plain film radiographs and intravenous pyelographic techniques were replaced in emergency rooms and office clinics by sonography and single-slice CT, beginning in the early 1990s [3,4,5].

Additional advances in imaging, including multidetector CT scanning, dual-energy CT scanning, improved sonographic equipment and scanning techniques, have further widened the use of imaging in stone disease. Imaging in suspected stone disease helps to confirm the diagnosis and exclude other pathologies (such as acute appendicitis, diverticulitis, ovarian torsion, etc.) with high accuracy [6,7]. Once the diagnosis of urolithiasis has been made, imaging provides anatomical, functional and physiological information about the stone and the collecting system, factors that help in managing therapeutic strategies.

Stones in the renal pelvis above the ureteropelvic junction are more often treated with shock wave lithotripsy (SWL), ureteroscopy, or percutaneous nephrolithotomy (PCNL). Larger stones and staghorn calculi are

Urinary Stones: Medical and Surgical Management, First Edition. Edited by Michael Grasso and David S. Goldfarb.

removed with PCNL. PCNL requires percutaneous ultrasonography (US) or fluoroscopically guided puncture of a renal calyx, tract dilation, and stone fragmentation-extraction. Stones in the ureter are usually treated via medical expulsive therapy, hydration, and pain control. Larger ureteral stones may require intervention with SWL or ureteroscopy with fragmentation-extraction. Imaging is therefore important both in the initial diagnosis of these stones in terms of location and size, and in follow-up of therapies to assess for resolution/complication.

This chapter will provide a brief overview of the various modalities available to the urologist in the diagnosis, management, and follow-up of urinary stones.

Conventional radiography/abdominal plain film

Traditionally, diagnosis of suspected renal stones was performed via a plain film radiograph, termed a radiograph of the kidneys, ureters, and bladder (KUB). Since the majority of urinary tract stones contain calcium, most stones that are sufficiently large (at least 2.6 mm in size) [8] should be visible on plain radiography. However, certain stone compositions, particularly radiolucent stones (such as uric acid or matrix stones), are not visible on KUB. The advantages of a KUB include its wide availability, minimal radiation exposure, and low cost. However, visualization of stones is limited by small size of the stones, overlying bowel gas/fecal retention in the colon, body habitus of the patient, and overlying bony strutures [9].

The sensitivity and specificity of KUB for detecting urinary tract calculi (when utilizing CT as the gold standard) have been reported as 45–59% and 71–77%, respectively [10]. Another limitation of plain film radiography is the lack of soft tissue detail of the viscera, limiting evaluation of the kidney, peri- and pararenal fascia, ureter, etc. Thus, it is not typically used for preoperative planning for percutaneous nephrolithotomy; instead, it is primarily used in planning fluoroscopically guided SWL, in follow-up of known radiopaque calculi (for patients who have elected for surveillance of their calculi), and for monitoring the status of stone fragments after SWL, ureteroscopy, and PCNL [11].

Ultrasound

Ultrasound is a popular modality for evaluation of the urinary tract. It does not utilize radiation and is thus a procedure of choice for children and pregnant patients with suspected urolithiasis. US is also the preferred imaging modality to detect hydronephrosis and hydroureter, although it may not reveal the cause of the obstruction [12].

In the setting of acute renal colic, measurement of the resistive index of the kidney may provide information about the true presence of obstruction, but the exact threshold for the resistive index (usually defined as greater than 0.7) is not precise. As background, in urinary tract obstruction, pathophysiological changes affecting the pressure in the collecting system and kidney perfusion occur. Ultrasound is very sensitive for the detection of collecting system dilation, but the collecting system may be dilated without obstruction. To differentiate these conditions, color Doppler sonography can be performed with measurement of the resistive index (RI) in the intrarenal arteries. True obstruction (except in the hyperacute stage) leads to intrarenal vasoconstriction with a consecutive increase of the RI above the upper limit of 0.7, whereas non-obstructive dilation does not cause an increase in the RI. Unfortunately, there is cross-over between other physiological conditions besides obstruction that may lead to an elevated RI, so that this measure in isolation has a relatively high variability between readers [13,14].

The sensitivity of US in detecting renal calculi varies widely in the literature, ranging from 12% to 93%, with the higher sensitivities of 93% reflecting the use of radiography or tomography as the reference standard, a flawed standard [10,15,16]. Further studies have shown a sensitivity of 77–79% when US was combined with KUB in evaluating ureteral colic [12,17]. Known weaknesses of sonography are in evaluating the midureter, secondary to overlying bowel gas, as well as in evaluating distal ureteral stones [11]. Transvaginal and transperineal sonographic techniques have better sensitivity for detecting distal ureteral stones than routine transabdominal sonography, but these techniques are operator dependent and are not routinely performed [18].

The size of stones is an important factor limiting the sensitivity of sonography; studies have shown that sonography demonstrates a sensitivity of 13% for detecting stones smaller than 3mm [15]. Another limitation of sonography is in estimating the size of the imaged stones; a common pitfall in sonography lies in estimating the edge of the stone, such that US tends to overestimate the stone size, which may have an effect on choice of intervention [19].

Intravenous urography/intravenous pyelography

Intravenous pyelography (IVP) previously served as the gold standard for the diagnosis and follow-up of urinary stones. This modality involves taking successive plain films targeted at the depth of the kidneys, after a bowel preparation has been administered, first with a scout radiograph, then at predetermined time points after the administration of hypertonic radiopaque contrast intravenously. The resultant high-resolution images demonstrate the kidneys in various stages of contrast enhancement, and demonstrate the excretion of the contrast into the collecting system of the kidney, thereby providing excellent anatomical detail of the minor and major calyces, infundibula, renal pelvices, and ureters [9]. A renal or ureteral stone is seen as a filling defect within the collecting system in this modality.

Advantages of this modality include its availability, its ability to estimate renal function, degree of obstruction, and its superior depiction of fine anatomy due to its high resolution (excellent demonstration of the cystic tubular ectasia of medullary sponge kidney, subtle calyceal diverticula, and subtle contrast extravasation) [20].

The disadvantages of IVP include its requirement for a bowel preparation for improved visualization of the kidneys, its requirement for intravenous contrast administration, the requirement for radiation, its poor depiction of intra-abdominal and pelvic organs, and its variable acquisition times (up to 108 min in one study) [21].

Furthermore, the sensitivity of IVP for detecting ureteral calculi varies from 59.1% to 64% in the literature, with a specificity of 92% [21,22].

Additionally, a meta-analysis of four studies involving 296 patients concluded that non-contrast helical CT was significantly better than IVP at diagnosing and excluding stones (pooled positive likelihood ratios for non-contrast CT and IVP were 23.15 and 9.32, respectively) [23].

Due to the better sensitivity and specificity of non-contrast (unenhanced) helical CT scans relative to IVP, this modality has been largely replaced by CT scans for the diagnosis of urolithiasis.

Computed tomography

Non-contrast helical CT is currently viewed as the optimal initial study for investigating patients with suspected urolithiasis [24,25].

Non-contrast CT was first described as useful in the investigation of stones in 1995, since when it has been repeatedly proven to have unparalleled accuracy in the diagnosis of urinary tract stones, with a reported sensitivity of 95–98% and a specificity of 96–100% [3,4,26,27,28,29,30].

Initially, all CT scans were performed utilizing single-slice, point and shoot technology (these are non-helical, non-spiral CT scanners). However, since 1998, when the first multidetector (also termed helical or spiral) CT scanners were introduced, almost all single-slice scanners have been replaced by multidetector scanners, ranging from two detectors to 128 detectors. These advances have allowed the resolution of CT scanners to dramatically improve, by acquiring data of subcentimeter slice thickness, allowing isotropic volume acquisition such that three-dimensional datasets can be generated by a single 1-min axial acquisition. Additionally, there have been advances in the postprocessing algorithms and workstations which generate multiplanar datasets. These advances have improved the diagnostic image quality of CT, such that the depiction of renal and ureteral stones, including the number, size, and location of the stones, skin-to-stone distance, and distance to the ureterovesicular junction, is easily made. Additionally, when axial images are reviewed in conjunction with high-resolution coronal reformatted images (generated from the isotropic thin slice axial acquisition), there is improved detection of stones [31,32].

With these advances in the depiction of small stones, there is also an improved ability of multidetector CT to assess the attenuation measurements and internal structure of stones, which again helps to predict response to therapy. Determination of stone composition is important for several reasons. Uric acid stones (which typically have Hounsfield unit [HU] values below 500) are usually treated with urinary alkalinization as a first-line treatment. Also, certain subtypes of calcium stones (HU values above 1700) and cysteine stones (HU values *in vitro* measuring from 600 to 1100) do not respond well to SWL [5,33,34]. Multidetector attenuation values thus allow for improved differentiation between calcium and uric acid stones using Hounsfield units.

While these studies have depicted an improved ability to differentiate uric acid stones from other stones, it is more difficult to differentiate between pure struvite and cysteine, calcium oxalate and brushite, and, most challenging, mixed composition stones [35,36,37]. Thus, there are persistent challenges in characterization of stone types with multidetector CT. More recently, the development of dual-energy CT has overcome some of these challenges in stone characterization [38].

Dual-energy CT is performed with either one (with rapid kilovolt peak switching between the low and high energy) or two X-ray tubes of low and high energy, with two corresponding 64-detector arrays in opposition at 90° angles [39,40]. The dual X-ray tubes allow for scanning at two different energies (typically 80 and 140 kVp), which allows the obtained data to be characterized for tissue content [41]. The tissue has variable X-ray attenuation at the low and high kVp energies, which the dual-energy software utilizes to determine the material being scanned. Thus, with dual-energy CT, it is possible to differentiate between pure uric acid, mixed uric acid, and calcified stones [42].

Thus, there are multiple advantages of unenhanced multidetector CT over other imaging modalities, including its wide availability, rapid acquisition time, lack of intravenous contrast material, accuracy in detecting stones, excellent soft tissue detail, and depiction of renal and extrarenal pathology [3,24]. In particular, CT scanning is useful for the diagnosis of unsuspected extrarenal pathology, particularly in patients with nonspecific abdominal pain mimicking pain from urolithasis (e.g. appendicitis, diverticulitis, ovarian torsion, aortic dissection, etc.).

There are disadvantages of CT scanning, predominantly related to the increased radiation dose of this modality relative to standard plain films and IVP (or ultrasound/MRI, which do not use radiation). The radiation dose delivered to a patient for a routine CT scan is approximately 8–16 milliSieverts (mSV) compared with 0.5–0.9 mSV for a plain film of the abdomen and 1.3–3.5 mSV for an IVP [43]. Newer reports with lower dose CT scans deliver radiation similar to that of abdominal plain films (0.5–2 mSV), and these studies have shown no change in accuracy in detecting stones compared with standard CT, with a sensitivity of 98% and specificity of 95% in the low-dose cohort [43,44]. While the long-term effects of repeated CT scans for patients who are habitual stone formers is not established, there is concern about the potential for increased malignancy (e.g. leukemia and thyroid cancer).

Magnetic resonance imaging

Magnetic resonance imaging is not sensitive for the detection of calcification, so it is of limited value in the evaluation or diagnosis of renal stone disease. However, in patients for whom radiation should be avoided (e.g. young patients, pregnant patients), MRI has utility in the diagnosis of obstructive stone disease, where it is usually used as an adjunct to sonography. Diagnosis of an obstructing stone on non-contrast MRI is usually seen on fluid-sensitive sequences as a dilated collecting system with increased signal (edema) surrounding the kidney/ureter; the stone (although usually not seen) may occasionally present as a signal void [45]. Regan et al. evaluated the efficacy of MR urography in the diagnosis of stone disease and concluded that it is highly accurate in identifying the level and degree of ureteric obstruction when compared with IVP [46].

Summary

Imaging of renal calculi is necessary to provide information about the presence of stones, their size and location, and to depict any associated complications. For the diagnosis of a suspected obstructing ureteral stone, a non-contrast helical CT is the current modality of choice. However, there are compelling indications for the use of ultrasound, IVP, and MR urography. Most follow-up of renal/ureteral stones is performed with abdominal plain films or ultrasound, in order to reduce radiation dose. Imaging of renal stones in the future may allow detailed and accurate identification of the stone composition, which has the potential to direct the management.

References

1. Scales CD Jr, Curtis LH, Norris RD, et al. Changing gender prevalence of stone disease. J Urol 2007; 177(3): 979–82.
2. Clark JY, Thompson IM, Optenberg SA. Economic impact of urolithiasis in the United States. J Urol 1995; 154(6): 2020–4.
3. Smith RC, Verga M, McCarthy S, Rosenfield AT. Diagnosis of acute flank pain: value of unenhanced helical CT. Am J Roentgenol 1996; 166(1): 97–101.
4. Smith RC, Rosenfield AT, Choe KA, et al. Acute flank pain: comparison of non-contrast-enhanced CT and intravenous urography. Radiology 1995; 194(3): 789–94.
5. Saw KC, McAteer JA, Monga AG, Chua GT, Lingeman JE, Williams JC Jr. Helical CT of urinary calculi: effect of stone composition, stone size, and scan collimation. Am J Roentgenol 2000; 175(2): 329–32.

6. Rosen MP, Siewert B, Sands DZ, Bromberg R, Edlow J, Raptopoulos V. Value of abdominal CT in the emergency department for patients with abdominal pain. Eur Radiol 2003; 13(2): 418–24.
7. Dalrymple NC, Verga M, Anderson KR, et al. The value of unenhanced helical computerized tomography in the management of acute flank pain. J Urol 1998; 159(3): 735–40.
8. Katz D, McGahan JP, Gerscovich EO, Troxel SA, Low RK. Correlation of ureteral stone measurements by CT and plain film radiography: utility of the KUB. J Endourol 2003; 17(10): 847–50.
9. Benway BM, Bhayani SM. Lower urinary tract calculi. In: Wein AJ, ed. *Campbell-Walsh Urology*, 10th edn. Philadelphia: Saunders Elsevier, 2011.
10. Levine JA, Neitlich J, Verga M, Dalrymple N, Smith RC. Ureteral calculi in patients with flank pain: correlation of plain radiography with unenhanced helical CT. Radiology 1997; 204(1): 27–31.
11. Nelson WK, Houghton SG, Milliner DS, Lieske JC, Sarr MG. Enteric hyperoxaluria, nephrolithiasis, and oxalate nephropathy: potentially serious and unappreciated complications of Roux-en-Y gastric bypass. Surg Obes Relat Dis 2005; 1(5): 481–5.
12. Ripolles T, Errando J, Agramunt M, Martinez MJ. Ureteral colic: US versus CT. Abdom Imaging 2004; 29(2): 263–6.
13. Mostbeck GH, Zontsich T, Turetschek K. Ultrasound of the kidney: obstruction and medical diseases. Eur Radiol 2001; 11(10): 1878–89.
14. Rud O, Moersler J, Peter J, et al. Prospective evaluation of interobserver variability of the hydronephrosis index and the renal resistive index as sonographic examination methods for the evaluation of acute hydronephrosis. BJU Int 2012; 110(8 Pt B): E350–6.
15. Fowler KA, Locken JA, Duchesne JH, Williamson MR. US for detecting renal calculi with nonenhanced CT as a reference standard. Radiology 2002; 222(1): 109–13.
16. Middleton WD, Dodds WJ, Lawson TL, Foley WD. Renal calculi: sensitivity for detection with US. Radiology 1988; 167(1): 239–44.
17. Catalano O, Nunziata A, Altei F, Siani A. Suspected ureteral colic: primary helical CT versus selective helical CT after unenhanced radiography and sonography. Am J Roentgenol 2002 Feb; 178(2): 379–87.
18. Glowacki LS, Beecroft ML, Cook RJ, Pahl D, Churchill DN. The natural history of asymptomatic urolithiasis. J Urol 1992; 147(2): 319–21.
19. Kampa RJ, Ghani KR, Wahed S, Patel U, Anson KM. Size matters: a survey of how urinary-tract stones are measured in the UK. J Endourol 2005; 19(7): 856–60.
20. Niall O, Russell J, MacGregor R, Duncan H, Mullins J. A comparison of noncontrast computerized tomography with excretory urography in the assessment of acute flank pain. J Urol 1999; 161(2): 534–7.
21. Wang JH, Shen SH, Huang SS, Chang CY. Prospective comparison of unenhanced spiral computed tomography and intravenous urography in the evaluation of acute renal colic. J Chinese Med Assoc 2008; 71(1): 30–6.
22. Sandhu C, Anson KM, Patel U. Urinary tract stones – Part I: role of radiological imaging in diagnosis and treatment planning. Clin Radiol 2003; 58(6): 415–21.
23. Worster A, Preyra I, Weaver B, Haines T. The accuracy of noncontrast helical computed tomography versus intravenous pyelography in the diagnosis of suspected acute urolithiasis: a meta-analysis. Ann Emerg Med 2002; 40(3): 280–6.

24. Ege G, Akman H, Kuzucu K, Yildiz S. Acute ureterolithiasis: incidence of secondary signs on unenhanced helical CT and influence on patient management. Clin Radiol 2003; 58(12): 990–4.
25. Heneghan JP, McGuire KA, Leder RA, DeLong DM, Yoshizumi T, Nelson RC. Helical CT for nephrolithiasis and ureterolithiasis: comparison of conventional and reduced radiation-dose techniques. Radiology 2003; 229(2): 575–80.
26. Boulay I, Holtz P, Foley WD, White B, Begun FP. Ureteral calculi: diagnostic efficacy of helical CT and implications for treatment of patients. Am J Roentgenol 1999; 172(6): 1485–90.
27. Fielding JR, Silverman SG, Samuel S, Zou KH, Loughlin KR. Unenhanced helical CT of ureteral stones: a replacement for excretory urography in planning treatment. Am J Roentgenol 1998; 171(4): 1051–3.
28. Fielding JR, Fox LA, Heller H, et al. Spiral CT in the evaluation of flank pain: overall accuracy and feature analysis. J Comput Assist Tomogr 1997; 21(4): 635–8.
29. Katz DS, Lane MJ, Sommer FG. Unenhanced helical CT of ureteral stones: incidence of associated urinary tract findings. Am J Roentgenol 1996; 166(6): 1319–22.
30. Hamm M, Wawroschek F, Weckermann D, et al. Unenhanced helical computed tomography in the evaluation of acute flank pain. Eur Radiol 2001; 39(4): 460–5.
31. Lin WC, Uppot RN, Li CS, Hahn PF, Sahani DV. Value of automated coronal reformations from 64-section multidetector row computerized tomography in the diagnosis of urinary stone disease. J Urol 2007; 178(3 Pt 1): 907–11; discussion 911.
32. Metser U, Ghai S, Ong YY, Lockwood G, Radomski SB. Assessment of urinary tract calculi with 64-MDCT: the axial versus coronal plane. Am J Roentgenol 2009; 192(6): 1509–13.
33. Kim SC, Burns EK, Lingeman JE, Paterson RF, McAteer JA, Williams JC Jr. Cystine calculi: correlation of CT-visible structure, CT number, and stone morphology with fragmentation by shock wave lithotripsy. Urol Res 2007; 35(6): 319–24.
34. Perks AE, Schuler TD, Lee J, et al. Stone attenuation and skin-to-stone distance on computed tomography predicts for stone fragmentation by shock wave lithotripsy. Urology 2008; 72(4): 765–9.
35. Mitcheson HD, Zamenhof RG, Bankoff MS, Prien EL. Determination of the chemical composition of urinary calculi by computerized tomography. J Urol 1983; 130(4): 814–19.
36. Motley G, Dalrymple N, Keesling C, Fischer J, Harmon W. Hounsfield unit density in the determination of urinary stone composition. Urology 2001; 58(2): 170–3.
37. Sheir KZ, Mansour O, Madbouly K, Elsobky E, Abdel-Khalek M. Determination of the chemical composition of urinary calculi by noncontrast spiral computerized tomography. Urol Res 2005; 33(2): 99–104.
38. Matlaga BR, Kawamoto S, Fishman E. Dual source computed tomography: a novel technique to determine stone composition. Urology 2008; 72(5): 1164–8.
39. Fletcher JG, Takahashi N, Hartman R, et al. Dual-energy and dual-source CT: is there a role in the abdomen and pelvis? Radiol Clin North Am 2009; 47(1): 41–57.
40. Flohr TG, McCollough CH, Bruder H, et al. First performance evaluation of a dual-source CT (DSCT) system. Eur Radiol 2006; 16(2): 256–68.

41. Johnson TR, Krauss B, Sedlmair M, et al. Material differentiation by dual energy CT: initial experience. Eur Radiol 2007; 17(6): 1510–17.
42. Primak AN, Fletcher JG, Vrtiska TJ, et al. Noninvasive differentiation of uric acid versus non-uric acid kidney stones using dual-energy CT. Acad Radiol 2007; 14(12): 1441–7.
43. Kluner C, Hein PA, Gralla O, et al. Does ultra-low-dose CT with a radiation dose equivalent to that of KUB suffice to detect renal and ureteral calculi? J Comput Assist Tomogr 2006; 30(1): 44–50.
44. Mulkens TH, Daineffe S, de Wijngaert R, et al. Urinary stone disease: comparison of standard-dose and low-dose with 4D MDCT tube current modulation. Am J Roentgenol 2007; 188(2): 553–62.
45. Lubarsky M, Kalb B, Sharma P, Keim SM, Martin DR. MR imaging for acute nontraumatic abdominopelvic pain: rationale and practical considerations. Radiographics 2013; 33(2): 313–37.
46. Regan F, Bohlman ME, Khazan R, Rodriguez R, Schultze-Haakh H. MR urography using HASTE imaging in the assessment of ureteric obstruction. Am J Roentgenol 1996; 167(5): 1115–20.

CHAPTER 14

Emergency Urinary Drainage Techniques Employed for an Obstructing Upper Urinary Tract Calculus With and Without Associated Sepsis

Sunil Mathur[1] *and Francis X. Keeley Jr*[2]

[1]Great Western Hospital, Swindon, UK

[2]Bristol Urological Institute, Bristol, UK

Introduction

Ureteral calculi can usually be managed with a period of observation or pharmacological management, with intervention reserved for the minority of stones that fail to pass spontaneously. In cases of ureteral obstruction associated with acute renal failure or the presence of an infected hydronephrosis, urgent decompression of the upper urinary tract is required in order to either restore renal function or prevent the onset of overwhelming sepsis [1]. Prolonged periods of obstruction, as well as leading to the complications of uremia and hyperkalemia, will result in permanent renal damage. The lack of antibiotic penetration into an infected hydronephrotic kidney can lead to pyonephrosis, a suppurative destruction of renal parenchyma resulting in significant loss of renal function. In the presence of infection, antibiotics alone will not reliably prevent progression to overwhelming sepsis and death. Drainage of the kidney is imperative.

There are two well-established methods of drainage of the upper urinary tract: percutaneous nephrostomy (PCN) and retrograde ureteral stenting. These do not involve the removal of the stone itself, and so avoid a prolonged procedure under general anesthetic in the potentially unstable patient.

Percutaneous nephrostomy was first described in 1955 by Goodwin as an alternative to open surgical drainage or primary nephrectomy [2]. In the technique's current form, a drainage tube ranging typically from 8 to 12 F is placed under local anesthetic or light sedation using ultrasound or fluoroscopic guidance by an interventional radiologist or urologist. The main

Urinary Stones: Medical and Surgical Management, First Edition. Edited by Michael Grasso and David S. Goldfarb.

advantage of the procedure is the high success rate in obtaining drainage, especially in a hydronephrotic kidney, with series demonstrating successful placement in 97–99% of cases [3,4,5]. In cases of infected hydronephrosis, this also allows direct sampling of infected urine from the kidney, which can occasionally provide additional microbiological information compared to samples from bladder urine samples [6]. Relative contraindications to PCN include coagulopathy, which increases the risk of hemorrhage following the procedure, or an unco-operative patient, which may necessitate the procedure being performed under a general anesthetic and thus negating one of its major advantages. Complications of PCN, while rare, can be significant. Transient minor hematuria occurs in almost all cases, but significant bleeding requiring transfusion or further intervention occurs in 1–4% of patients [7,8,9]. Injury to adjacent organs such as colon or pleura can occur, but are rare, both at around 0.2%. Overall procedure-related mortality is 0.05–0.3% [9].

Retrograde ureteral catheterization was initially reported in 1967 [10]. The procedure is carried out by a urologist using a cystoscope usually under a general anesthetic with fluoroscopic guidance, although placement under local anesthetic is possible even in the urgent setting [11,12]. Retrograde catheters tend to have smaller lumens than nephrostomy tubes, 6–7 F being commonly employed. Complication rates from ureteral catheterization are less widely reported than for nephrostomy. Major complications such as significant bleeding or damage to adjacent organs almost never occur. The most common complication of ureteral stenting is failure to successfully place the stent. While older studies looking at obstruction from all causes show low technical success rates [13,14], more recent data and data looking at stones in particular indicate a more favorable outcome, possibly due to more modern instrumentation. A success rate of 94% was found in a study for acute intrinsic obstruction, of which 52 of 61 cases were obstruction due to stone [15]. In another study on acute obstruction due to stone, success rates of 98% under general anesthetic and 91% under local anesthetic were obtained [11].

Which procedure should be used for emergency drainage of the obstructed kidney?

Arguments in favor of both techniques exist. It has been suggested that the wider bore tube of a nephrostomy provides better drainage than a narrow ureteral stent, or that stent placement allows for earlier hospital discharge without the need for a second procedure to internalize drainage with antegrade stent placement. However, there seems to be little clear evidence in the literature as to which method of upper tract drainage is to be preferred. There are two randomized trials comparing PCN with ureteral stenting in urinary tract stone disease, one involving patients with infected hydronephrosis and one involving patients with obstruction and a variety of complicating factors [12,16].

Pearle et al. conducted a trial in which 42 patients presenting to emergency departments with ureteral or ureteropelvic junction stones along with clinical signs of infection (white blood cell count raised over 17,000 per mm^3 or temperature greater than 38 °C) were randomly allocated to receive PCN or ureteral stenting [16]. PCN was performed under local anesthetic and sedation. Ureteral stenting was performed under general or regional anesthesia in 76% and intravenous sedation in the remainder. Technical success rates were high. All retrograde catheters were successfully placed. One nephrostomy attempt failed and was converted to a ureteral stent. One nephrostomy tube was dislodged after the patient had recovered from sepsis and been discharged from hospital, but before definitive treatment of their stone was undertaken. The study was powered to detect a 1-day difference in the primary outcome of time to normalization of temperature and white count. There was no statistically significant difference between the two groups on this basis. There were also no significant differences in secondary clinical outcomes as measured by time to normal temperature (PCN 2.3 days, stent 2.6 days), time to normal white count (PCN 2.0 days, stent 1.7 days) or length of hospital stay (PCN 4.5 days, stent 3.2 days). The one difference that was noted was the disparity in cost between the two methods of management, with ureteral stenting costing twice as much as PCN. The paper concluded that both techniques were effective.

Mokhmalji et al. studied patients with stone-induced hydronephrosis in addition to either raised temperature (greater than 38 °C), raised serum creatinine (greater than 1.7 mg/dL), stone size greater than 15 mm, or persistent pain [12]. Forty patients were randomized between PCN and ureteral stenting, with 11 in each group of 20 having signs of infection. Both procedures were carried out under local anesthetic. Technical success was mixed. Ureteral catheterization was not possible in four male patients, in two cases because of inability to tolerate the procedure and in two because of prostatic enlargement. They went on to have nephrostomies placed. All nephrostomies were successful. It is possible that a higher success rate could have been achieved for stenting if the procedure were carried out under general anesthetic. The authors report that patients treated with stents required longer courses of intravenous antibiotics, with the criteria for prescribing antibiotics being for 3 days beyond the resolution of fever, but the finding is not statistically significant. They also reported that stents remained in place for longer than nephrostomies, but it is unclear why this was. Quality of life questionnaires given 2–4 weeks after the procedure showed a greater negative impact from ureteral stenting than PCN, although differences were small. The paper concluded in favor of the superiority of PCN, although the results described do not seem consistent with such a strong endorsement.

Some findings were inconsistent between the two studies. Pearle et al. found longer procedure times, greater fluoroscopy times and higher analgesic use in PCN, while Mokhmalji et al. found the opposite, likely reflecting differing local practices rather than fundamental properties of the two techniques.

A non-randomized retrospective case review of outcomes following emergency drainage of infected hydronephrosis was carried out by Yoshimura et al. [17]. Thirty-five renal units were stented and 24 had nephrostomies placed, with some patients presenting on more than one occasion during the 10-year study period. No information is given on the criteria for choosing PCN or stenting in these patients, although those undergoing PCN tended to have larger stones (9.7 versus 2.6 mm) and were also older. Of all hospital admissions for treatment of upper urinary tract calculi, 12% required drainage for urinary tract sepsis. This was strictly defined as meeting the criteria for the systemic inflammatory response syndrome [18] in the presence of a positive urine culture, or significant pyuria if previous antibiotics had been prescribed. There was no difference in most outcome parameters between the two groups. Equal proportions required intensive care management and peak inflammatory marker levels were similar. Those undergoing stenting had more severe thrombocytopenia and more rapid progression of inflammation, but recovered earlier. This study was not primarily designed to compare outcomes between PCN and stenting and no firm conclusions can be drawn.

Once a patient has recovered from renal dysfunction or sepsis, they will be left to manage with a nephrostomy or ureteral stent while awaiting stone passage or definitive management. It is well recognized that ureteral stents are associated with a significant impact on health-related quality of life compared to those not stented following uncomplicated ureteroscopy [19,20]. Studies comparing quality of life between those with ureteral stents and those with nephrostomies inserted for stone disease have shown no significant difference between the two [21]. Stents result in significant lower urinary tract symptoms, while nephrostomy tubes require maintenance, leak and can become dislodged. Both can cause significant discomfort. No preference can be given to stenting or PCN on a quality of life basis.

In summary, there is no evidence from the literature to favor either ureteral stenting or PCN as a superior treatment for urinary obstruction for acute renal failure or infected hydronephrosis. The slightly higher technical success rate for PCN is offset by the more significant complications, and there are no differences in clinical outcomes or quality of life.

Despite this lack of evidence, there are trends among medical professionals as to which procedure is preferred. A postal questionnaire survey in the United Kingdom conducted among 227 urologists and radiologists has shown a preference for PCN in patients without a coagulopathy, at least in the setting of infected hydronephrosis [22]. When asked for their preferred method of draining the urinary tract for acute renal failure, 53% of radiologists and 55% of urologists preferred PCN to ureteral stenting. In the setting of obstruction in the clinically septic patient, 78% of radiologists and 88% of urologists preferred PCN. In contrast, a survey of hospital discharge summaries in the United States has shown very different results [23]. Of the 113,459 patients who had urgent drainage of the upper urinary tract for infection and urolithiasis, 87.7% underwent stenting. The use of PCN had declined significantly over the study period between 1999 and 2009, suggesting the practice is falling from favor. In this survey, those undergoing PCN had worse outcomes than those having stents, but with only discharge summary data to work from, it is more likely that this reflected PCN being reserved for those patients with more severe sepsis rather than it being an inferior technique.

In many cases the choice between PCN and ureteral stenting will be based on the availability of local resources or the characteristics of individual patients rather than any perceived benefit of one procedure over another. Critically unwell patients can pose anesthetic risks, but are also difficult to position for PCN insertion. While it may be safe to resuscitate a patient in renal failure overnight and drain their kidney during working hours, especially if advanced to the point where dialysis is required in any case, an infected hydronephrosis requires immediate drainage. This means the choice of procedure will depend on the availability of interventional radiologists or urologists at that time in a particular hospital. Staffing levels in operating suites and radiology departments may determine where they are best managed. Not all hospitals will have 24-h cover for interventional radiology procedures, while they will have emergency operating rooms.

In the longer term, as nephrostomy tubes can dislodge, many urologists would wish to convert their patients to a ureteral stent before discharge in any case, thus exposing them to a second procedure which would not have been needed if they were stented acutely. For some upper ureteral or ureteropelvic junction stones, a PCN may provide a convenient access point for a future percutaneous nephrolithotomy, although planning a convenient access route during an emergency PCN procedure is not always possible.

In conclusion, on current evidence, clinicians can be reassured that they may safely choose whichever upper urinary tract drainage method is most easily provided in their facility, as the outcome for their patients is likely to be equally good (Figure 14.1).

Technical aspects

All patients are appropriately resuscitated and, in the case of infected hydronephrosis, broad-spectrum intravenous antibiotics are given according to local microbiology department guidelines after cultures have been obtained. A coagulation screen is performed.

In our institution, PCN is the preferred initial management option in those without contraindications. This is performed under a local anesthetic or conscious sedation using a combination of ultrasound and fluoroscopy guidance. The patient is positioned prone on the fluoroscopy table and the skin prepared and draped. The kidney is identified on ultrasound and an entry point into the collecting system is selected. This is usually a posterolateral approach into one of the posterior calyces, as they tend to lie along a relatively avascular plane between the regions supplied by the anterior and posterior divisions of the renal artery. After infiltration of the proposed track with local anesthetic, a small incision is made in the skin. A 19 gauge sheathed needle

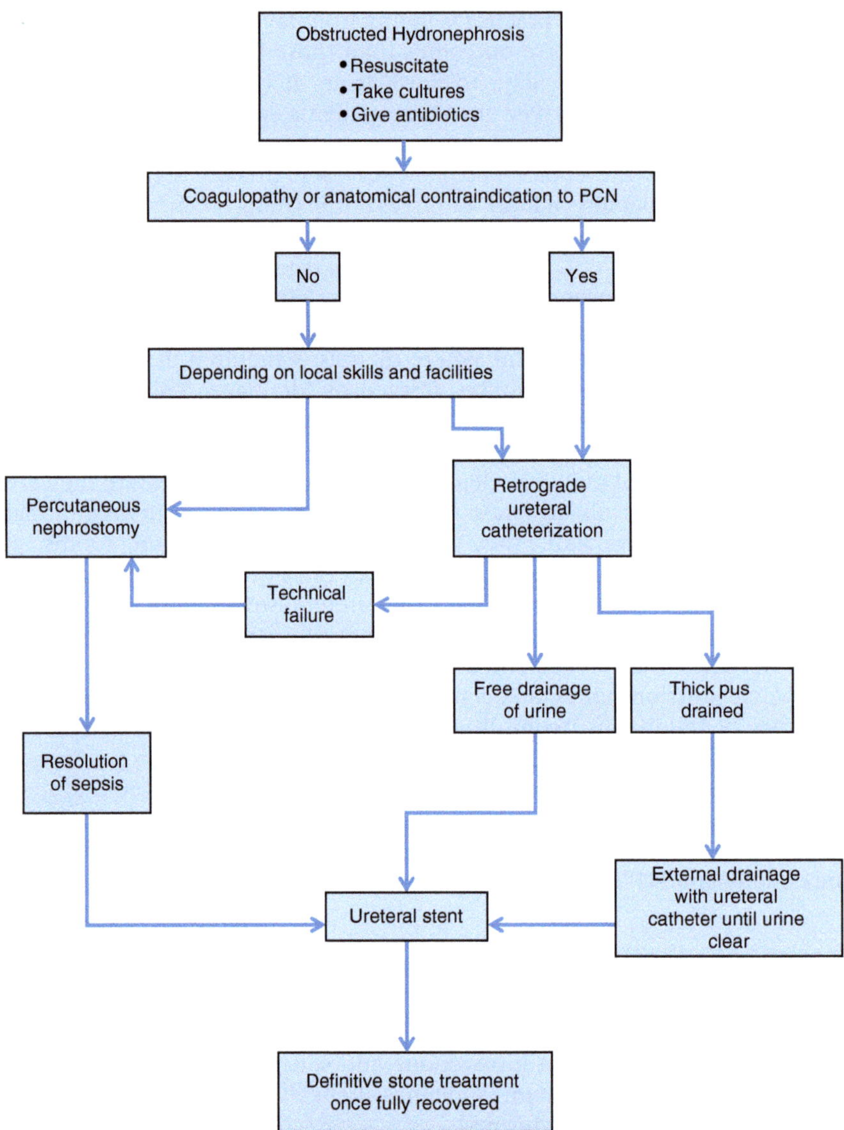

Figure 14.1 Algorithm for management of obstructive hydronephrosis.

is passed into the collecting system. In the obstructed system urine will usually drain through the needle when the collecting system is punctured. A small volume of contrast medium may be injected to confirm position on fluoroscopy if required. A 0.035 inch guidewire can then be coiled in the renal pelvis. Sequential dilation of the track is performed with fascial dilators until a 10F pigtail locking nephrostomy tube can be placed. The tube is securely fixed to the skin. Drained urine is sent for culture.

Formal nephrostogram and antegrade placement of a ureteral stent is delayed for 48 h or until the patient is stable and afebrile. The placement of an antegrade stent is especially useful if ureteroscopy is planned to treat the obstructing stone after the resolution of infection and the patient prefers not to have an indwelling nephrostomy. Less commonly, a nephrostomy is maintained to allow for percutaneous nephrolithotomy and/or antegrade ureteroscopy.

In the setting of obstruction, nephrostomy placement is typically made easier by the presence of hydronephrosis. Occasionally, the collecting system is not particularly dilated despite obstruction, making PCN more challenging. Other complicating factors include anatomical variants such as horseshoe or pelvic kidneys. In these cases or if the patient has an uncorrected bleeding diathesis, PCN is contraindicated.

If a nephrostomy cannot be placed, due to contraindications or availability of staff or equipment, a retrograde ureteral stent is inserted cystoscopically. We perform this under a general anesthetic with fluoroscopic guidance. The patient is placed in the lithotomy position, appropriately prepared and draped. A 0.035 inch guidewire is inserted into the ureteral orifice through a rigid cystoscope and Albarran bridge. This is advanced under fluoroscopy until coiled in the collecting system. We tend not to perform a retrograde pyelogram in the setting of sepsis provided the guidewire passes easily and into an appropriate position on fluoroscopy. This is to avoid the risk of overdistending the collecting system causing urinary extravasation and bacteremia. If insertion is not straightforward, however, a small volume of contrast should be instilled into the ureteral orifice through an open-ended ureteral catheter. This catheter can then be advanced to the site of the stone and used to stabilize a guidewire inserted through it, which should then pass the obstruction. An angle-tipped hydrophilic guidewire may be helpful in this situation; however, it must be replaced by a more secure PTFE guidewire as soon as access to the renal pelvis is obtained in order to reduce the risk of displacement.

Once a guidewire is securely placed, a relatively large-caliber (8 F) ureteral catheter is advanced over the guidewire above the obstruction into the renal pelvis and the guidewire removed to allow for drainage. This urine is sent off for culture and sensitivity analysis. If the urine is thick and foul-smelling, a single-pigtail catheter can be placed to allow for temporary external drainage of the infected kidney. The catheter can be flushed in the postoperative period with small volumes of saline to ensure adequate drainage, which is not always secure with an indwelling ureteral stent. Once the urine becomes clear and sepsis resolves, a stent can be placed using fluoroscopy with or without cystoscopy until definitive treatment is appropriate.

If the urine draining through the ureteral catheter is relatively clear, placement of a ureteral stent can be safely carried out. This is accomplished by advancing a 24 or 26 cm 6 F double-pigtail stent over the guidewire until the proximal tip can be coiled in the renal pelvis, ensuring a reasonable length is still present within the bladder as viewed through the cystoscope. Shorter stents are inadvisable if the renal pelvis and upper ureter are particularly dilated. Turbid urine will tend to drain through and around the stent. A urethral Foley catheter is placed at the end of the procedure. Placement of a stent may be complicated due to impacted stones or tortuosity of the ureter. An extra-stiff guidewire is occasionally needed to straighten out the ureter and allow for the stent to pass an impacted stone.

References

1. Türk C, Knoll T, Petrik A, Sarica K, Straub M, Seitz C. Guidelines on urolithiasis. European Association of Urology. Available at: www.uroweb.org/gls/pdf/20_Urolithiasis_LR%20March%2013%202012.pdf.
2. Goodwin WE, Casey WC, Woolf W. Percutaneous trocar (needle) nephrostomy in hydronephrosis. J Am Med Assoc 1955; 157: 891–4.
3. Rana AM, Zaidi Z, El-Khalid S. Single centre review of fluoroscopy-guided percutaneous nephrostomy performed by urologic surgeons. J Endourol 2007; 21: 688–91.
4. Radecka E, Magnusson A. Complications associated with percutaneous nephrostomies. A retrospective study. Acta Radiol 2004; 45: 184–8.
5. Wah TM, Weston MJ, Irving IC. Percutaneous nephrostomy insertion: outcome data from a prospective multi-operator study at a UK training centre. Clin Radiol 2004; 59: 255–61.
6. Watson RA, Esposito M, Richter F, Irwin RJ Jr, Lang EK. Percutaneous nephrostomy as adjunct management in advanced upper urinary tract infection. Urology 1999; 54: 234–9.
7. Farrell TA, Hicks ME. A review of radiologically guided percutaneous nephrostomies in 303 patients. J Vasc Interv Radiol 1997; 8: 769–74.
8. Sim LS, Tan BS, Yip SK, et al. Single centre review of radiologically-guided percutaneous nephrostomies: a report of 273 procedures. Ann Acad Med Singapore 2002; 31: 76–80.
9. Ramchandani P, Cardella JF, Grassi CJ, et al. Quality improvement guidelines for percutaneous nephrostomy. J Vasc Interv Radiol 2001; 12: 1247–51.
10. Zimskind PD, Fetter TR, Wilkerson JL. Clinical use of long-term indwelling silicone rubber ureteral splints inserted cystoscopically. J Urol 1967; 97: 840–4.
11. Sivalingam S, Tamm-Daniels I, Nakada SY. Office-based ureteral stent placement under local anesthesia for obstructing stones is safe and efficacious. Urology 2013; 81: 498–502.
12. Mokhmalji H, Braun PM, Martinez Portillo FJ, Siegsmund M, Alken P, Kohrmann KU. Percutaneous nephrostomy versus ureteral stents for diversion of hydronephrosis caused by stones: a prospective, randomized clinical trial. J Urol 2001; 165: 1088–92.
13. Pocock RD, Stower MJ, Ferro MA, Smith PJ, Gingell JC. Double J stents. A review of 100 patients. Br J Urol 1986; 58: 629–33.
14. Smedley FH, Rimmer J, Taube M, Edwards L. 168 double J (pigtail) ureteric catheter insertions: a retrospective review. Ann R Coll Surg Engl 1988; 70: 377–9.
15. Yossepowitch O, Lifshitz DA, Dekel Y, et al. Predicting the success of retrograde stenting for managing ureteral obstruction. J Urol 2001; 166:1746–9.

16. Pearle MS, Pierce HL, Miller GL, et al. Optimal method of urgent decompression of the collecting system for obstruction and infection due to ureteral calculi. J Urol 1998; 160: 1260–4.
17. Yoshimura K, Utsunomiya N, Ichioka K, et al. Emergency drainage for urosepsis associated with upper urinary tract calculi. J Urol 2005; 173: 458–62.
18. Bone RC, Balk RA, Cerra FB, et al. Definitions for sepsis and organ failure and guidelines for the use of innovative therapies in sepsis. The ACCP/SCCM Consensus Conference Committee. American College of Chest Physicians/ Society of Critical Care Medicine. Chest 1992; 101: 1644–55.
19. Joshi HB, Stainthorpe A, MacDonagh RP, Keeley FX, Timoney AG, Barry MJ. Indwelling ureteral stents: evaluation of symptoms, quality of life and utility. J Urol 2003; 169: 1065–9.
20. Nabi G, Cook J, N'Dow J, McClinton S. Outcomes of stenting after uncomplicated ureteroscopy: systematic review and meta-analysis. BMJ 2007; 334: 544–5.
21. Joshi HB, Adams S, Obadeyi OO, Rao PN. Nephrostomy tube or 'JJ' ureteric stent in ureteric obstruction: assessment of patient perspectives using quality of life survey and utility analysis. Eur Urol 2001; 39: 695–701.
22. Lynch M, Anson K, Patel U. Percutaneous nephrostomy and ureteric stent insertion for acute renal deobstruction. Consensus based guidelines. Br J Med Surg Urol 2008; 1: 120–5.
23. Sammon JD, Ghani KR, Karakiewicz PI, et al. Temporal trends, practice patterns, and treatment outcomes for infected upper urinary tract stones in the United States. Eur Urol 2013; 64: 85–92.

CHAPTER 15

Endoscopic Management of Lower Urinary Tract Calculi: Tips and Tricks

Christopher M. Dixon[1] *and Sean Fullerton*[2]
[1]Lenox Hill Hospital, New York, NY, USA
[2]New York Medical College, New York, NY, USA

Introduction

Lower urinary tract calculi represent about 5% of urinary calculus disease [1,2] and include primary and secondary bladder stones as well as prostatic and urethral calculi. Urinary diversion procedures such as various continent diversions and orthotopic neobladders are included. Although the treatment of most lower tract stones is straightforward, there are some challenging clinical scenarios that can be more effectually managed with the help of some "tips and tricks."

The tools available to the urologist for managing urinary calculi continue to expand. Endoscopic techniques and principles used to manage upper tract calculi can also be applied to the lower tract in many cases. For example, access to the bladder or a continent urinary diversion may be limited for anatomical reasons. The use of flexible scopes, percutaneous techniques, ureteroscopes, and imaging modalities in addition to the conventional rigid telescopes may be helpful in solving a particular clinical problem. The standard in most urology settings for fragmenting bladder stones has become the holmium laser, but other modalities including electrohydrolic lithotripsy (EHL), ultrasonic lithotripsy, pneumatic lithotripsy, shock wave lithotripsy, and mechanical lithotripsy (cystolitholapaxy) have all been used [3,4]. Worldwide access to holmium laser technology has not been achieved largely due to cost. This chapter will also provide some useful information in common and uncommon situations. While this chapter discusses "endoscopic management," it should be understood that even in today's minimally invasive surgical world, there are situations when lower tract calculi are most appropriately managed by simply making a cystotomy, reaching into the bladder and removing the stones intact [5,6].

Urinary Stones: Medical and Surgical Management, First Edition. Edited by
Michael Grasso and David S. Goldfarb.

Standard endoscopic techniques

Holmium laser

For bladder stones that are too large to simply irrigate or extract from the bladder, standard rigid cystoscopy using a holmium laser is generally the preferred treatment method. Anesthesia is required and the urine should be free of infection. A rigid cystoscope or continuous-flow cystoscope is preferred. Virtually all stones can be fragmented with the holmium laser. Machines that deliver higher wattage may allow more efficient treatment by allowing a higher rate of energy delivery. A larger laser fiber, 1000 μm, is also preferred to improve efficiency. An appropriately sized open-ended ureteral catheter can be used as a stabilizing sheath for the laser fiber if necessary. Laser safety credentialing is standard.

The stone is visualized endoscopically and the fiber placed in direct contact with the stone to initiate fragmentation (Figures 15.1, 15.2). Several strategies are used to fragment the stone, varying the power and delivery rate to optimize the procedure. The surgeon can choose to fragment the stone into several large pieces and then work on each piece separately, or try to maintain the stone as long as possible by fragmenting from the periphery of the stone circumferentially toward the center (Figure 15.3).

In addition to rate and power adjustments, the efficiency and speed of the procedure can be improved by maintaining visualization with proper irrigant flow and fragmenting during the drainage phase as long as visualization can be maintained. Frequent bladder irrigation with the bulb evacuator will remove fragments and avoid unnecessary lasing time.

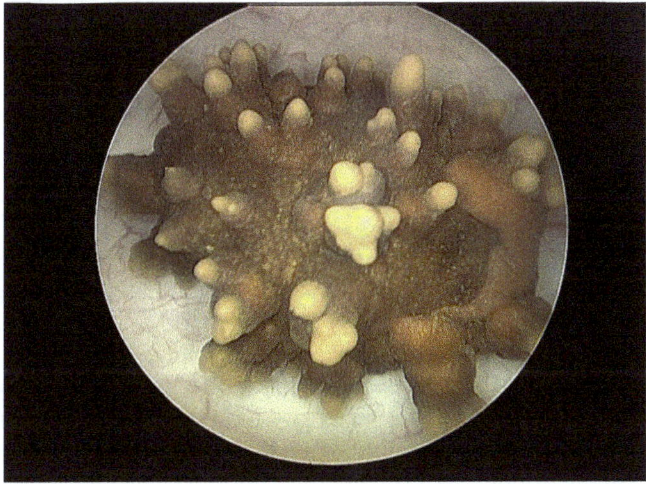

Figure 15.1 Endoscopic view of a classic "Jack stone" within the bladder (calcium oxalate).

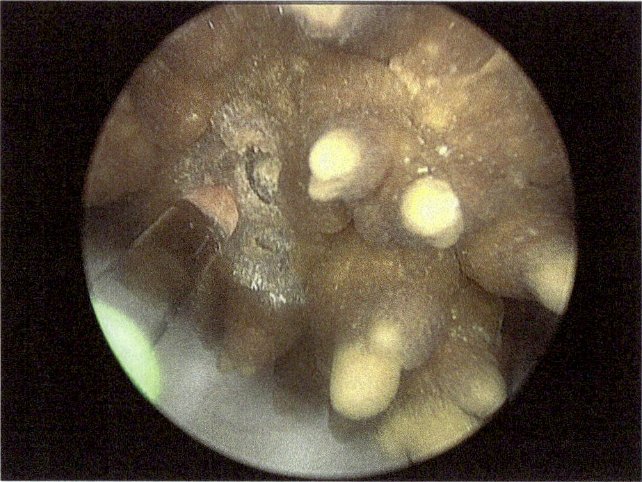

Figure 15.2 Proper endoscopic position of the 1000 μm laser fiber in contrast with the stone. The fiber is properly positioned just outside the scope to prevent scope or lens damage. The green fiber insulation is just visible. Note the lithotripsy has just started.

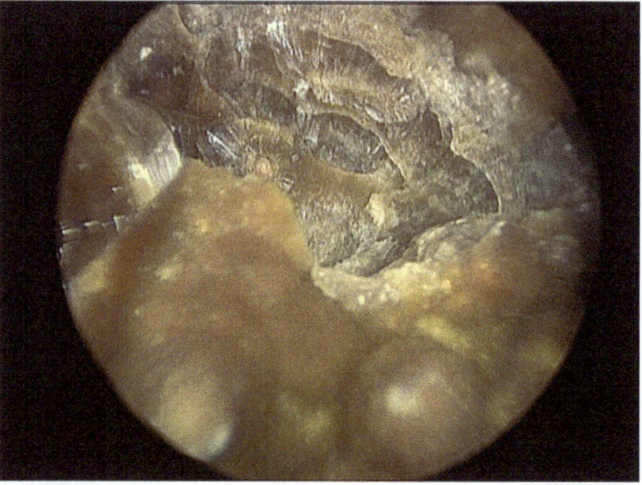

Figure 15.3 Fragmentation is being performed by laser lithotripsy approaching the stone's center and protecting the bladder by the outer stone shell.

Care must be taken as the holmium laser will damage the cystoscopic lens, perforate or incise the bladder or anything that comes in contact with it while activated (including guidewires). At high rates (>15/min), the fiber becomes a "scalpel" and the operator should be able to quickly disengage the laser should visualization suddenly diminish (irrigant runs out) or the patient moves due to light anesthesia.

If a stone is located in a diverticulum, it is best to move it into the bladder before lithotripsy, if possible. The diverticular wall is very thin (no muscularis propria) and it is much more likely that the bladder will be perforated should the active laser come in contact with the diverticular wall.

Cystolitholapaxy

This refers to the mechanical crushing of bladder stones and was commonly used prior to the advent of more efficient methods such as EHL and the holmium laser. Traditionally, the stone was engaged by a heavy lithotrite that would simply crush the stone by mechanical force between two metal jaws. The crushing force is supplied by the surgeon squeezing the device [7]. There is almost no reason to consider this option; however, a rather subdued form of litholapaxy can sometimes be helpful. This situation occurs when there are large, multiple "eggshell calcifications" as occur from the Foley balloon of an indwelling catheter. These types of calcifications are often too big and are shaped like "flakes," making them difficult to irrigate through the cystoscope sheath. While the laser will certainly fragment these "eggshells," a rigid grasper (lithotrite of sorts) can be used to rapidly crush the flakes into small pieces that are quickly irrigated. Using the laser to break these flakes into smaller pieces is tedious.

At the conclusion of these procedures, all fragments should be removed. This should be endoscopically confirmed, particularly if there are bladder diverticula or heavy trabeculations.

Bladder calculi

Bladder outlet obstruction (BOO)

Bladder calculi secondary to bladder outlet obstruction is the most common clinical scenario seen today [8]. The cause of the obstruction is most typically due to benign prostatic hyperplasia (BPH). Traditionally, the presence of bladder calculi was an indication to perform simultaneous stone removal and a prostate procedure to relieve the obstruction. The etiology was believed to be urinary stasis. With the widespread use of office bladder scan machines to measure postvoid residual volumes, questions regarding the relationship between urinary stasis and bladder calculi formation have risen. Many men with BPH have measurable urinary residuals yet only a small percentage develop bladder calculi. Recently, Childs et al. studied the pathogenesis of bladder calculi and urinary stasis [9]. In their prospective, comparative analysis, they suggested that patients with bladder stones were more likely to have a history of renal calculi and that multiple lithogenic factors, including metabolic abnormalities, may be important in addition to urinary stasis in the pathogenesis of bladder calculi.

In managing patients with outlet obstruction, the relevant clinical question is not so much removing the stones but whether or not to surgically intervene by performing a prostate procedure. The surgical risks of endoscopic stone removal are minimal compared to prostate procedures, particularly as prostate size increases and the procedure becomes more complicated. Although medical therapy for BPH has been shown to reduce the clinical progression of BPH, specifically symptom progression, urinary retention and the need for BPH-related surgery [10], this has not been established for bladder calculi, at least in part because it is such an uncommon event and would require an impractical sample size to study properly.

In uncomplicated cases of outlet obstruction due to BPH, it is reasonable to consider endoscopic stone removal without concomitant prostate surgery. With more complicated scenarios or more severe cases of BOO, for example, bladder stones with retention and/or hydronephrosis, common surgical sense dictates that an outlet procedure be performed [11].

Spinal cord injury

For a variety of reasons, the spinal cord-injured patient is at increased risk of both upper and lower urinary tract calculi [12,13,14]. Many of these patients are managed by intermittent catheterization or indwelling catheters which are frequently associated with active urinary infection or bacterial colonization. Prior to endoscopic treatment, every effort should be made to treat with culture-specific antibiotics to minimize the risk of procedure-induced sepsis.

In patients with transverse spinal cord injuries, typically above the sixth thoracic vertebra, monitoring for autonomic dysreflexia should be performed when distending the bladder such as occurs during endoscopic removal of bladder calculi. This syndrome of sympathetic discharge can result in life-threatening hypertension of rapid onset. Endoscopic procedures on the bladder should be done under a regional anesthetic or carefully monitored conditions.

Urinary diversion calculi

Calculi may form within continent urinary diversions and orthotopic neobladders due to urinary stasis, infection, retained mucus or anastomotic staples acting as a nidus for stone formation.

In these situations, calculi may be more difficult to treat due to access issues and stone location. Usually these are very capacious reservoirs, sometimes making it difficult to reach the stone. Flexible scopes may be helpful in these situations, as well as when there is concern that the continence mechanism could be adversely affected by larger, conventional rigid scopes. If access via the efferent limb or urethra is not possible or the stone is not reachable, percutaneous methods can be used. Care should be taken to be certain there is no overlying bowel in the planned percutaneous pathway. CT scanning preoperatively can help plan the percutaneous location [15]. Percutaneous access into the reservoir can be done with ultrasound guidance and the tract dilated using standard techniques. Oftentimes the old suprapubic tube site is acceptable because the reservoir has adhered to that location. The risk is inadvertent extravasation into the peritoneum or percutaneous injury to the intestines or adjacent organs. If uncertainty still remains, a standard open procedure should be performed.

If the etiology of stone formation can be determined, corrective measures may be worth attempting [16]. Irrigation of the reservoir, confirming adequate emptying, and eliminating infection are all simple measures that should be evaluated. Permanent sutures or staples used in the creation of the reservoir should be removed if it can be done without compromising the continence mechanism or being harmful in some other way.

Special situations

Trauma

Occasionally, months following traumatic rupture of the bladder due to external violence and pelvic fracture, bone fragments, spicules, or even orthopedic hardware will penetrate the bladder wall and either form additional stones or be taken for a bladder calculus. In this setting, there are several clues that will make diagnosis clear. The trauma history should raise suspicion and most often this occurs after an extraperitoneal bladder rupture that has been managed by catheter drainage alone. Plain radiographs and ultrasound may be confusing but computed tomography (CT) imaging and cystoscopy should be diagnostic and easily distinguish this situation from a classic bladder stone.

In these situations, a cystolithotomy and resection of the abnormal bone fragment (or orthopedic hardware) and bladder repair is required. Endoscopic management is useful in making the diagnosis but not in the treatment of this problem.

"Forgotten stent"

A retained or "forgotten" double-J ureteral stent can be challenging and often requires multiple procedures [17]. The bladder portion of the stone can be very large but usually can be rapidly fragmented with the holmium laser. If desired, once the stent is exposed, it can be cut with the laser to facilitate removal. Large stones may be adherent to the bladder which may limit visibility and risk bladder injury. In such cases, cystolithotomy may be preferred.

Unusual presentations

There are many unusual cases that have been associated with lower tract calculi, including erosions of an intrauterine device [18], calcified tumors including sarcomas [19,20], encrusting cystitis from *Corynebacterium* [21], and many self-inflicted foreign body devices in the psychiatric patient [8].

Prostatic urethral calculi

Prostatic calculi

True prostatic calculi form within the prostate tissue and are generally small and incidentally discovered on prostate imaging or at the time of transurethral prostate surgery. Most are composed of calcium phosphate and do not require any specific treatment.

Rarely, large calculi are seen embedded into the prostate and can be treated endoscopically. These may or may not be associated with BPH. Chronic infection, particularly with urease-producing bacteria, may cause such stones. Tuberculosis and schistosomiasis (in endemic areas) should be considered in these situations [22,23].

Endoscopic management is the best approach but may require several procedures to eradicate the stones. A combination of laser lithotripsy and transurethral resection may be required. The embedded stone can be fragmented and overlying tissue vaporized or incised with the holmium laser. Since the stone is contained within the prostate tissue, it is less mobile and can be more effectively fragmented. It may be adherent to the tissue which can cause bleeding and limit visibility. If the visibility and/or anatomy becomes unclear it may be prudent to abort the procedure and plan another attempt so as to prevent any complications related to urinary control or sexual function.

Post radiation

Transurethral resection or laser vaporization following radiation therapy for prostate cancer may lead to dystrophic calcification within the prostatic urethra. This is occasionally severe and difficult to resolve. It does not appear to occur if transurethral surgery is performed before radiation therapy providing there has been enough time for healing and re-epithelialization. It appears to be related to necrotic, coagulated, or poorly vascularized tissue in contact with the urinary environment. Although there is limited experience with this problem, repeated resection down to "fresh" tissue may allow re-epithelialization. This type of calcification becomes "part of the tissue" but can be scraped off the prostatic urethra initially without using any current. The risk of urinary incontinence and erectile dysfunction following repeated resections must also be considered.

Metal urethral stent

Expandable, endoscopically deployable metal alloy stents have been used for select patients with BPH and urethral stricture disease.

If the metal tines of the stent remain exposed to urine, stones will inevitably form and may cause symptoms of infection or obstruction. The clinical problem is dealing with these stones but not dislodging the stent in the process. This is particularly important because the Urolume™ (American Medical Systems) is no longer available for implant. Because the stones usually take some time to form (months to years), most of the stent is well embedded and covered with urothelium. The exposed portions of the stent are usually located at one end or the other. If it was implanted for BPH, it may have been placed or migrated with a small portion projecting into the bladder lumen. Rarely has it completely migrated into the bladder and remained long enough to form a stone of any significance. Most of these stones are <1 cm in size and are usually attached to the stent.

Endoscopically clearing the stones from the stent should be done carefully. If the stent has been overgrown with recurrent scar tissue, this must be dealt with first. Electroresection, staying within the lumen of the stent, can be done to clear the tissue ingrowth. This is best done with a pediatric resectoscope which can easily be maneuvered inside the stent lumen. Holmium laser resection is not recommended to remove the scar tissue because it will also cut the wires of the stent. Once the scar is cleared, however, the holmium laser is an excellent tool to fragment any stones as well as remove the portions of the stent that protrude from the urothelium in order to minimize stone reformation. The wire tines will cut very easily with the laser and any small pieces can be irrigated from the bladder along with the stones. Flexible scopes can also be used, including adult and pediatric sizes if necessary.

In the uncommon situation of a stent that has migrated into the bladder and remained long enough to calcify, standard holmium techniques can be used to fragment the stone and cut the stent into smaller pieces. A grasper and rigid cystoscope (or resectoscope sheath) can be used to engage the stent pieces and remove them. The stent should be brought through the rigid sheath, not the unprotected urethra.

New devices

With increasing innovation, various devices have been used within the urethra. Most recently, the Urolift® system is being developed for the treatment of BPH. This is a permanently implanted device that is designed to retract the lateral lobes of the prostate, thereby increasing the urethral lumen and reducing outlet obstruction. The urethral side of the implant epithelializes. Stone formation has not been reported but the device is still being studied in clinical trials [24,25,26].

Anterior urethral calculi

Urethral calculi include migrant stones from the bladder that become lodged in the urethra, those related to retained devices and those occurring in relation to urethral anomalies or previous reconstruction.

Migrant stones

Migrant urethral stones typically present with obstructive symptoms and may be palpable. If endoscopic manipulation is necessary, standard techniques used for removing ureteral stones can be employed. The use of a pediatric cystoscope facilitates working in the penile urethra and gentle, proximal urethral occlusion prevents proximal migration. Alternatively, the stone can be flushed or carefully manipulated back into the bladder and treated.

Urethral reconstruction

Stone formation following urethral reconstruction may occur due to obstruction, stasis, and/or infection. Although less common today, urethral reconstruction in the past often included the use of hair-bearing skin. The residual "urethral hair" serves as a nidus for infection and sometimes stone formation. Efforts to remove the hair should be considered. Urethral diverticula are uncommon but may occur after urethral reconstruction due to redundant flaps or distal obstruction leading to high-pressure voiding. Stone formation within the urethral diverticula may occur. Endoscopic management of this situation is generally not recommended except in cases where infection requires draining. Ultimately, open surgery is required to remove the stone and diverticulum and reconstruct the urethra. Care must be taken not to injure the reconstructed urethra resulting in the need for a more complicated urethroplasty in the future.

Summary

The vast majority of lower tract calculi can be managed endoscopically due to improved endoscopic access methods and in large part the use of holmium laser technology, which will fragment all stones with minimal injury to surrounding tissues. Where available, it has largely replaced the other modalities used in the past to treat lower tract calculi. Occasionally, more complex situations occur that require innovation and the use of new and established surgical stone removal techniques. The etiology of the stone should be investigated and corrective measures taken if practical.

References

1. Schwartz BF, Stoller ML. The vesical calculus. Urol Clin North Am 2000; 27(2): 333–46.
2. Papatsoris AG, Varkarakis I, Dellis A, et al. Bladder lithiasis: from surgery to lithotripsy. Urol Res 2006; 34(3): 163–7.
3. Philippou P, Moraitis K, Masood J, et al. The management of bladder lithiasis in the modern era of endourology. Urology 2012; 79(5): 980–6.
4. Wadhwa SN, Hemal AK, Sharma RK. Intracorporeal lithotripsy with the Swiss lithoclast. Br J Urol 1994; 74(6): 699–702.
5. Gallego VD, Beltran PJ, Perez MM, et al. Giant bladder lithiasis: case report and bibliographic review. Arch Esp Urol 2011; 64(4): 383–7.
6. Richter S, Ringel A, Sluzker D. Combined cystolithotomy and transurethral resection of prostate: best management. Urology 2002; 59(5): 688–91.
7. Mebust WK. Transurethral surgery: vesical lithoplaxy and lithotripsy. In: Walsh PC, Retik AB, Stamey TA, et al., eds. *Campbell's Urology*, 6th edn. Philadelphia: Saunders, 1992, pp. 2918–19.
8. Ho KV, Segura JW. Lower urinary tract calculi. In: Wein AJ, Kavoussi LR, Novick AC, et al., eds. *Campbell's Urology*, 9th edn. Philadelphia: Saunders, 2007, pp. 2663–73.
9. Childs MA, Mynderse LA, Rangel LJ, et al. Pathogenesis of bladder calculi in the presence of urinary stasis. J Urol 2013; 189: 1347–51.
10. McConnell JD, Roehrborn CG, Bautista OM, et al. The long-term effect of doxazosin, finasteride, and combination therapy on the clinical progression of benign prostatic hyperplasia. N Engl J Med 2003; 349(25): 2387–98.

11. Shah HN, Heade SS, Shah JN, et al. Simultaneous transurethral cystolithotripsy with holmium laser enucleation of the prostate: a prospective feasibility study and review of literature. BJU Int 2007; 99(3): 595–600.
12. Cameron AP, Rodriguez GM, Schomer KG. Systematic review of urological followup after spinal cord injury. J Urol 2012; 187(2): 391–7.
13. Gormley EA. Urologic complications of the neurogenic bladders. Urol Clin North Am 2010; 37(4): 601–7.
14. Welk B, Fuller A, Razvi H, et al. Renal stone disease in spinal-cord-injured patients. J Endourol 2012; 26(8): 954–9.
15. Catalá V, Sola M, Samaniego J, et al. CT findings in urinary diversion after radical cystectomy: postsurgical anatomy and complications. Radiographics 2009; 29(2): 461–76.
16. Stickler DJ, Fenely RC. The encrustation of blockage of long-term indwelling bladder catheters: a way forward in prevention and control. Spinal Cord 2010; 48(11): 784–90.
17. Veltman Y, Shields JM, Ciancio G, et al. Percutaneous nephrolithotomy and cystolithalapaxy for a "forgotten" stent in a transplant kidney: case report and literature review. Clin Transplant 2010; 24(1): 112–17.
18. Mustafa M. Erosion of an intrauterine contraceptive device through the bladder wall causing calculus: management and review of the literature. Urology Int 2009; 82(3): 370–1.
19. Pant-Purhit M, Lopez-Beltran A, Montironi R, et al. Small cell carcinoma of the urinary bladder. Histol Histopathol 2010; 25(2): 217–21.
20. Grubisic I, Lenicek T, Tomas D, et al. Primary osteosarcoma of bladder diverticulum mimicking intradiverticular calculus: a case report. Diagnost Pathol 2011; 6: 37.
21. Pagnoux C, Bérezné A, Damade R, et al. Encrusting cystitis due to Corynebacterium urealyticum in a patient with ANCA-associated vasculitis: a case report and review of the literature. Semin Arthritis Rheumatol 2011; 41(2): 297–300.
22. Khalaf I, Shokeir A, Shalaby M. Urologic complications of genitourinary schistosomiasis. World J Urol 2012; 30(1): 31–8.
23. Vilana R, Corachan M, Gascon J, et al. Schistosomiasis of the male genital tract: transrectal sonographic findings. J Urol 1997; 158(4): 1491–93.
24. Woo H, Chin P, McNicholas T, et al. Safety and feasibility of the prostatic urethral lift: a novel, minimally invasive treatment for lower urinary tract symptoms (LUTS) secondary to benign prostatic hyperplasia (BPH). BJU Int 2011; 108: 82–8.
25. Chin PT, Bolton DM, Jack G, et al. Prostatic urethral lift: two year results after treatment for lower urinary tract symptoms secondary to benign prostatic hyperplasia. Urology 2012; 79(1): 5–11.
26. Barkin J, Giddens J, Incze P, et al. UroLift system for relief of prostate obstruction under local anesthesia. Can J Urol 2012; 19(2): 6217–22.

CHAPTER 16
Ureteroscopy

Israel Franco[1] *and Lesli Nicolay*[2]
[1]New York Medical College, Maria Fareri Children's Hospital, Valhalla, NY, USA
[2]Loma Linda University Medical Center, Loma Linda, CA, USA

Since Ritchey described his experience with endoscopic management of a distal ureteral stone in 1988 [1], ureteroscopy has dramatically evolved as a feasible treatment modality in pediatric urolithasis. Over the last 20–30 years, advances in technology such as improved optics, miniaturized scopes, and the development of smaller ancillary instruments, including the holmium:YAG laser, have expanded the indications for ureteroscopy usage in the treatment of stones for the pediatric population.

Early retrospective studies have established that ureteroscopy can be safely performed in prepubertal children, reaching similar treatment efficacy to that of adults [2,3,4]. Al Busaidy's study of 43 prepubertal children undergoing ureteroscopy demonstrated that it is applicable to even the youngest children, with a reported 21% of treated children being under the age of 2 years and the youngest being 6 months old [5]. In a study comparing ureteroscopy to shock wave lithotripsy (SWL) for the treatment of distal ureteral stone treatment, de Dominicis and colleagues randomized 31 children to undergo either ureteroscopy or SWL with stone-free rates of 94% verses 43%, respectively, after one treatment [2]. Such success has not only proven ureteroscopy to be feasible but has lead to it being defined as the treatment of choice for children with distal ureteral stones [6,7].

In contrast, SWL has traditionally been the first line of therapy for most upper tract ureteral stones up to 15 mm and historically only SWL failures would be considered for upper tract ureteroscopy treatment [8]. However, the pendulum of stone management appears to be shifting towards expanding use for ureteroscopy in pediatric stone management. As more practitioners are performing ureteroscopy for the management of urolithiasis in children, many have reported data in various pediatric populations supporting the notion that ureteroscopy can also be safe and effectively used in the management of children with upper tract stones [9,10,11,12,13,14]. In a reviewed collection of literature, overall stone-free rates were reported to be 84–100% with acceptable complication rates comparable to the adult population [15].

Urinary Stones: Medical and Surgical Management, First Edition. Edited by Michael Grasso and David S. Goldfarb.

In one of the largest series, Kim and colleagues examined their data on 167 children undergoing flexible ureteroscopies, with 60% of stones found in the upper urinary tract, and 86% of those upper tract stones located intrarenally in the lower pole [16]. The results demonstrated clearance rates for stone burdens less than 10mm to be 100%, and only slightly decreased to 97% when stone burdens were greater than 10mm. Of note, however, on initial attempt to obtain retrograde access, 57% (95 of 167) could not do so and required placement of a ureteral stent for passive dilation for a period of 1–2 weeks. In contrast, Lesani and Palmer reported their experience with ureteroscopy access on 24 prepubertal children using graduated 4.5F to 6F or 8F rigid scopes [17]. Each procedure was performed without placement of a preoperative stent for passive dilation or performing active dilations at the time of the initial procedure. Twenty of the 24 (83%) children underwent successful rigid ureteroscopy while the remaining four (17%) were converted to flexible endoscopy and successfully completed without any intraoperative or postoperative complications and 100% of the children were rendered stone free.

With ever-broadening treatment indications, current recommendations suggest that it is reasonable to consider primary ureteroscopic management of stones up to 2cm [15]. A study supporting such recommendations reviewed 23 children with mean stone burdens of 17mm resulting in stone-free rates of 75% for renal pelvis calculi and 100% for polar stones [13]. However, there are limitations to treating large upper tract stone burdens. Tanaka and colleagues observed the outcomes of 50 children undergoing ureteroscopy for upper tract calculi. They reported that 71% of upper tract stones greater than 10mm required more than one procedure to obtain a stone-free state and that the stone-free rate for seven individuals with more complex stones, described as stones involving more than one calyx, was 14% [18].

As larger stone burdens are being attempted with ureteroscopic treatment, the utility of ureteral access sheaths has also been considered for children. Singh and colleagues reported their experience with eight children using ureteral access sheaths for stone treatment [19]. They confirmed the findings of the adult population that access sheaths not only enable treatment of large stones by facilitating repetitive upper tract access, but also reduce intrarenal pressures, decrease operative times, and improve stone-free rates. In young boys, the use of a sheath can reduce trauma to the urethra and potentially minimize the risk of stricture formation later on.

Accessing the upper tract can be one of the most challenging aspects of ureteroscopy and there is no unanimous consensus as to the best method of approach. Some advocate always placing a pretreatment stent for up to 8 weeks prior to definitive treatment while others place a stent only at the time of failed retrograde access [20]. The disadvantage to this approach is that the child will be exposed to an additional anesthetic. Conversely, we favor active dilations using either balloon dilation or co-axial dilators, enabling access at the time of treatment. However, this technique is not as commonly used in the pediatric population. The potential disadvantages with this technique are the risk of causing transient vesicoureteral reflex as well as ureteral perforation and stricture; however, such risks are thought to be relatively low and we have not experienced them [8]. After stone treatment, leaving an indwelling stent is equally as controversial. This decision is typically left up to the experience of the surgeon, considering factors such as operative time, number of scope passes into the ureter, and visible damage to the ureteral mucosa and ureteral edema. Additionally, a stent can be left in place with a string to prevent another anesthetic, and then removed in the clinic or by the parents.

Despite encouraging data on ureteroscopy, the results and utility should be interpreted with caution since there is a lack of prospective randomized studies which compare the various stone treatment modalities. Additionally, there is no consensus on how a stone-free status should be defined, adding further uncertainty to the interpretations and data comparisons that have been reported. Furthermore, some of the studies previously mentioned include individuals older than 18 years of age.

Relative contraindications to ureteroscopy include staghorn calculi, individuals with anatomical anomalies, prior failed endoscopic therapy, or a history of reconstructive surgery such as a bladder neck closure or cross-trigonal ureteral reimplant [15].

Most postpubertal children have close to adult body habitus and mass, allowing ureteroscopy to be approached similar to that of adults.

Equipment

It is essential in the pediatric population to have the appropriate sized ureteroscopic equipment that is not only familiar to all the operative staff, but also must be meticulously maintained. These instruments are small and fragile and require delicate handling during the sterile cleaning process to prevent the equipment from becoming damaged. Instruments must be routinely inspected to repair and replace worn parts as well as keeping each aspect of the instrument in optimal operating condition. In addition, prior to any surgical procedure, all required instruments must be pulled and inspected to ensure both availability and proper functionality. Inspection should include looking through all scopes to make sure there are no cracked lenses or damaged optics and manually deflecting all flexible ureteroscopes to confirm retained deflection.

There are two categories of ureteroscopes: the semi-rigid ureteroscope and the flexible ureteroscopy. The semi-rigid ureteroscope consists of an outer metal sheath that can range in size from 4.5 F to 10 F with working ports of 2.4–5 F. This scope is somewhat malleable, allowing for limited bending, provides a less distorted image with improved irrigation, and is more durable compared to the flexible scopes. The semi-rigid ureteroscope is ideal for use in the distal ureter; it can be more difficult to pass proximally, but in experienced hands it can be made to reach the kidney. In contrast, the flexible ureteroscope has a 6.8 F outer sheath and 1.8–3.5 F working port. Its advantage is that it has flexible properties that enable tip deflection up to 270°, making this an excellent tool for treating proximal and intrarenal stones. The disadvantage of the flexible ureteroscope is that it can be easily damaged if not used or maintained properly, and is more difficult to pass up into the ureter. When advancing the flexible ureteroscope into the ureter or passing wires and/or lasers through the working port, the scope must be in a straight and undeflected position to prevent damage to the scope.

Additional endourological equipment may include:

- rigid cystoscopes – 7.5–13 F
- guidewires and glidewires – 0.018, 0.025 and 0.035
- double J ureteral stent – 3, 4.8 and 6 F (internal diameter)
- open-ended catheters – 3–5 F
- balloon and co-axial ureteral dilators
- ureteral access sheaths – 9.5–11 F
- holmium:YAG laser.

Ureteroscopy technique

A preoperative urine culture demonstrating no bacterial growth is mandatory and must be obtained prior to every ureteroscopy. It is important to perform all ureteroscopic procedures under general anesthetic with paralytic agents to minimize the risk of movement that would potentially cause a catastrophic ureteral injury or perforation. Prophylactic IV antibiotics, aminoglycoside +/− ampicillin or first/second-generation cephalosporin dosed by weight of the child should be given within 60 min of endoscopy [21].

With the child in the lithotomy position, rigid cystoscopy (7.5 F or 17 F) may be performed to identify and inspect the bladder and ureteral orifices. The ureteral orifice is initially intubated either with a guidewire or open-ended ureteral catheter. Once the open-ended catheter (3 or 4 F) is in the distal aspect of the ureter, a retrograde ureteropyelogram can be performed with the aid of fluoroscopy to identify the location of the stone as well as mapping the anatomy of the renal pelvis. Next, a guidewire is advanced through the open-ended catheter until the wire is coiled in the renal pelvis, which is visually confirmed on fluoroscopy. If there is any difficulty passing the guidewire, an angled or straight hydrophilic glidewire may be used instead. A glidewire is much softer than other wires and able to maneuver around even impacted stones without the concern for perforation as with standard guidewires. Once a glidewire is in the renal pelvis, it can be exchanged for a standard or stiff wire through an open-ended catheter and may then function as a safety or working wire.

Access into the ureter can be attempted by direct passage of the semirigid or flexible ureteroscope aided by fluoroscopy to visualize the entry of the scope into the ureter. Direct visualization of the ureter is essential for passage of the rigid scope and in scopes which have an oblong shape, i.e.

Storz scopes, it is best to turn the scope 90° to facilitate entry into the ureter. Additionally, hydrodistension of the ureter can also help with passage of the rigid scope. If the ureteral orifice is tight and has not been prestented, co-axial dilation with 8/10 F dilators or balloon dilation may be used to help gain entry into the ureter. Some have reported a preference for co-axial dilation due to the tactile feedback providing a sense of resistance when using co-axial dilators compared to balloon dilation. If much resistance or difficulty is encountered during attempted dilation, it may be prudent to place a ureteral stent and plan to return for a second procedure rather than attempting to dilate more aggressively which can lead to ureteral injury and perforation. On the other hand, we have used balloon dilation almost exclusively and have not encountered any form of increased incidence of reflux or urinary tract infections (UTIs) related to transient reflux. Rarely, balloon dilation is not feasible and we will then stent the ureter and return a few weeks later and have always been successful with balloon dilation at that time.

Whether a semi-rigid or a flexible ureteroscope is used is based on the size and location of the stone as well as surgeon preference. However, regardless of which ureteroscope is used, it is important to maintain a safety wire to secure ureteral access throughout the procedure. For the flexible ureteroscope, in addition to the safety wire it is necessary to have a working wire to advance the flexible ureteroscope over to gain access into the ureter. The ideal wire for passing a flexible scope is a superstiff wire. This helps prevent kinking or bending as the scope goes up the ureter and can allow the scope to pass over bends in the ureter much more easily than softer wires. In cases where there is a large stone burden in the upper tract, a ureteral access sheath (9.5–12 F) may be used to facilitate repetitive re-entry of the flexible ureteroscope into the ureter and expedite stone removal. Isotonic irrigation solutions warmed to body temperature should be used during the entire procedure to prevent metabolic disturbances such as hyponatremia and hypothermia.

Holmium:YAG laser is the preferred energy source for stone fragmentation, but others are available such as ultrasonic lithotripsy or electrohydraulic lithotripsy. Care must be taken to keep an adequate space between the scope and the laser fiber or electroydraulic lithotripter since the ensuing shock wave and heat can damage these small fragile scopes. Small residual stone fragments may be extracted by baskets such as the flat or helical Nitinol tipless baskets (1.7–3 F). Judicious care must be taken while attempting removal of only small fragments to avoid entrapment of larger stone fragments in the ureter, ultimately risking ureteral avulsion. Whether a postoperative stent is left in place is up to the discernment of the surgeon. Factors to consider are duration of procedure, number of scope passes, need for ureteral dilation, and presence of ureteral trauma. If a stent is placed, it is reasonable to consider leaving a string in place and plan for stent removal at home by the parent or in the clinic after 3–7 days. If a stent is left without a string, it can be removed with a short anesthetic procedure.

Limitations and complications

If a simple ureteral perforation is identified, it is important to stop the procedure promptly and place a temporary ureteral stent. However, more significant injuries, including ureteral avulsion, may require immediate open repair and fortunately are only rarely reported. A large multi-institutional study from Turkey examined factors leading to complications in 642 children undergoing ureteroscopy. In this series, they reported the overall complication rate to be 8.4%, and the complications ranged from hematuria, pain, and UTI to obstruction and ureteral perforation requiring additional procedures. However, most complications were low grade and self-limiting. Multivariate analysis identified only operative time as being significantly associated with and affecting complication rates. Age, stone burden, stenting, ureteral orifice dilation or experience were not associated with the complication rate [22].

Percutaneous nephrolithotomy

Percutaneous nephrolithotomy (PCNL) was initially performed in adults and has since been established as a feasible treatment for large stone burdens. However, many practitioners were hesitant to perform PCNL in children due to concerns of using large, adult-sized instruments along with unknown long-term sequelae from performing such procedures on developing kidneys.

The first pediatric PCNL series, performed on seven patients described by Woodside and colleagues in 1985, reported encouraging results [23]. Larger series continued to support its success and feasibility [24]. However, most early series avoided performing PCNL on children less than 5 years of age due to concerns about potential injury to the kidney and associated compications [14]. Gunes and colleagues' data on PCNL treatment for staghorn calculi in children demonstrated that children younger than 7 years of age had a higher incidence of complications compared to older children [25]. However, many other studies have since reported acceptable outcomes, suggesting that both safety and efficacy can be maintained while using adult size instruments to perform PCNL on even very young children [26,27,28,29].

Early studies also explored the concerns of renal damage occurring as a result of PCNL being performed on the developing renal parenchyma. Nuclear renal scans were performed to evaluate the effects of PCNL in children. There was no evidence of PCNL leading to detrimental effects on renal parenchyma either by causing renal scarring or decreasing renal function [24,30]. In contrast to these studies, another report showed that renal scarring was observed in 5% of patients after PCNL. However, it should be noted that no preoperative scan was performed to enable the conclusion that the scarring was new and had occurred as a direct result of the procedure [31].

Despite the feasibility of PCNL using large, adult sized instruments on children, Jackman and colleagues engineered the Mini-PERC™ consisting of a 13 F ureteral outer sheath and 11 F inner sheath as an alternative to the adult sized intraments [32]. Miniaturizing the access has the theoretical advantages of decreasing tract injury to renal parenchyma, thus theoretically decreasing blood loss, increasing maneuverability and decreasing hospital stay. Their initial outcomes demonstrated stone-free rates of greater than 85% in children with a mean age of 3.4 years having stone burdens ≤2 cm [32,33]. The potential disadvantages of using smaller access include limited visibility in situations of bleeding, prolonged operative times and loss of stone extraction efficiency of very large stone burdens resulting from a smaller access tract. However, Dogan proposes that in selected cases, particularly those presenting with large stone burdens, using adult instruments might be more beneficial in optimizing stone clearance efficiency, decreasing operative time and exposure to fluoroscopy without increasing complication risk [34].

In reviewing the current literature, overall stone-free rates after PCNL are reported to range from 68% to 100%. However, achieving the higher stone-free rates may require the use of multiple access tracts and staged procedures in some instances [8,14,26]. An alternative to staged PCNL monotherapy is combining PCNL with either SWL or ureteroscopy for individuals with very large stone burdens.

There is no unanimous agreement on absolute indications for PCNL as the primary treatment modality used in children with urolithasis; rather there are only relative indications, which are similar to guidelines used in adults and include upper tract stone burdens greater than 15 mm, lower pole stone greater than 10 mm, stones resistant to SWL, stones composed of cysteine or struvite, and upper collecting system stones that have failed ureteroscopy. Additionally, individuals with abnormal anatomy or impaired urinary clearance or those who have undergone lower tract reconstruction such as cross-trigonal ureteral reimplants, bladder neck closure, or diversion will be best approached by PCNL [8,14,35,36].

As previously mentioned, complication rates from pediatric PCNL are similar to rates seen in adults. The type of potential complications may be quite broad and must be discussed prior to the procedure. However, the two most common complications encountered are bleeding, with possible need for transfusion in up to 24% of patients, and postoperative fever with or without UTI. Other complications include sepsis, extravasation, prolonged urine leak, and injury to surrounding structures causing pneumothorax, hydrothorax, and bowel injury. Factors affecting the risk of complications appear to be length of procedure, larger stone burdens, and increased number of tract dilations [14,35,37].

Percutaneous nephrolithotomy technique

When preparing for PCNL, certain steps must be taken to ensure a safe and effective procedure. First, every patient must have a negative preoperative urine culture. Particularly in cases of an infectious stone, a full antibiotic course following culture sensitivities must be administered and a repeat urine culture obtained after the completed treatment. Secondly, all radiological images must be judiciously reviewed. It is essential that the differentiation between staghorn calculi and medullary sponge kidney be determined. Medullary sponge kidney can be associated with nephrocalcinosis, but the important distinction is that the calcification will be outside the collecting system. Management for medullary sponge kidney is often through medical methods and it is not responsive to endoscopic treatment.

Prior to surgery, broad-spectrum IV antibiotics such as ampicillin and gentamicin should be given. The operating room should be prewarmed to keep the child's body as warm as possible for the duration of the procedure. Positioning is extremely important and should be done after the patient has been placed under general anesthesia. Initially, the child should be placed in the lithotomy position or for small children a "frog leg" position will enable cystoscopy with the advancement of an open-ended ureteral catheter into the collecting system to aid in localization and mapping of the upper tract for access. Once the ureteral catheter is in place, a Foley is inserted and left to gravity drainage. The ureteral stent is secured to the catheter to prevent the stent from becoming dislodged. The stent is then connected to a short sterile IV tube and it will eventually be draped sterilely into the field.

Next, the patient is repositioned into the prone position, taking care to pad all pressure points. Towel rolls or gel blocks are positioned vertically along the lateral aspect of the chest and abdomen in order to elevate the patient, creating a more natural position with the torso at approximately 30° to the bed. In children with spina bifida, contractures, and other spinal or bony structure abnormalities, positioning can be very difficult, hardware can interfere with fluoroscopic imaging and anatomy can be distorted, making access and potential for injury to surrounding structures even greater. In presurgical planning for a PCNL, it is important to know the extent of the patient's torso and extremities mobility in order to properly plan for variations in positioning and approaches. Additionally, one must be mindful of latex precautions in these individuals. The sterile connecting tubing is brought up into the field and it is connected to the dye-filled syringe, which will allow for visualization of the calyceal system. The initial image is captured and saved for reference throughout the procedure.

In deciding the appropriate calyx to access, it is best to choose one that will provide the shortest and most direct tract. For full staghorns and complex stones, multiple tracts may be needed, both to access the lower pole as well as a supracoastal approach into a posterior calyx for stones located in the upper pole. The advantage of the upper pole access is that in addition to enabling access to the superior calyx, it allows access to the renal pelvis, ureter and lower pole with minimal torque compared to other calyx approaches (Figure 16.1).

After the appropriate calyx has been selected, an 18 gauge spinal needle is used. With the needle perpendicular to the skin and using the 12th rib as a general landmark, the needle is advanced to the targeted calyx opacified by contrast which has been injected through the ureteral catheter and

(a)

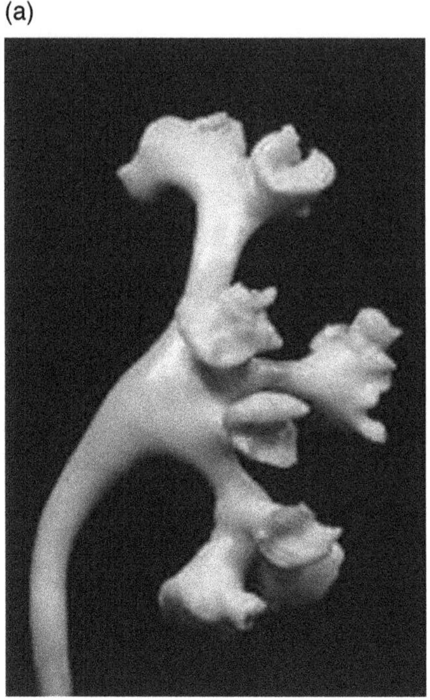

(b)

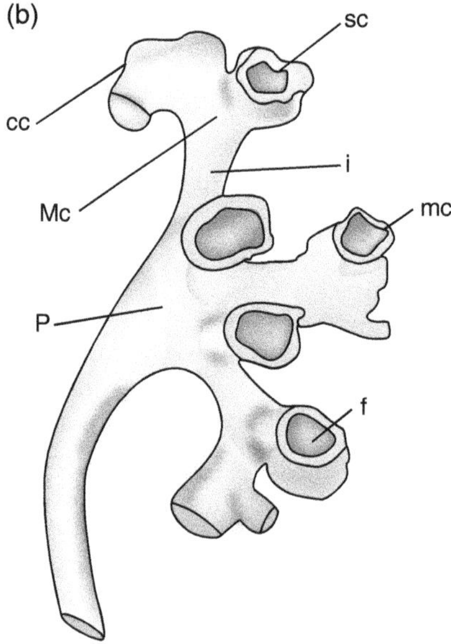

Figure 16.1 (a) Anterior view of left renal pelvicalyceal endocast from an injection-corrosion technique. (b) Schematic of left renal endocast with anatomical labels. cc, complex calyx; f, calyceal fornix; i, infundibulum; Mc, major calyx; mc, minor calyx; P, renal pelvis; sc, single calyx. Source: Sampaio FJB, Zanier JFC, Aragao AHM et al. Intrarenal access:3-dimensional anatomical study. J Urol. 1992: 148:1769–73. Reproduced with permission of Elsevier.

visualized by fluoroscopic guidance. Initially, the fluoroscopic head is placed at 90° to enable identification of the desired calyx, then the it is rotated to 30° from the vertical plan of the table to determine the depth of the puncture (Figures 16.2, 16.3, 16.4, 16.5). Urine or irrigation fluid should be aspirated from the needle to confirm the collecting system position. To

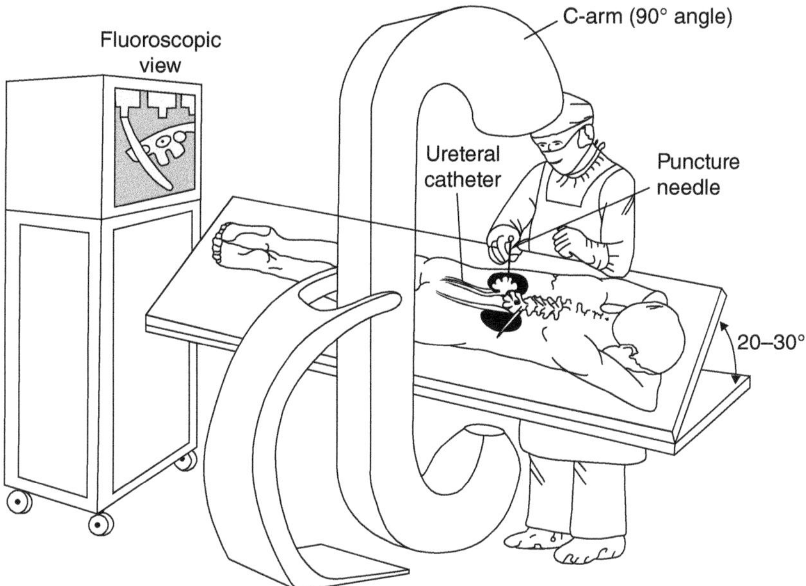

Figure 16.2 Proper adjustment of the fluoroscopic image at the start of the procedure is essential. Orientate the picture on the screen so that it corresponds exactly to the way the patient is lying and from the perspective the surgeon is looking at the patient.

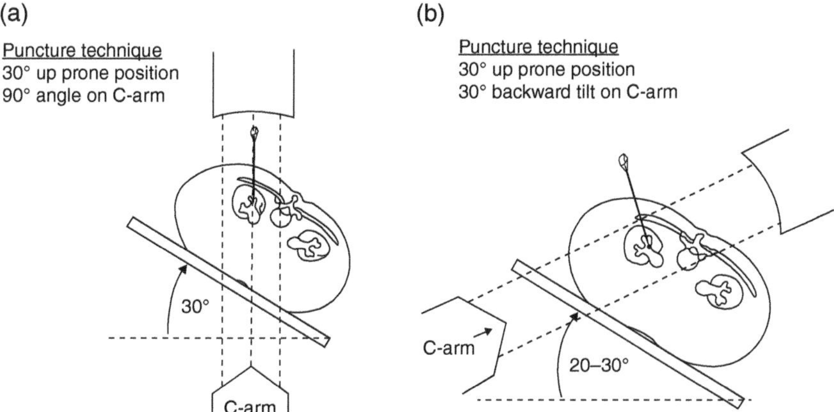

Figure 16.3 (a) Puncture technique with the patient in the 30° up prone position. (b) Rotate the fluoroscopic arm from 90° to 30° to provide the target calyx and depth of penetration.

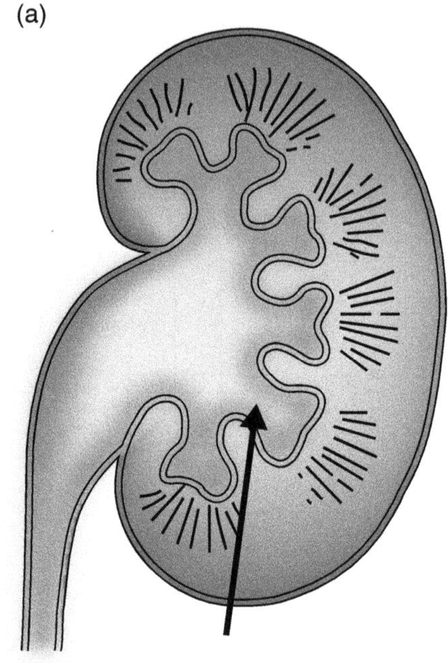

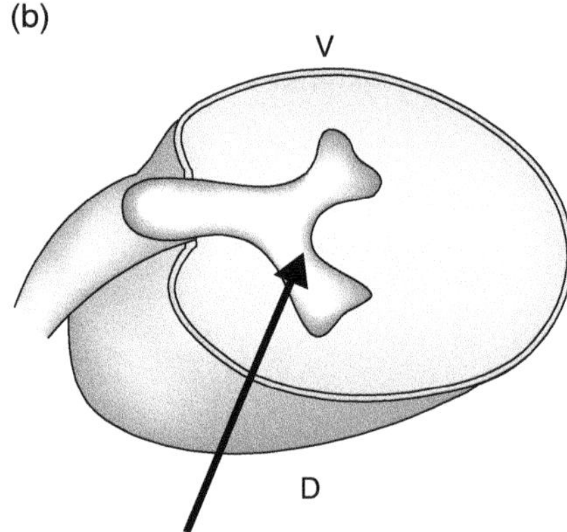

Figure 16.4 (a) Posterior and longitudinal view of right kidney demonstrating an incorrect puncture through the calyceal infundibulum (*arrow*). This puncture should not be done due to the risk of vascular injury. (b) Superior and transverse view of the right kidney also illustrating the incorrect puncture approach into the right calyceal infundibulum. Source: *Smith's Textbook of Endourology*, 3rd edn. Oxford: John Wiley & Sons Ltd, 2012. Reproduced with permission of John Wiley & Sons Ltd.

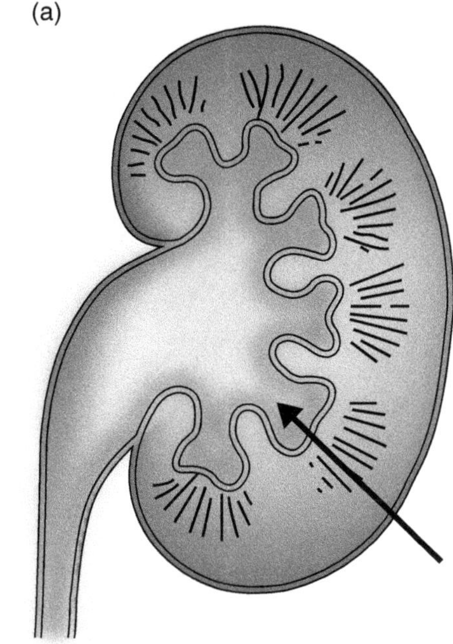

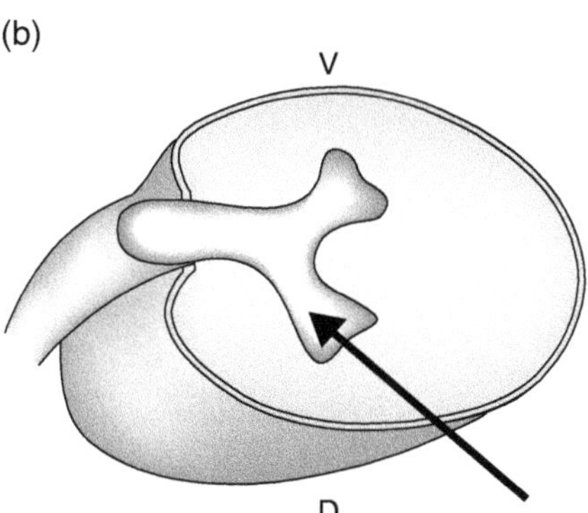

Figure 16.5 (a) Posterior and longitudinal view of right kidney demonstrating a puncture through the calyceal fornix (*arrow*). This puncture is safe and provides minimal risk of vascular injury. (b) Superior and transverse view of the right kidney also illustrating a puncture approach into the right calyceal fornix. Source: *Smith's Textbook of Endourology*, 3rd edn. Oxford: John Wiley & Sons Ltd, 2012. Reproduced with permission of John Wiley & Sons Ltd.

avoid injury to the kidney, the needle must always be pulled back out of the renal cortex prior to redirecting the needle (Figures 16.6, 16.7). An alternative to fluoroscopy is ultrasound guidance to localize the desired calyx with the benefit of minimal radiation exposure. Ultrasound can also

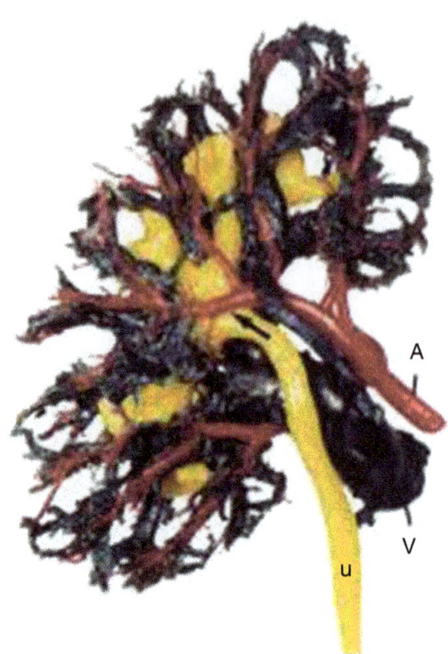

Figure 16.6 Posterior view of a left renal endocast and intrarenal arteries and veins. A, renal artery; V, renal vein; U, ureter. Source: Sampaio, FJB, Uflanker R, eds. *Renal Anatomy Applied to Urology, Endourology and Interventional Radiology*. Thieme, 1993. Reproduced with permission of Thieme Publishing Group.

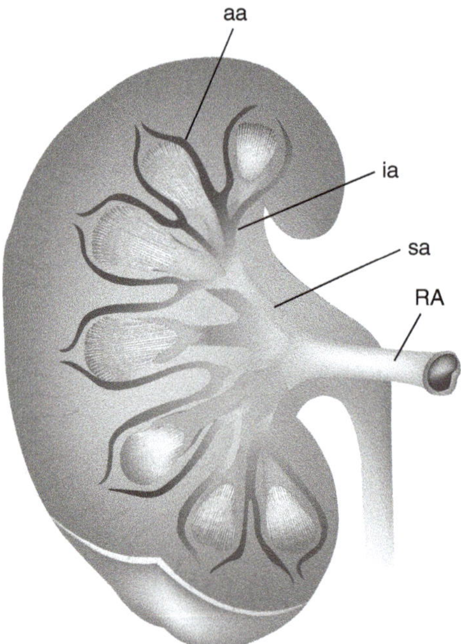

Figure 16.7 A renal diagram depicting the intrarenal structures. aa, arcuate artery; ia, interlobar (infundibular) artery; Ra, renal artery; sa, segmental artery. Source: Sampaio, FJB, Uflanker R, eds. *Renal Anatomy Applied to Urology, Endourology and Interventional Radiology*. Thieme, 1993. Reproduced with permission of Thieme Publishing Group.

be used if opacifying the collecting system is not feasible due to a complete obstruction.

Understanding the anatomical relationships of the kidney to adjacent structures is key to minimizing potential complications. For example, a puncture too lateral to either kidney may enter the bowel whereas a puncture too medial on the right may lead to an inferior vena cava injury. Additionally, it should be noted that the 12th rib in children is softer than that of adults, making it possible to inadvertently pierce or chip the rib if the surgeon is not fully aware of the location of the needle during puncture.

After the needle is confirmed to be in a good position in the desired calyx, a flexible-tipped guidewire is passed through the needle into the collecting system and down the ureter into the bladder. A Kumpe or Cobra catheter (Figures 16.8, 16.9) can be passed over the flexible guidewire to help direct the wire around difficult angles of the kidney, enabling easier navigation into the bladder. The puncture site in the skin is enlarged with a #11 blade and a dual-lumen 6–10 F catheter is passed over the wire into the ureter to enable passage of an Amplatz stiff wire into the bladder to act as the working wire.

Tract dilation can be performed by a variety of methods, depending on surgeon preference. Typically, the patient's age, anatomy and stone burden as well as the size of the working instruments are taken into consideration. Amplatz serial dilation can be used over the working wire followed by sheath placement under fluoroscopic guidance. However, in pediatric patients the kidney can be more mobile than in adults, potentially causing the kidney to be pushed away by the dilators rather than penetrating the

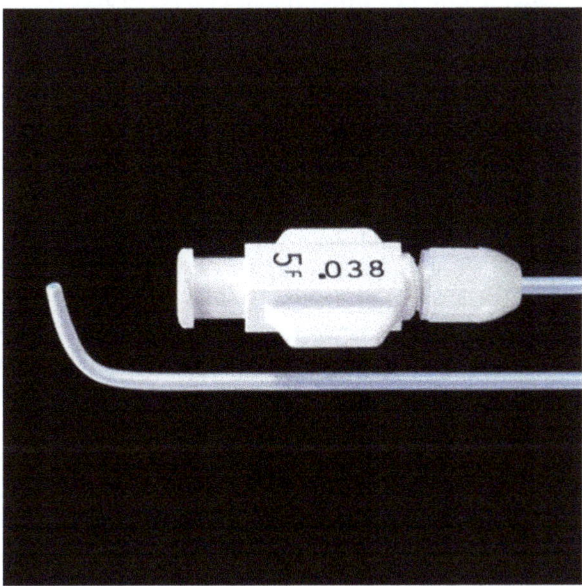

Figure 16.8 Kumpe catheter Source: Cook Urological Inc., Reproduced with permission of Cook Urological Inc, Bloomington, IN, USA.

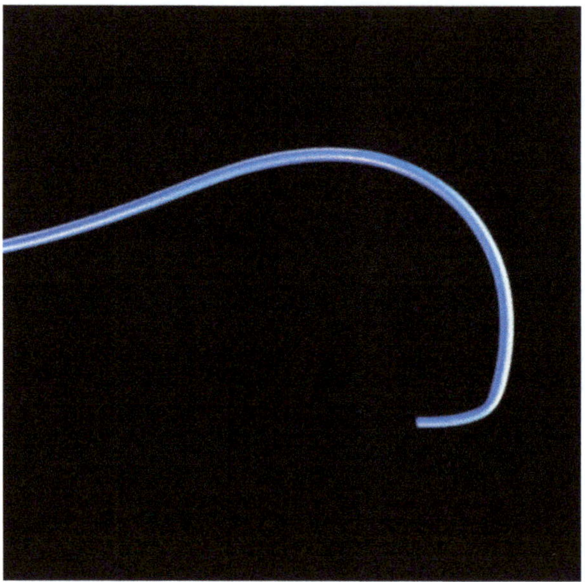

Figure 16.9 Cobra catheter Source: Cook Urological Inc., Reproduced with permission of Cook Urological Inc, Bloomington, IN, USA.

tract into the kidney appropriately. The Docimo Mini-PERC™ Entry set (Cook Urological Inc., Bloomington, IN) is a peel-away introducer that is passed over a guidewire under direct fluoroscopic visualization and results in a 13 F outer sheath and 11 F inner shealth for renal access (Figure 16.10). This approach requires the use of only pediatric sized equipment. Still another technique is using balloon dilation with either the Nephromax™ (Boston Scientific Corp., Natick, MA) or the Ultraxx™ (Cook Urological Inc., Bloomington, IN), which can dilate the tract up to 30 F. The balloon is inflated under fluoroscopic guidance and a sheath is passed over the inflated balloon. If smaller instruments are to be used, an 18 F ureteral balloon catheter can be employed with an appropriate sized sheath and this will work the same as the larger 30 F set (Figure 16.11).

After securing access, nephroscopy and stone treatment can then be performed. Nephroscopes as small as 15 F with a 6 F working channel are available. In addition, 7–9.5 F off-set cystoscopes with 5 F working channels and 7–9 F flexible ureteroscopes can be used through the Mini-PERC. Energy sources including electrohydraulic lithotripsy (EHL), holmium:YAG laser and ultrasonic lithotripsy can all be used. However, one advantage of ultrasonic lithotripsy is that in addition to fragmenting the stone, it also works with suction to evacuate the broken stone particles. This is extremely useful and helps reduce multiple passes in and out of the kidney. It also minimizes the risk of steinstrasse developing in the distal ureter.

Children are more sensitive than adults to both temperature changes and fluid shifts. Therefore, operative times should be limited to minimize environmental exposures leading to hypothermia. Additionally, all

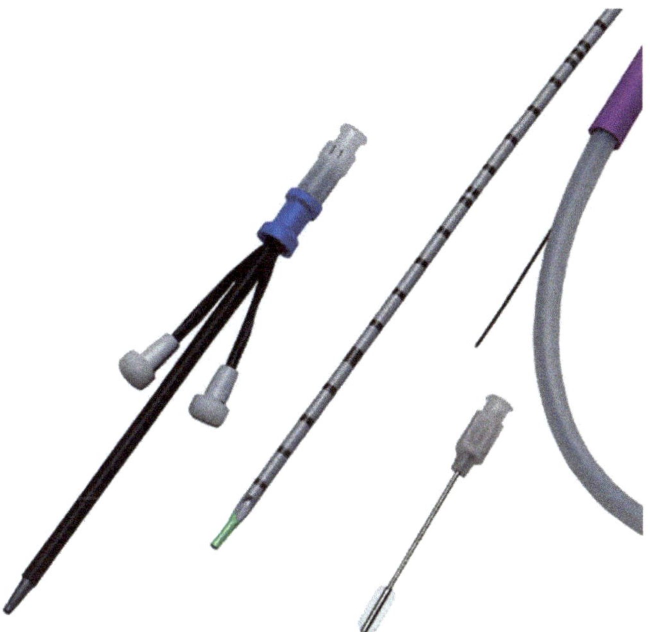

Figure 16.10 Docimo Mini-PERC™ Entry set Source: Cook Urological Inc., Reproduced with permission of Cook Urological Inc, Bloomington, IN, USA.

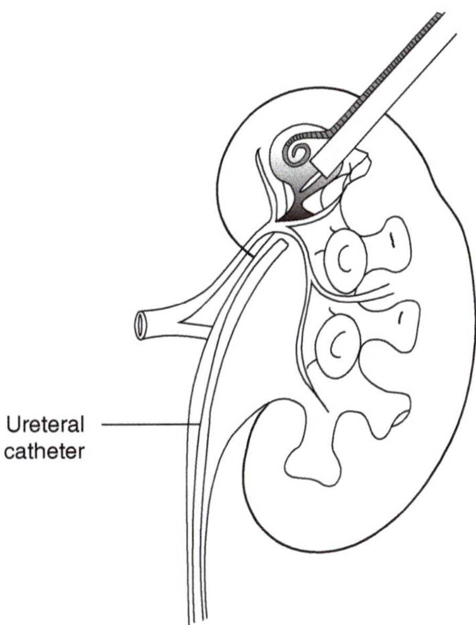

Figure 16.11 Calyceal anatomy with an upper pole access sheath and ureteral catheter in position.

irrigation fluids must be isotonic, warmed, and run with lower irrigation pressures to reduce the risk of hyponatremia.

Stent placement is left up to the discretion of the surgeon. Bilen and colleagues reported their success on 28 renal units treated with tubeless PCNL using the Mini-PERC, leaving only a ureteral catheter for diversion on preschool age children [38]. The mean age was 3.0 years (range 0.58–6 years) and mean stone burden was 1.9 cm. Outcomes were then compared to age-matched children undergoing standard PCNL. They reported that in the ubeless group, despite larger stone burdens, they had better stone-free rates, shorter operative times, and shorter hospital stays. Another recent, prospective randomized series of 23 patients under the age of 14 years reported data on completely tubeless PCNLs without any diversion, not even the ureteral catheter. Their findings also indicate the tubeless approach to be safe in selected pediatric patients with reports of decreased hospital stay and less analgesic use without an increase in complication rates [39]. Despite these promising data, larger prospective studies still need to be done.

Summary

Despite initial concern about performing PCNL in children and particularly the very young, PCNL has not only proven to be safe and effective, but has become an essential tool in the armamentarium of stone treatment for children. With the proven success of both adult and pediatric sized instruments, the case may be tailored to the surgeon's preference, equipment options and availability. Pediatric urologists must develop the skills and efficiency to perform PCNL with the growing number of children presenting with complex and large stone burdens.

References

1. Ritchey M, Patterson DE, Kelais PP, Segura JW. A case of pediatric ureteroscopic lasertripsy. J Urol 1988; 139(6): 1272–4.
2. De Dominicis M, Matarazzo E, Capozza N, et al. Retrograde ureteroscopy for distal ureteric stone removal in children. Br J Urol 2005; 95: 1049–52.
3. Bassiri A, Ahmadnia H, Darabi MR, Yonessi M. Transureteral lithotripsy in pediatric practice. J Endourol 2002; 16: 257–60.
4. Schuster TG, Russell KY, Bloom D, Koo HP. Ureteroscopy for the treatment of urolithiasis in children. J Urol 2002; 167: 1813–16.
5. Minevich E, Defoor W, Reddy P, et al. Ureteroscopy is safe and effective in prepubertal children. J Urol 2005; 174(1): 276–9.
6. Al Busaidy SS, Prem AR, Medhat M. Paediatric ureteroscopy for ureteric calculi: a 4-year experience. Br J Urol 1997; 80: 797–801.
7. Wu Hy, Docimo SG. Surgical management of children with urolithiasis. Urol Clin North Am 2004; 31(3): 589–94.

8. Hwang K, Mason MD, Peters CA. Clinical Practice: surgical approaches to urolithiasis in children. Eur J Pediatr 2011; 170: 681–8.
9. Tan AH, Al-Omar M, Denstedt JD, Razvi H. Ureteroscopy for pediatric urolithiasis: an evolving first-line therapy. Urology 2005; 65(1): 153–6.
10. Smaldone MC, Cannon GM, Wu HY, et al. Is ureteroscopy first line treatment for pediatric stone disease? J Urol 2007; 178(5): 2128–31.
11. Koura AC, Ravish IR, Amarkhed S, et al. Ureteroscopy stone management in prepubertal children. Pediatr Surg Int 2007; 23: 1123–6.
12. Cannon GM, Smaldone MC, Wu HY, et al. Ureteroscopic management of lower-pole stones in a pediatric population. J Endourol 2007; 21(10): 1179–82.
13. Dave S, Khoury AE, Braga L, Farhat WA. Single-institutional study on the role of ureteroscopy and retrograde intrarenal surgery in treatment of pediatric renal calculi. Urology 2008; 72(5): 1018–21.
14. Smaldone MC, Docimo SG, Ost MC. Contemporary surgical management of pediatric urolithiasis. Urol Clin North Am 2010; 37: 253–67.
15. Thomas JC. How effective is ureteroscopy in the treatment of pediatric stone disease? Urol Res 2010; 38: 333–5.
16. Kim SS, Kolon TK, Canter D, et al. Pediatric flexible ureteroscopic lithotripsy: the Children's Hospital of Philadelphia experience. J Urol 2008; 180: 2616–19.
17. Lesani OA, Palmer JS. Retrograde proximal rigid ureteroscopy and pyeloscopy in prepubertal children: safe and effective. J Urol 2006; 176: 1570–3.
18. Tanaka ST, Makari JH, Pope JC, et al. Pediatric ureteroscopic management of intrarenal calculi. J Urol 2008; 180: 2150–4.
19. Singh A, Shah G, Young J, et al. Ureteral access sheath for management of pediatric renal and ureteral stones: a single center experience. J Urol 2006; 175: 1080–2.
20. Hubert K, Palmer JS. Passive dilation by ureteral stenting before ureteroscopy: eliminating the need for active dilation. J Urol 2005; 174: 1079–80.
21. Wolf JS, Bennett CJ, Dmochowski RR, et al. Best practice policy statement on urologic surgery antimicrobial prophylaxis. J Urol 2008; 179: 1379–90.
22. Dogan HS, Onal B, Satar N, et al. Factors affecting complication rates of ureteroscopic lithotripsy in children: results of multi-institutional retrospective analysis by pediatric stone disease study group of Turkish Pediatric Urology Society. J Urol 2011; 186: 1035–40.
23. Woodside JR, Stevens GF, Stark GL, et al. Percutaneous stone removal in children. J Urol 1985; 134: 1166–7.
24. Mor Y, Elmasry YE, Kellett MJ, et al. The role of percutaneous nephrolithotomy in the management of pediatric renal calculi. J Urol 1997; 158: 1319–21.
25. Gunes A, Yahya UM, Yilmaz U, et al. Percutaneous nephrolithotomy for pediatric stone disease – our experience with adult-sized equipment. Scand J Urol Nphrol 2003; 37: 477.
26. Zeren S, Satar N, Bayazit Y, et al. Percutaneous nephrolithotomy in the management of pediatric renal calculi. J Endourol 2002;16: 75–8.
27. Salah MA, Toth C, Khan AM, et al. Percutaneous nephrolithotomy in children: experience with 148 cases in a developing country. World J Urol 2004; 22(4): 277–80.
28. Samad L, Aquil S, Zaidi Z. Paediatric percutaneous nephrolithotomy: setting new frontiers. BJU Int 2006; 97(2): 359–63.
29. Bilen CY, Kocak B, Kitirci G, et al. Percutaneous nephrolithotomy in children: lessons learned in 5 years at a single institution. J Urol 2007; 177: 1867–71.

30. Dwaba MS, Shokeir AA, Hafez AT, et al. Percutaneous nephrolithotomy in children: early and late anatomical and functional results. J Urol 2004; 172: 1078–81.
31. Samad L, Qureshi S, Zaidi Z. Does percutaneous nephrolithotomy in children cause significant renal scarring? J Pediatr Urol 2007; 3: 36–9.
32. Jackman SV, Hedican SP, Petters CA, Docimo SG. Percutaneous nephrolithotomy in infants and preschool age children: experience with a new technique. Urology 1998; 52(4): 697–701.
33. Jackman SV, Docimo SG, Cadeddu JA, et al. The "mini-perc" technique: a less invasive alternative to percutaneous nephrolithotomy. World J Urol 1998; 16: 371–4.
34. Dogan B, Atmaca AF, Canda AE, et al. Efficiency of percutaneous nephrolithotomy in pediatric patients using adult-type instruments. Urol Res 2012; 40(3): 259–62.
35. Dogan HS, Tekgul S. Minimally invasive surgical approaches to kidney stones in children. Curr Urol Rep 2012; 13: 298–306.
36. Farhat WA, Kropp BP. Surgical treatment of pediatric urinary stones. AUA Update Series 2007; 26(3): 22–7.
37. Ozden E, Mercimek MN, Yakupoglu YK, et al. Modified Clavien classification in percutaneous nephrolithotomy: assessment of complications in children. J Urol 2011; 185: 264–8.
38. Bilen CY, Gunay M, Ozden E, et al. Tubeless mini percutaneous nephrolithotomy in infants and preschool children: a preliminary report. J Urol 2010; 184: 2498–503.
39. Aghamir SMK, Salavati A, Aloosh M, et al. Feasibility of totally tubeless percutaneous nephrolithotomy under the age of 14 years: a randomized clinical trial. J Endourol 2012; 26(6): 621–4.

CHAPTER 17

Extracorporeal Shock Wave Lithotripsy in Children: Renal Stones

Jordan Gitlin and Kai-wen Chuan
North Shore-Long Island Jewish Health System, New Hyde Park, NY, USA

Introduction

The emergence of extracorporeal shock wave lithotripsy (ESWL) during the early 1980s transformed the minimally invasive nature of treating adult urinary stone disease. This trend toward employing endourological or extracorporeal approaches as first-line treatment is paralleled in the pediatric realm. In 1986, Newman et al. [1] reported the first series of ESWL experience in a pediatric population. They performed ESWL in 15 children between 3 and 17 years old for the treatment of upper urinary tract calculi and found that success was achieved in 93% of the cases (72% stone free and 21% insignificant fragments) without major complications. Since then, technological advances have led to the development of many different generations of lithotripters with features aiming to maximize the safety and portability of this treatment modality, while maintaining efficacy and improving complication rates. Recently, Onal et al. [2] analyzed the change in practice pattern in managing pediatric stone disease in a local Turkish urological center and clearly demonstrated a decreasing role for open surgery in this context. They found that of the 783 procedures performed between June 1987 and October 2010, 75.9% were open surgery before the introduction of ESWL, 29.7% after ESWL, and 6.1% after the introduction of percutaneous nephrolithotomy (PCNL).

Compared to treating adult patients with ESWL, special considerations regarding renal development, renal function, radiation exposure, rate of retreatment, and body habitus and positioning are of even greater importance in pediatric patients. As discussed by Ost and Schneck [3], ESWL monotherapy in children generally has superior success rates compared to adults, owing to softer stone composition, smaller relative stone volumes,

Urinary Stones: Medical and Surgical Management, First Edition. Edited by Michael Grasso and David S. Goldfarb.

increased ureteral complicance for fragment passage, and smaller body volume to facilitate shock transmission. In addition, Gofrit et al. [4] reported in 2001 that the pediatric ureter is at least as efficient as the adult for transporting stone fragments after ESWL. While ESWL has not been approved by the Food and Drug Administration (FDA) for use in children, it is not only a widely accepted treatment option but also one that brings encouraging results, particularly in the management of renal and proximal ureteral stones.

Renal functional outcomes after extracorporeal shock wave lithotripsy

Several reports published in the 1990s did not demonstrate meaningful renal functional changes in children after undergoing ESWL [5,6,7,8]. More contemporary data appear to be consistent. In 2001, Villanyi et al. [9]studied the biological effect of ESWL on the function of immature kidneys by following 65 children who were treated for stones over a 5-year period. Immediately before and at various time points after ESWL up to 3 months, serum and urinary electrolyte parameters, urinary enzyme activity, and the excretion of β2-microglobulin were measured. A significant elevation in the urinary excretion of aspartate transaminase (AST), alkaline phosphatase, lactate dehydrogenase (LDH), and β2-microglobulin was observed, indicating proximal tubular dysfunction and cell destruction. However, these enzyme levels returned to baseline within 15 days. Based on these results, the authors concluded that ESWL can induce functional damage, but the effects were transient. An effort should be made to minimize the number of shocks and energy intensity used. They recommended that an interval between two consecutive ESWL treatments should be at least 15 days.

In 2007, Wadhwa et al. [10] assessed renal functional outcome in 14 patients less than 13 years of age with dimercaptosuccinic acid (DMSA) scan and glomerular filtration rate (GFR) before ESWL and at 3- and 6-month follow-up. No renal units developed *de novo* scars on follow-up DMSA, and none of the children developed new-onset hypertension, proteinuria, or alteration in kidney size.

As some of the renal functional consequences from cellular damage, such as hypertension, may not manifest clinically immediately after ESWL, long-term follow-up is of particular importance. Over a 7-year period, Lottmann et al. [11] aimed to evaluate the potential effects on renal parenchyma using renal scintigraphy in 19 infants (range 5–24 months) done before and at least 6 months after the last session of ESWL. At mean follow-up of 36 months (range 8 months to 8 years), no hypertension was recorded, no acquired parenchymal damage was detected with conventional imaging, and no new real scars were seen on scintigraphy.

In a prospective fashion, Vlajkovic et al. [12] followed a larger series of 84 children of an older age (mean age 9.1 years) with renal functional scans and GFR measurements prior to, immediately after, and 3 months after ESWL. Repeat evaluation was again performed after an observation period of 12–67 months (mean 38 months). They found that while GFR was significantly lower immediately after ESWL compared to pretreatment measurements (107 versus 118 mL/min), these values returned to baseline at the 3-month visit and remained stable at the end of the observation period. This study again showed that ESWL is a safe treatment modality in pediatric stone patients without long-term demonstrable functional effects on the growing kidneys.

Intraoperative monitoring and surgical techniques

Anesthesia perspective

In order to better target stones and optimize shock wave delivery, it is often necessary to limit patient movements, which can represent a unique challenge in the pediatric population. For that reason, general anesthesia is administered in the majority of small children undergoing ESWL. With the development of modern, portable lithotripters that allow ESWL to be performed in the office or ambulatory setting, intravenous sedation has been reported to be successful in older, more co-operative children.

Several prospective randomized studies exist in the literature comparing the effects of different anesthetic agents on the recovery time, hemodynamic variables, and complications in children under going ESWL. Koruk et al. [13]compared dexmedetomidine-ketamine and midazolam-ketamine combinations in this setting, and found that patients in the dexmedetomidine group had a statistically significant shorter eye-opening time (9.3 versus 16.2 min), shorter verbal response time (12.8 versus 19.2 min), and shorter co-operation time (17.1 versus 23.3 min) while maintaining equal hemodynamic stability. With a similar study design, Eker et al. [14]reported that when compared to placebo, administration of intravenous paracetamol 30 min before the procedure reduced the amount of propofol-ketamine needed to achieve a Wisconsin sedation score of 1 or 2 (arouses to no consciousness or slowly to consciousness with sustained painful stimulus) and significantly shortened recovery time from 29.6 to 19.4 min. Lastly, Aldridge et al. [15] suggested that post-ESWL vomiting in children can be reduced more effectively with increased intraoperative analgesia than intraoperative antiemetic medications.

Case reports of ESWL-induced lung injuries have been previously described in the literature [16] and the clinical presentation usually includes hemoptysis. As a result, shock-absorbing Styrofoam sheets and altered mode of mechanical ventilation have been proposed as ways to protect lungs and manipulate lung-renal excursions during ESWL.

Ungated ESWL

Ungated ESWL is associated with cardiac arrhythmias in adults. The first report on the incidence of arrhythmias in children undergoing ungated ESWL came from Rhee and Palmer [17] in 2006. They evaluated eight consecutive children between 3.5 and 17 years of age (median age 13.5) undergoing 10 ESWL procedures for renal stones. Six (75%) patients received 3000 shocks, and the remaining two patients received 800 and

2200 shocks, respectively. No patients developed cardiac arrhythmias or other intraoperative complications or required conversion to gated ESWL, and the overall stone-free rate was 90%. Similar encouraging results were later demonstrated by Shouman et al.[18] in a larger series of 27 patients at a younger median age of 5 years. The median stone size in this series was 9.9 mm, and the average number of shocks delivered was 2500 per session. After 69 ungated ESWL sessions, again no cardiac arrhythmias or conversion to gated ESWL were seen.

The total number of patients included in these reports was small. While the safety of ungated ESWL in children was suggested, it was not definitively established. Therefore, we recommend that gated ESWL be performed whenever possible.

Indications for prestenting

After reviewing currently available literature, it appears that no strong evidence exists at this time advocating for or against pre-ESWL stent placement in children. In fact, the most recent AUA guidelines for the treatment of ureteral stones advise against the standard use of ureteral stents in adults. The theoretical benefits of prestenting in facilitating stone fragment passage and preventing steinstrasse need to be weighed against the potential side-effects of stent-related discomfort. While the decision to proceed with pre-ESWL stent is often a function of surgeon preference, common indications include stone in a solitary kidney, staghorn calculi, pre-existing ureteral obstruction, and anomalous anatomy.

Number and intensity of shocks

In an article published in the American Urological Association Update Series 2007, Farhat and Kropp [19] reported consensus practice patterns in treating children with ESWL regarding shock wave number and intensity. Treatment sessions should start at low-power settings, generally 17–22 kV depending on the machine used, and gradual incremental energy increase should apply in order to prevent stone migration. There are regional differences on limit of total shocks, but typically less than 3000 shock waves are delivered per session unless the patient is very young (less than 2000 shocks) or the fragmentation of stone, as evidenced by intraoperative imaging, is rapidly satisfactory. When comparing the outcome of ESWL in children and adults, Kurien et al. [20] reported that equivalent stone-free rate and efficacy quotient can be achieved in children using significantly few shocks (950 versus 1262) and less energy (11.83 versus 12.36).

Predictors of extracorporeal shock wave lithotripsy success

Size

Regarding stone size as a predictor for outcome after ESWL, results vary across series, with earlier reports showing lack of association and later reports showing worse outcome with increased stone size and burden. In 2003, Ather and Noor [21] analyzed the impact of renal stone size on stone clearance in 151 pediatric patients using the *International Classification of Diseases*, 9th edition (ICD-9) codes and ESWL registry. They found that the mean stone size in the treatment failure group was 15.9 mm and 14 mm in the stone-free group, indicating that treatment outcome is not adversely affected by increased stone size.

In contrast, Tan et al. [22] reported in 2006 that increased stone diameter and burden were the most significant factors that adversely affect the stone-free rate for renal pelvic stones after reviewing the records of 85 children treated with ESWL, stratified by stone location. More specifically, Habib et al. [23] reported in 2012 that the ESWL failure rate in children was significantly higher in stones greater than 3 cm in size and that the rate of auxiliary procedures increased in stones greater than 2 cm in size.

Therefore, it appears that stone size may have a greater impact on success rate when it is over 2 cm in diameter.

Location

Compared to stone size, the data on stone location as a predictor for ESWL outcome are more consistent, with the majority of studies pointing to lower pole as an unfavorable factor associated with lower stone clearance. In a retrospective review series, Ather et al. [24] investigated the effect of intracalyceal distribution of renal stones 20 mm or greater in size on fragment clearance. In four out of 21 pediatric patients who failed ESWL in this setting, two had stones exclusively in the lower pole calyx while the other two had stones in both lower pole calyx and renal pelvis. Based on this result, the authors recommended that large lower pole and partial staghorn stones with a major component in the lower pole calyx should be approached by a percutaneous method for removal and not ESWL. Focusing only on lower pole stones, Ozgur et al. [25] further identified mean lower pole infundibular length (but not width) and lower infundibulopelvic angle as factors significantly influencing stone clearance.

Age

While there are an abundant number of studies that examine stone-related factors, such as size and location, as predictors for stone clearance after ESWL, few exist that examine patient-related factors. Recently, Goktas et al. [26] evaluated the outcome of ESWL in children with renal stones in an age-dependent manner. One hundred and sixty-four children were divided into two groups based on age: Group I (n = 133, 0–6 years old) and Group II (n = 31, 7–15 years old).They found that the younger children had a significantly higher stone-free rate after the first session (67.6% versus 38.7%) and lower average number of ESWL sessions applied (1.6 versus 2.9), indicating younger age as a favorable predicator for shorter interval to stone-free status and fewer treatments needed to do so.

Nomogram

In recent years, validated nomograms for several diseases, such as prostate cancer, have gained popularity as predictive tools that can provide patient-specific risk estimation in an objective and evidence-based manner. In a parallel effort, Onal et al. [27] reported in early 2013 the first study-generated nomogram table and scoring system for predicting the stone-free rate after ESWL in children. These nomograms (Tables 17.1, 17.2) take into consideration age, gender, previous history of ipsilateral stone treatment, stone location, and stone burden, and they can provide useful information for clinicians when counseling patients and parents in the preoperative setting. This study was internally validated using the bootstrap method.

Outcomes in contemporary large series

The existing body of data reporting the complication, safety, and stone-free rates in the pediatric cohorts is largely descriptive in nature. The variability in lithotripter type, numbers of shocks administered, stone location, stone size, and definition of success makes direct comparisons among studies difficult to interpret. Table 17.3 summarizes the results of contemporary large series published in or after the year 2000 and including 100 or more patients. The average stone-free rate is approximately 80%, with a wide range of retreatment rates, with more recent studies showing a lower need for retreatment.

Special groups

Infants

After several previous studies demonstrated comparable results of ESWL in older children when compared to adults, McLorie et al. [28] devised the first study focusing on its use in children under the age of 3.5 years. Thirty-four children (36 renal units) with an average age of 23.4 months (range 6–40 months) underwent ESWL for an average stone size of 13 mm (range 4–22 mm). Overall success rate was 86%, with 66% achieved after a single session, and no major acute or long-term complications were noted. The authors also reported that modifications of the commercially available positioning device improved coupling and localization in smaller patients.

In 2007, Ramakrishnan et al. [29] reported another infant series with approximately half the average age and twice the patient number compared to McLorie's series. A total of 74 patients with an average age of 14.5 months (range 3–24 months) were treated by ESWL for an average renal stone size of 18.2 mm or an average ureteral stone size of 9.4 mm. At 3-month follow-up, there was an overall success rate of 97%, including 88% who were stone free and 9% who were asymptomatic with clinically insignificant residual fragments. Retreatment rate was 35%, and major complications occurred in five (7%) patients, including two complete ureteral obstruction

Table 17.1 Nomogram table for boys predicting the cumulative probability of stone-free status according to number of treatment sessions

History of previous treatment	Age at presentation	Number of session	Stone burden, cm^2		
			G1 (≤1)	G2 (1.1–2.0)	G3(>2.0)
			(%)	(%)	(%)
No	≤5 years	1	53	34	20
		2	75	53	34
		3	90	72	50
		4	94	78	57
	5–10 years	1	47	29	17
		2	69	47	29
		3	86	66	44
		4	91	73	51
	>10 years	1	42	26	15
		2	63	42	26
		3	81	60	39
		4	87	67	45
Yes	≤5 years	1	36	22	12
		2	57	36	22
		3	75	53	34
		4	81	60	39
	5–10 years	1	32	19	11
		2	51	32	19
		3	69	48	30
		4	76	54	35
	>10 years	1	28	16	9
		2	45	28	16
		3	64	42	26
		4	71	49	30

Source: Onal B, Tansu N, Demirkesen O, et al. 2013 [27]. Reproduced with permission of John Wiley & Sons, Ltd.

Table 17.2 Nomogram table for girls predicting the cumulative probability of stone-free status according to number of treatment sessions

History of previous treatment	Stone location	Age at presentation	Number of session	Stone burden, cm²		
				G1 (≤1)	G2 (1.1–2.0)	G3(>2.0)
				(%)	(%)	(%)
No	Pelvis or Upper Ureter	≤5 years	1	72	40	18
			2	98	79	46
			3	99.8	93	66
			4	99.9	99.4	87
		5–10 years	1	57	28	12
			2	92	64	33
			3	98	83	51
			4	99.9	96	73
		>10 years	1	42	19	8
			2	81	48	23
			3	94	68	37
			4	99.5	88	58
	Calix	≤5 years	1	62	32	14
			2	94	69	37
			3	99.3	86	55
			4	99.9	97	78
		5–10 years	1	46	22	10
			2	85	53	26
			3	96	73	41
			4	99.8	91	62
		>10 years	1	33	15	6
			2	71	39	18
			3	88	57	29
			4	98	80	47
	Mid or Lower Ureter	≤5 years	1	37	17	7

History of previous treatment	Stone location	Age at presentation	Number of session	Stone burden, cm^2		
				G1 (≤1)	G2 (1.1–2.0)	G3(>2.0)
				(%)	(%)	(%)
			2	75	43	20
			3	91	62	32
			4	99.0	84	52
		5–10 years	1	26	11	5
			2	60	30	13
			3	80	47	22
			4	95	69	38
		>10 years	1	18	7	3
			2	45	21	9
			3	65	34	15
			4	86	54	26
	Multiple	≤5 years	1	29	12	5
			2	64	34	15
			3	83	51	25
			4	96	74	41
		5–10 years	1	20	8	3
			2	49	23	10
			3	69	37	17
			4	89	58	29
		>10 years	1	13	5	2
			2	35	16	7
			3	53	26	11
			4	76	43	20
Yes	Pelvis or Upper Ureter	≤5 years	1	71	39	18
			2	97	77	45
			3	99.8	92	64
			4	99.9	99.2	85

(*Continued*)

Table 17.2 (continued)

History of previous treatment	Stone location	Age at presentation	Number of session	Stone burden, cm²		
				G1 (≤1)	G2 (1.1–2.0)	G3(>2.0)
				(%)	(%)	(%)
		5–10 years	1	55	27	12
			2	91	62	32
			3	98	81	49
			4	99.9	95	71
		>10 years	1	41	19	8
			2	79	47	22
			3	93	67	35
			4	99.4	87	56
	Calix	≤5 years	1	60	30	13
			2	93	67	36
			3	99.2	85	53
			4	99.9	97	76
		5–10 years	1	45	21	9
			2	83	51	25
			3	95	71	39
			4	99.7	90	61
		>10 years	1	32	14	6
			2	69	37	17
			3	87	56	28
			4	97	78	46
	Mid or Lower Ureter	≤5 years	1	35	16	7
			2	74	41	19
			3	90	60	31
			4	98	82	50
		5–10 years	1	25	11	5
			2	58	29	13
			3	78	45	21

History of previous treatment	Stone location	Age at presentation	Number of session	Stone burden, cm²		
				G1 (≤1)	G2 (1.1–2.0)	G3(>2.0)
				(%)	(%)	(%)
			4	94	68	36
		>10 years	1	17	7	3
			2	43	20	9
			3	63	33	15
			4	84	52	26
	Multiple	≤5 years	1	28	12	5
			2	63	32	15
			3	82	49	24
			4	96	72	40
		5–10 years	1	19	8	3
			2	47	22	10
			3	67	36	16
			4	87	57	28
		>10 years	1	13	5	2
			2	34	15	7
			3	52	25	11
			4	74	42	20

Source: Onal B, Tansu N, Demirkesen O, et al. 2013 [27]. Reproduced with permission of John Wiley & Sons, Ltd.

with sepsis, one partial obstruction, and two febrile urinary tract infections. Long-term follow-up data were available in 39 (52.7%) patients, and eight developed recurrent stones, two had stone growth, and one had mild hypertension without significant renal functional deterioration.

Overall, ESWL appears to be a relatively safe and effective treatment option for infants with stone disease.

Congenital anomalies

Data regarding the effectiveness of ESWL in treating stones located in a congenitally anomalous system vary. In 2006, Al-Tawheed [30] examined 25 patients with kidneys that were horseshoe in nature, ectopic, malrotated, duplicated, polycystic, or hypoplastic, who underwent ESWL with an average stone burden of 1.44 cm^3. Overall, 77.4% of renal units were completely cleared of stones, 6.5% were partially cleared, and 16.1% failed. The most prevalent anomaly in this series was horseshoe kidney, and there were nine patients with a total of 13 such renal units. Poor urine drainage and stasis are believed to be the major causes of stone formation rather than metabolic or genetic causes in this population [31]. Ten renal units (76.9%) were deemed successfully treated with ESWL, and those who failed subsequently required either open surgery or PCNL. Al-Tawheed et al. found their outcome to be comparable to patients with normal kidneys and concluded that most stones in kidneys with congenital anomalies may be successfully treated by ESWL as the first-line therapy.

By contrast, Nelson et al. [32] observed a statistically significant difference in the stone-free rate between children without and with a history of anatomical urological conditions or surgery, at 67% and 12.5%, respectively ($p<0.0001$). Accordingly, this group of authors advocated, and we agree, that children with congenital renal anomalies or previous genitourinary surgical history are best treated with modalities other than ESWL for their stones, such as PCNL.

Staghorn calculi

To evaluate the efficacy and parenchymal consequences of ESWL for staghorn calculi in children, Lottmann et al.[33] examined the outcomes of 16 young patients (5.5 months to 2 years old) and seven older patients (6–11 years old) who were treated for either complete (6) or partial (17) staghorn calculi. They found that infection was the main etiology behind stone formation and that in 21 (91.3%) patients, the stone burden was more than 20 mm. For the younger and older cohorts, retreatment rates were 31.3% and 42.8%, respectively. Overall stone-free rate was 82.6%. No steinstrasse or pyelonephritis was noted, and no parenchymal scarring attributable to ESWL was observed in the 6-month postprocedure DMSA scan.

In 2003, Al-Busaidy et al. [34] reported a similar overall stone-free rate of 79% at 3 months after ESWL in 42 children (9 months to 12 years old) with staghorn calculi. The cohort was substratified by pre-ESWL prophylactic ureteral stent status (19 without and 23 with). While the two subgroups were comparable in terms of age, stone size, and number of shocks, the authors reported that the unstented group had a statistically significant increase in major complications (21% versus 0%) requiring auxiliary procedures and longer hospital stay. They concluded that ESWL monotherapy was efficient in treating staghorn calculi in children and that its safety can be improved with pre-ESWL stenting.

More recently, Shouman et al. [35] from Egypt determined, in a prospective study, the safety and efficacy of ESWL as monotherapy for renal stones >25 mm in children. Twenty-four children with an average age of 7 years (range 2–14 years) underwent 53 ESWL sessions for an average stone size of 31 mm (range 25–35 mm). After delivering 3489 shocks on average per session with gradual incremental energy increase from 14 to 20 kV, an overall stone-free rate of 83.3% was achieved, as defined by no radiographic evidence of stone by post-treatment ultrasonography or kidney, ureter, and bladder plain films (KUB). The results were not stratified by stone composition. This study showed results consistent with previous work that ESWL is a high-effective first-line treatment for children with large renal stones. However, it is worth noting that the average number of shocks administered each session in this study exceeded the 2500 shocks outlined in the premarket FDA-approved study protocol for the Dornier company in 1983.

Inferior calyceal calculi

In order for stone fragments to pass from the lower pole after ESWL, they must be able to navigate the infundibulopelvic angle, which is relatively more difficult due to the sharp turn compared to other calyces. As a result, it is generally recognized in the adult population that the use of ESWL for treating stones in this location may be less efficacious, particularly for more sizeable stones. In 2012, Mandal et al. [36] retrospectively evaluated the effectiveness of ESWL for inferior calyceal stones less than or equal to 20 mm in size in 230 children and compared the results to their adult cohort of 1006 patients. All the perioperative parameters examined showed a favorable trend in children across the board, with higher stone-free rate (82.2% versus 40%), lower failure rate (0.8% versus 12.2%), lower retreatment rate (31% versus 65%), lower auxiliary procedure rate (5.2% versus 16.2%), and lower complication rate (5.6% versus 15%). The authors cited a few possible explanations to account for these differences based on anatomy and physics. First, the pediatric ureter is shorter, more elastic, and more distensible than that of an adult [37] and these features can promote easier fragment passage and prevent ureteral impaction. Second, the small body volume of a child translates into less energy loss as the shock waves travel through tissue, thereby facilitating energy delivery. Lastly, the lower kilo-voltage used in children may fragment stones into finer pieces and facilitate their passage. While ESWL for inferior calyceal stones in adults may remain suboptimal, it appears to be a reasonable option for children.

Cystine calculi

Stone composition is a known factor affecting the outcome of lithotripsy, and cystine stones are among the harder ones to break. Not surprisingly, the stone-free rate at 3 months after ESWL was found to be lower at 50% by Slavkovic et al. [38] when treating six children with cystine nephrolithiasis. In addition, these investigators noted that cystine stones located in the renal pelvis or ureter had a higher likelihood of elimination than those located in the renal calyces. In this particular group of patients, combination therapy with medical dissolution for retained fragments was effective.

Radiolucent calculi

Uric acid stones comprise a significant proportion of urinary stones, and their radiolucent nature does not preclude them from being effective targets of ESWL, especially when combined with medical therapy in the form of urinary alkalization. Mokhless et al. [39] were able to achieve 100%

stone-free rate in 24 children with average age of 6.3 years (range 2–12), who had radiolucent stones ranging from 12 to 65 mm, after 3 months of using combined ESWL and oral potassium citrate.

Summary

For the management of pediatric patients with upper tract renal urinary stones, ESWL is a valuable tool in the surgical armamentarium. It is a feasible, effective, and safe treatment modality across a wide spectrum of patient age, stone size, location, and composition. Children, compared to adults, have anatomical features that better facilitate stone fragmentation and passage after ESWL and therefore require fewer shocks and lower energy for comparable stone clearance. Factors predicting success or failure of the procedure are similar to those identified in the adult literature, and a newly developed nomogram is now available to provide risk estimation tailored to a specific individual. Current data do not highlight any evidence of long-term renal functional compromise on pediatric kidney after ESWL, but continued monitoring of blood pressure should be advocated.

Extracorporeal shock wave lithotripsy in children: ureteral stones

Extracorporeal shock wave lithotripsy for ureteral stones in children was first described by Newman et al. [1] in 1986. Since then, ESWL has become an accepted treatment option for the management of ureteral stones, in both adults and children as noted by the AUA Nephrolithiasis Guideline Panel [40]. However, it should be noted again that at the present time, ESWL is not FDA approved for use in children.

As in adults, when children present with ureteral stones, the first line of therapy should be observation with medical expulsive therapy (MET) or observation alone. Mokhless et al. [41] recently evaluated 61 children with ureteral stones up to 12 mm in size. With observation alone, they found a 64% rate of spontaneous passage and an average expulsion time of 14.5 days. However, when children were treated with α-blockers, there was an 87.8% stone-free rate, and the stone expulsion time decreased to 8.2 days. This 23% improvement in stone passage compares to similar results seen in adults receiving MET [42].

For the ureteral stone that does not pass spontaneously, or with MET, ESWL is a very reasonable option, particularly in children. As per d'Addessi [43], the pediatric ureter may have some inherent benefits with regard to stone passage following ESWL. These include a shorter ureter and a smaller body volume. Because of this, the shock waves can be transmitted with little loss of energy. Most importantly, though, the pediatric ureter is more elastic and distensible to allow passage of fragments. This was confirmed by Gofrit et al. [4] who found a 95%

stone-free rate in children following ESWL for renal stones, versus 78.9% in adults, again suggesting the improved ability of the pediatric ureter to pass stone fragments.

Is ESWL for ureteral stones safe?

In children, there is concern about the shock waves hitting surrounding structures. Several studies have addressed these specific issues. McCullough et al. [44] subjected rat ovaries to 1500 shocks at 20 kV. They then sectioned the ovaries and found no histological differences in either treated or untreated ovaries. Taking this evaluation even further, they performed unilateral oophorectomies, and subjected the remaining, contralateral ovaries to ESWL. All animals were allowed to mate, and all became pregnant. There were no differences in litters or fetal weights between the rats which received ESWL and those which did not. This suggests that ESWL does not cause damage to the ovaries in rats. Erturk [45] evaluated 10 women who were treated for distal ureteral stones with ESWL. They found that all women who later attempted to become pregnant following ESWL were able to do so, with 11 healthy babies being born. However, at this time, ESWL is not FDA approved for use in the distal ureter in women of child-bearing age.

In men, distal ureteral ESWL has been shown to cause a transient but reversible impairment in semen quality [46,47,48]. Both microscopic and macroscopic hemospermia can be seen, as well as decreased sperm density and motility. This is likely from transient damage to the seminal vesicles or ejaculatory ducts. These changes were not seen in men having upper tract ESWL, when the shock waves were directed away from the bony pelvis. However, all changes in sperm quality were transient and returned to normal by 3 months following ESWL. This suggests that any damage to semen from ESWL is transient and short-lived.

Is ESWL for ureteral stones effective?

The adult literature can provide some insight into the differences in ESWL and ureteroscopy for ureteral stones. The recent Cochrane review of ESWL versus ureteroscopy for ureteric calculi in adults found that "Ureteroscopy provided better stone free rates, but patients had to stay in the hospital longer, and there was a higher risk of complications" [49]. Patients following ESWL recovered faster, had fewer auxiliary procedures.

With regard to children, the EUA/AUA Nephrolithiasis Clinical Guideline Panel published its findings on the management of ureteral calculi in children. They did issue the caveat that, "The number of patients and available data were small, and did not support meaningful comparisons among treatment groups." However, they did report that ureteral ESWL may be more effective than what is seen in adults, due to the inherent benefits of the pediatric ureter, as described earlier.

While the number of studies available was small, ESWL compared favorably to ureteroscopy (URS) for proximal stones (81% ESWL stone free

Table 17.3 Comparison of ESWL and ureteroscopy for treatment of ureteral stones in children

Location	ESWL	Ureteroscopy
Proximal ureter	**81**%	**57**%
	<10 mm 90%	
	>10 mm 63%	
Mid ureter	**82**%	**80**%
	<10 mm 80%	
	>10 mm 96%	>10 mm 78%
Distal ureter	**80**%	**92**%
	<10 mm 86%	<10 mm 86%
	>10 mm 83%	

Source: Preminger GM, Tiselius HG, Assimos DG, et al. 2007 [40]. Reproduced with permission of Elsevier.

versus 57% URS). For midureteral stones, the numbers were similar (82% ESWL versus 80% URS). Interestingly, for midureteral stones greater than 10 mm, ESWL success approached 96%, compared to 78% for ureteroscopy. For distal stones, ureteroscopy appeared to offer improved success, with 92% stone-free rates, versus 80% for ESWL. Again, improved stone-free rates were seen when stones less than 10 mm were treated with ESWL – 86% stone free. Table 17.3 shows the stone-free rates for children based on stone location. Of note, with ESWL, approximately 1.3 primary procedures were required to render these patients stone free, compared to one primary procedure in the ureteroscopy group.

Complication rates were low, and did not seem to differ based on stone location. Ureteroscopy appeared to be associated with greater postoperative bleeding, but less postoperative pain. There was a 2% risk of obstruction, 2% risk of urinary tract infection (UTI), 1% risk of stricture, and 4% risk of sepsis within the ESWL group. These all compared favorably to ureteroscopy. Aboumarzouk et al. recommended that "Both ESWL and ureteroscopy are effective in this population. Treatment choices should be based on the child's size and urinary tract anatomy" [49].

More recently, Lu et al. [50] studied 115 children undergoing ESWL for ureteral stones. They had 53 proximal, 16 mid, and 43 distal ureteral stones, with a mean size of 7.4 mm and an average age of 7 years. Stone-free rates at 3 months were 94.8%, with a 15.7% retreatment rate. Patients were treated in both the supine and prone positions, and general anesthesia was only used in 26% of children. The overall stone-free rates at 3 months based on location were: proximal stones 96.2%, midureteral stones 87.5%, and distal ureteral stones 95.7%.

When the results were broken down based on size and location, stones less than 1 cm had the greatest stone-free rates and lowest need for retreatment. The retreatment rates were again highest for midureteral stones. Retreatment rates for proximal and distal stones less than 1 cm were 5.6% and 9.4% respectively. In this study, patients were retreated approximately 2 weeks from the initial therapy. The authors found that stone disintegration and clearance after ESWL were easier and earlier than in adults. This was attributed to the shorter, more elastic ureter. The authors also felt that the shock wave was less dampened as it traversed the smaller body of a child, leading to greater disintegration.

Even though the midureteral stone-free rates were lower, they were higher compared to results in adults. These authors felt that the success was enhanced because the bony pelvis in children has less density compared to adults, allowing easier localization and improved penetration of shock waves. Complications were rare, but 25% of patients did have gross hematuria post procedure. These authors felt that ESWL should be considered first-line treatment for ureteric stones in the pediatric age group. They did, however, warn that ESWL is not approved by the FDA for use in children, and that this needs to be discussed when counseling parents.

Muslumagolu et al. [51] evaluated 192 children having ESWL for ureteral stones. They used a standard technique starting at 13 kV and increasing up to 18 kV, with a maximum of 3500 shocks. They found an overall stone-free rate of 91%, but a 49% need for retreatement. When broken up based on location, the success was similar for each location (90–94%), but midureteral stones had the highest number of retreatments (80%), which may have been due to difficulties in localization. Complications were rare, and no patient developed dermal ecchymosis. Interestingly, 26% of patients did not receive any anesthesia. The remaining patients were split evenly, with 38% needing intravenous sedation and 35% requiring general anesthesia.

For the passage of stones following ESWL, α-blockers have been shown to be effective in adults. While there are no studies in children, the evidence is convincing. Zhu et al. [52] performed a meta analysis of seven randomized trials including 484 adults with both renal and ureteral stones who had ESWL and either did or did not receive tamsulosin. They found that there was a 19% pooled risk benefit with regard to clearance rate in the α-blocker group. There was an 8-day mean difference for expulsion times (favoring tamsulosin), and a lower pain and analgesia need for patients receiving tamsulosin.

What are the risk factors for ESWL failure?

Habib et al. [23] provide the only data looking at risk factors for children and ureteral stones treated with ESWL. There were 18 patients with upper ureteral stone, and they found that size greater than 1.35 cm was the greatest predictor of failure.

The remaining studies looking at risk factors for ESWL failures for ureteral stones have been done in adults. Pareek et al. [53] found that

ESWL success was related to lower Hounsfield units (HU) as seen on CT scan (577 HU versus 910). Delakas et al. [54] identified the following factors as being involved in ESWL failures: distal ureteral stones (located in the bony pelvis), stone size >1 cm, obstruction, and obesity (in adults). Salman et al. [55] had a large series of 468 adult patients, and found an 84% success for ureteral stones treated with ESWL but 50% required retreatment. They identified negative factors leading to ESWL failure: patients with stones in the distal ureter, stones with a transverse diameter of greater than 8 mm, and patients who were prestented.

Conclusion

Extracorporeal shock wave lithotripsy is a reasonable treatment option for the management of ureteral stones in children, with success rates above 80% for most stones. While some patients may require retreatment, the procedure is relatively non-invasive, safe, and low risk. Patients with coagulopathy, obstruction, active infection, or non-functioning kidneys should be excluded.

Key points

The procedure

- Check prothrombin time and partial thromboplastin, complete blood count and platelet count.
- Stop all aspirin and non-steroidal anti-inflammatory drugs 2 weeks before procedure.
- Check urinalysis and urine culture.
- Localize stone on ESWL machine before induction of anesthesia.
- Start therapy at low power, and increase – observe for fragmentation.
- Expect and prepare patients and parents for gross hematuria post procedure.
- Consider α-blockers post procedure.

The pediatric ureterShort

- Elastic
- Distensible
- Smaller body habitus may allow shock waves to be transmitted with little loss of energy

ESWL in children

- Safe and effective
- Lower risk of steinstrasse compared to adults
- Presenting is usually not necessary
- Effective in large renal stones

AUA Nephrolithiasis Guideline Panel 2007 statement on ESWL in children

"Both ESWL and ureteroscopy are effective in this population. Treatment choices should be based on the child's size and urinary tract anatomy. The small size of the pediatric ureter favors the less invasive approach to ESWL."

References

1. Newman DM, Coury T, Lingeman JE, et al. Extracorporeal shock wave lithotripsy experience in children. J Urol 1986; 136(1): 238–40.
2. Onal B, Citgez S, Tansu N, et al. What changed in the management of pediatric stones after the introduction of minimally invasive procedures? A single-center experience over 24 years. J Pediatr Urol 2013a; www.ncbi.nlm.nih.gov/pubmed/23313064 (epub ahead of print).
3. Ost MC, Schneck FX. Surgical management of pediatric stone disease. In: Wein AJ, Kavoussi LR, Novick AC, Partin AW, Peters CA, eds. *Campbell-Walsh Urology*. Philadelphia: Saunders, 2011, p. 3671.
4. Gofrit ON, Pode D, Meretyk S, et al. Is the pediatric ureter as efficient as the adult ureter in transporting fragments following extracorporeal shock wave lithotripsy for renal calculi larger than 10 mm? J Urol 2001; 166(5): 1862–4.
5. Corbally MT, Ryan J, Fitzpatrick J, et al. Renal function following extracorporeal lithotripsy in children. J Pediatr Surg 1991; 26(5): 539–40.
6. Thomas R, Frentz JM, Harmon E, et al. Effects of extracorporeal shock wave lithotripsy on renal function and body height in pediatric patients. J Urol 1992; 148: 1064–6.
7. Sarica K, Kupei S, Sarica N, et al. Long-term follow-up of renal morphology and function in children after lithotripsy. Urol Int 1995; 54: 95–8.
8. Goel MC, Baserge NS, Babu RV, et al. Pediatric kidney: functional outcome after extracorporeal shock wave lithotripsy. J Urol 1996; 155: 2044–6.
9. Villanyi KK, Szekely JG, Farkas LM, et al. Short-term changes in renal function after extracorporeal shock wave lithotripsy in children. J Urol 2001; 166(1): 222–4.
10. Wadhwa P, Aron M, Bal CS, et al. Critical prospective appraisal of renal morphology and function in children undergoing shockwave lithotripsy and percutaneous nephrolithotomy. J Endourol 2007; 21(9): 961–6.
11. Lottmann HB, Archambaud F, Traxer O, et al. The efficacy and parenchymal consequences of extracorporeal shock wave lithotripsy in infants. BJU Int 2000; 85(3): 311–15.
12. Vlajkovic M, Slavkovic A, Radovanovic M, et al. Long-term functional outcome of kidneys in children with urolithiasis after ESWL treatment. Eur J Pediatr Surg 2002; 12(2): 118–23.
13. Koruk S, Mizrak A, Gul R, et al. Dexmedetomidine-ketamine and midazolam-ketamine combincation for sedation in pediatric patients undergoing extracorporeal shock wave lithotripsy: a randomized prospective study. J Anesth 2010; 24(6): 858–63.
14. Eker HE, Cok OY, Ergenoglu P, et al. IV paracetamol effect on propofol-ketamine consumption in pediatric patients undergoing ESWL. J Anesth 2012; 26(3): 351–6.
15. Aldridge RD, Aldridge RC, Aldridge LM. Anesthesia for pediatric lithotripsy. Paediatr Anaesth 2006; 16(3): 236–41.
16. Tiede JM, Lumpkin EN, Wass CT, Long TR. Hemoptysis following extracorporeal shock wave lithotripsy: a case of lithotripsy-induced pulmonary contusion in a pediatric patient. J Clin Anesth 2003; 15: 530–3.
17. Rhee K, Palmer JS. Ungated extracorporeal shock wave lithotripsy in children: an initial series. Urology 2006; 67(2): 392–3.
18. Shouman AM, Ghoneim IA, ElShenoufy A, et al. Safety of undated shockwave lithotripsy in pediatric patients. J Pediatr Urol 2009; 5(2): 119–21.

19. Farhat WA, Kropp BP. Surgical treatment of pediatric urinary stones. AUA Update Series 2007; 26(3): 22–8.
20. Kurien A, Symons S, Manohar T, et al. Extracorporeal shock wave lithotripsy in children: equivalent clearance rates to adults is achieved with fewer and lower energy shock waves. Br J Urol 2009; 103(1): 81–4.
21. Ather MH, Noor MA. Does size and site matter for renal stones up to 30 mm in size in children treated by extracorporeal lithotripsy? Urology 2003; 61(1): 212–15.
22. Tan MO, Kirac M, Onaran M, et al. Factors affecting the success rate of extracorporeal shock wave lithotripsy for renal calculi in children. Urol Res 2006; 34(3): 215–21.
23. Habib EI, Morsi HA, Elsheemy MS. Effect of size and site on the outcome of extracorporeal shock wave lithotripsy of proximal urinary stones in children [published online ahead of print]. J Pediatr Urol 2013; 9(3): 323–7.
24. Ather MH, Noor MA, Akhtar S. The effect of intracalyceal distribution on the clearance of renal stones greater or equal to 20 mm in children after extracorporeal lithotripsy. BJU Int 2004; 93(6); 827–9.
25. Ozgur Tan M, Karaoglan U, Sen I, et al. The impact of radiological anatomy in clearance of lower calyceal stones after shock wave lithotripsy in pediatric patients. Eur Urol 2003; 43(2): 188–93.
26. Goktas C, Akca O, Horuz R, et al. Does child's age affect interval to stone-free status after SWL? A critical analysis. Urology 2012; 79(5): 1138–42.
27. Onal B, Tansu N, Demirkesen O, et al. Nomogram and scoring system for predicting stone-free status after extracorporeal shock wave lithotripsy in children with urolithiasis. BJU Int 2013; 111(2): 344–52.
28. McLorie GA, Pugach J, Pode D, et al. Safety and efficacy of extracorporeal shock wave lithotripsy in infants. Can J Urol 2003; 10(6): 2051–5.
29. Ramakrishnan PA, Medhat M, Al-Bulushi YH, et al. Extracorporeal shockwave lithotripsy in infants. Can J Urol 2007; 14(5): 3684–91.
30. Al-Tawheed AR, Al-Awadi KA, Kehinde EO, et al. Treatment of calculi in kidneys with congenital anomalies: an assessment of the efficacy of lithotripsy. Urol Res 2006; 34(5): 291–8.
31. Smith JE, van Arsdalen KN, Hanno PM, et al. Extracorporeal shockwave lithotripsy treatment of calculi in horseshoe kidneys. J Urol 1989; 412: 683–6.
32. Nelson CP, Diamond DA, Cendron M, et al. Extracorporeal shock wave lithotripsy in pediatric patients using a late generation portable lithotripter: experience at Children's Hospital Boston. J Urol 2008; 180(4): 1865–8.
33. Lottmann HB, Traxer O, Archambaud F, et al. Monotherapy extracorporeal shock wave lithotripsy for the treatment for staghorn calculi in children. J Urol 2001; 165(6): 2324–7.
34. Al-Busaidy SS, Prem AR, Medhat M. Pediatric staghorn calculi: the role of extracorporeal shock wave lithotripsy monotherapy with special reference to ureteral stenting. J Urol 2003; 169(2): 629–33.
35. Shouman AM, Ziada AM, Ghoneim IA, et al. Extracorporeal shock wave lithotripsy monotherapy for renal stones > 25 mm in children. Urology 2009; 74(1): 109–11.
36. Mandal S, Sankhwar SN, Singh MK, et al. Comparison of extracorporeal shock wave lithotripsy for inferior calyceal calculus between children and adults: a retrospective analysis – why do results vary? Urology 2012; 80(6); 1209–13.
37. Goktas C, Akca O, Horuz R, et al. SWL in lower calyceal calculi: evaluation of the treatment results in children and adults. Urology 2011; 78(6): 1402–6.

38. Slavkovic A, Radovanovic M, Siric Z, et al. Extracorporeal shock wave lithotripsy for cystine urolithiasis in children: outcome and complications. Int Urol Nephrol 2002–2003; 34(4): 457–61.
39. Mokhless IA, Sakr MA, Abdeldaeim HM, et al. Radiolucent renal stones in children: combined use of shock wave lithotripsy and dissolution therapy. Urology 2009; 73(4): 772–5.
40. Preminger GM, Tiselius HG, Assimos DG, et al. EAU/AUA Nephrolithiasis Guideline Panel. 2007 guideline for the management of ureteral calculi. J Urol 2007; 178(6): 2418–34.
41. Mokhless I, Zahran AR, Youssif M, et al. Tamsulosin for the management of distal ureteral stones in children: a prospective randomized study. J Pediatr Urol 2012; 8(5): 544–8.
42. Parsons JK, Hergan LA, Sakamoto K, et al. Efficacy of alpha-blockers for the treatment of ureteral stones. J Urol 2007; 177(3): 983–7.
43. D'Addessi A, Bongiovanni L, Sasso F, et al. Extracorporeal shockwave lithotripsy in pediatrics. J Endourol 2008; 22(1): 1–12.
44. McCullough DL, Yeaman LD, Bo WJ, et al. Effects of shock waves on the rat ovary. J Urol 1989; 141(3): 666–9.
45. Erturk E, Ptak AM, Monaghan J. Fertility measures in women after extracorporeal shockwave lithotripsy of distal ureteral stones. J Endourol 1997; 11(5): 315–17.
46. Sayed MA. Semen changes after extracorporeal shockwave lithotripsy for distal-ureteral stones. J Endourol 2006; 20(7): 483–5.
47. Andreessen R, Fedel M, Sudhoff F, et al. Quality of semen after extracorporeal shock wave lithotripsy for lower urethral stones. J Urol 1996; 155(4): 1281–3.
48. Martínez Portillo FJ, Heidenreich A, Schwarzer U, et al. Microscopic and biochemical fertility characteristics of semen after shockwave lithotripsy of distal ureteral calculi. J Endourol 2001; 15(8): 781–4.
49. Aboumarzouk OM, Kata SG, Keeley FX, et al. Extracorporeal shock wave lithotripsy (ESWL) versus ureteroscopic management for ureteric calculi. Cochrane Database Syst Rev 2012; 5: CD006029.
50. Lu J, Sun X, He L, et al. Efficacy of extracorporeal shock wave lithotripsy for ureteral stones in children. Pediatr Surg Int 2009; 25(12): 1109–12.
51. Muslumanoglu AY, Tefekli AH, Altunrende F, et al. Efficacy of extracorporeal shock wave lithotripsy for ureteric stones in children. Int Urol Nephrol 2006; 38(2): 225–9.
52. Zhu Y, Duijvesz D, Rovers MM, Lock TM. Alpha-blockers to assist stone clearance after extracorporeal shock wave lithotripsy: a meta-analysis. BJU Int 2010; 106(2): 256–61.
53. Pareek G, Armenakas NA, Panagopoulos G, et al. Extracorporeal shock wave lithotripsy success based on body mass index and Hounsfield units. Urology 2005; 65(1): 33–6.
54. Delakas D, Karyotis I, Daskalopoulos G, et al. Independent predictors of failure of shockwave lithotripsy for ureteral stones employing a second-generation lithotripter. J Endourol 2003; 17(4): 201–5.
55. Salman M, Al-Ansari AA, Talib RA, et al. Prediction of success of extracorporeal shock wave lithotripsy in the treatment of ureteric stones. Int Urol Nephrol 2007; 39(1): 85–9.

CHAPTER 18

Extracorporeal Shock Wave Lithotripsy: Generators and Treatment Techniques

Jessica E. Paonessa and James E. Lingeman
Indiana University School of Medicine, Indianapolis, IN, USA

Introduction

Surgical management of urinary calculi prior to the 1980s involved various open surgical techniques associated with significant morbidity and lengthy hospital stays. In the 1980s, the range of treatment options for stones was expanded to include extracorporeal shock wave lithotripsy (ESWL), ureteroscopy, and percutaneous nephrolithotomy [1,2]. ESWL was quickly approved by the FDA and gained rapid popularity among patients, providers, and payers.

The first human was treated with ESWL on 20 February 1980 by Dr Christian Chaussy, using an HM1 lithotripter produced by the German aerospace firm, Dornier [1,3,4]. However, the first commercially available lithotripter (HM3) was not introduced until 1984 [1,3]. That same year, Dr James Lingeman performed the first ESWL procedure in North America [5]. The widespread, rapid acceptance of ESWL can be attributed to its non-invasiveness, low morbidity, and excellent initial success rates (stone-free rates near 90%).

As ESWL evolved, newer generation lithotripters emerged offering the benefits of decreased cost, portability, and convenience. While newer devices proved to be more convenient, an increasing number of problems were identified [6,7]. Coupling issues first became apparent with the development of dry head lithotripters [8,9,10]. Efforts to achieve high peak pressures and narrow focal zones were found to produce greater tissue trauma and lower success rates [11,12,13]. The ability to treat stones at a faster rate was an attractive means of shortening procedure times, but later research demonstrated that stones break more completely at a slower treatment rate [14,15,16,17,18,19,20,21].

A great deal of research has been conducted in order to better understand how shock waves break stones as well as the advantages and disadvantages of the various generator types. Advances in our understanding

Urinary Stones: Medical and Surgical Management, First Edition. Edited by Michael Grasso and David S. Goldfarb.

of shock wave technology have revealed that the technique of shock wave delivery can have a dramatic impact on treatment success [11,22].

The demands of clinical practice make it difficult for most urologists to stay current on the large body of literature involving ESWL. However, it is important for the urologist to have a basic understanding of the principles of ESWL and a working knowledge of techniques to improve shock wave efficiency. This chapter aims to provide a concise review of ESWL principles including mechanisms of stone comminution, shock wave generators, and factors influencing ESWL outcomes. With a better understanding of ESWL, the urologist will be prepared to treat patients using the safest and most efficient methods.

Mechanisms of stone comminution

A shock wave is a short acoustic pulse (lasting ~5 μsec) generated by an energy source (Figure 18.1) [6]. Each wave begins with a positive pressure wave followed by a negative pressure wave. The positive component (or compressive phase) is characterized by an almost instant rise to a peak positive pressure of about 30–110 MPa, depending on the lithotripter and the setting. The negative component (or tensile phase) is of longer duration and lower amplitude (−5 to −15 MPa) [6,7].

Multiple theories have been developed to explain how shock waves break stones. Below is a brief summary of the established and most likely mechanisms resulting in stone fragmentation.

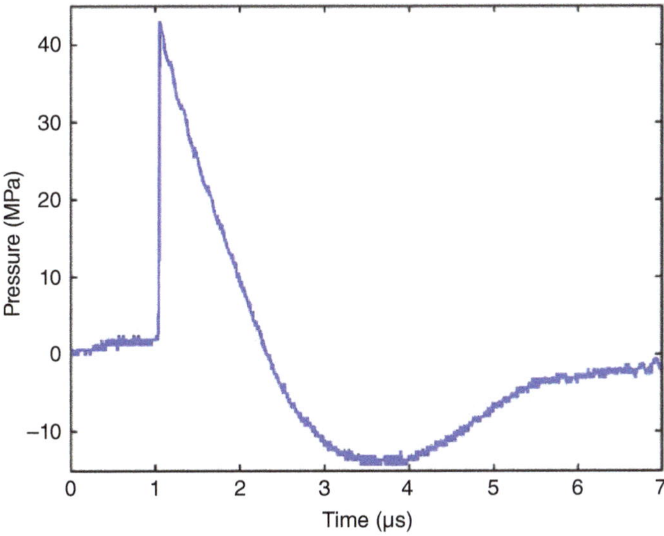

Figure 18.1 A pressure waveform measured at the focus of an electrohydraulic lithotripter (Dornier HM3). Source: Cleveland 2007 [6]. Reproduced with permission of PMPH- USA.

Spallation

According to this theory, shock waves enter the proximal surface of the stone, travel through the stone and are reflected at its distal surface. Tension is highest in the distal part of the stone, which causes a *spall fracture* to occur. Breakage occurs from inside and produces the initial spall fracture near the back wall of the stone [6,7,20].

Tear and shear forces

Impedance changes at the stone–urine interface create pressure gradients, which lead to the development of shear and tensile stresses in the stone. Pressure inversion occurs as shock waves are reflected, resulting in tensile stress which causes fragmentation at both proximal and distal ends of the stone. A similar action occurs within the stone at the interface of stone crystals and organic binders [6,7,23].

Cavitation

The negative pressure tail of the shock wave generates small bubbles in the fluid surrounding the stone. As the bubbles collapse, microjets of fluid impact the surface of the stone, causing cavitation-induced erosion. The collapsing bubbles also discharge secondary shock waves, which have an amplitude similar to that of the focused shock wave. Cavitation damage is greatest at the surface of the stone facing the incoming shock wave [6,7,20,23,24].

Quasi-static squeezing

Acoustic waves travel faster through the stone than through the fluid surrounding the stone, resulting in shear stresses. In order for quasi-static squeezing to be effective, the focal zone must have a larger diameter than that of the stone [7,11,24,25].

Dynamic squeezing

This theory hypothesizes that squeezing waves on the outside of the stone induce further shear waves within the stone, resulting in stone fragmentation [7,25].

Fatigue

All renal calculi have small imperfections which become areas of "stress concentrations" during exposure to repetitive shock waves. The sites of imperfection develop into microcracks which expand into macrocracks as subsequent shock waves are applied. The progressive evolution of cracks is the primary characteristic of fatigue and can take place anywhere in the stone [6,7,26].

Shock wave generators

Lithotripters are classified based on the energy source used to produce shock waves. The three principal types of generators are electrohydraulic, electromagnetic, and piezoelectric. Regardless of the type of generator used, all lithotripters share some basic characteristics: an energy source, a shock wave focusing mechanism, a coupling medium, and a system for localizing the target [22].

Electrohydraulic generators

These utilize a spark source to create shock waves (Figure 18.2). The spark source is positioned at the focus (F1) of an ellipsoidal reflector. Energy from the spark source is reflected off the walls of the ellipsoidal reflector, which focuses the acoustic energy to the *focal point,* a region in space, otherwise known as F2. Proper positioning of the spark source at F1 is critical for focusing the shock wave. Reduced ability to focus the shock wave can occur if the spark source is misaligned by even a few millimeters [3,6].

Advantages	Disadvantages
Broad focal zone	Substantial variation in the amplitude of the shock wave from shock to shock
Low peak positive pressures	Shifting in the position of the focal zone
Efficient stone comminution	Electrode (spark plug) has a short lifespan

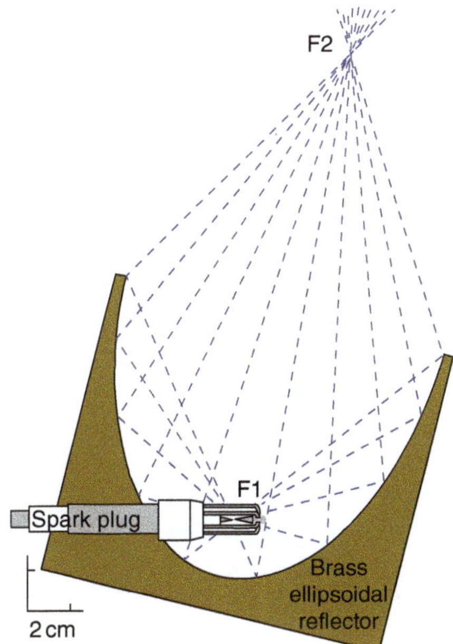

Figure 18.2 The focusing design of a Dornier HM3 electrohydraulic lithotripter. A spark plug is located at the focus (F1) of an ellipsoidal reflector. Energy from the spark plug is reflected and focused to the second focus of the ellipsoidal reflector (F2). Source: Cleveland 2007 [6]. Reproduced with permission of PMPH- USA.

Electromagnetic generators

These utilize a magnetic field to create shock waves. An electrical coil is placed adjacent to a metal plate. When a short electrical pulse is applied to the coil, a repulsive force acts on the metal plate, which produces a shock wave. The metal plate can be flat or cylindrical. Two focusing mechanisms are used in electromagnetic lithotripters, depending on the configuration of the metal plate (Figure 18.3). A flat plate generates a plane wave which is focused by an acoustic lens. A cylindrical plate generates a cylindrical wave which is focused by a parabolic reflector [3,6].

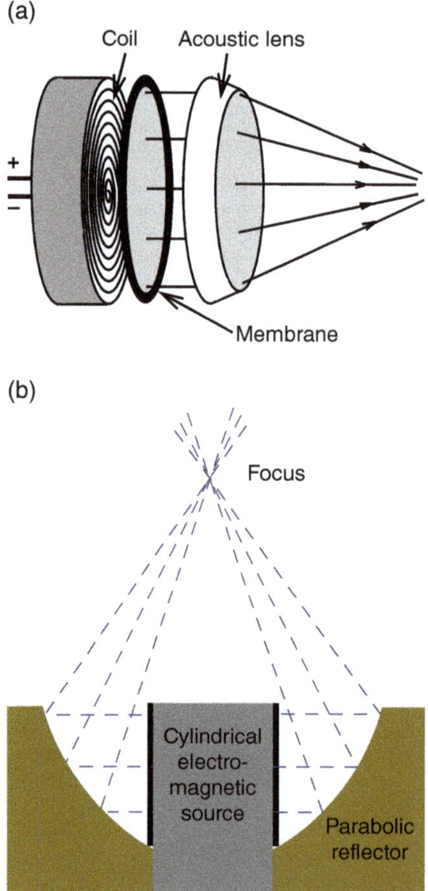

Figure 18.3 The two focusing mechanisms employed in electromagnetic lithotripters. (a) In a Siemens or Dornier lithotripter, a membrane is driven by a coil to produce a plane wave, which is then focused by an acoustic lens. (b) In a Storz lithotripter, a coil excites a cylindrical membrane, which generates a wave that is focused by a parabolic reflector. Source: Cleveland 2007 [6]. Reproduced with permission of PMPH- USA.

Advantages	Disadvantages
Minimal variation in the amplitude of the shock wave from shock to shock No electrode to replace Efficient stone comminution	Narrower focal zone Higher peak positive pressures

Piezoelectric generators

These utilize ceramic crystals to create shock waves. Piezoceramic elements are arranged on the inner surface of a spherical dish. When electricity is applied to the piezoceramic elements, the crystals are distorted and produce an ultrasonic wave. The focal point is located at the center of the radius of curvature of the sphere (Figure 18.4) [3,6].

Advantages	Disadvantages
Minimal variation in the amplitude of the shock wave from shock to shock No electrode to replace	Narrowest focal zone Higher peak positive pressures Reduced efficiency of stone comminution

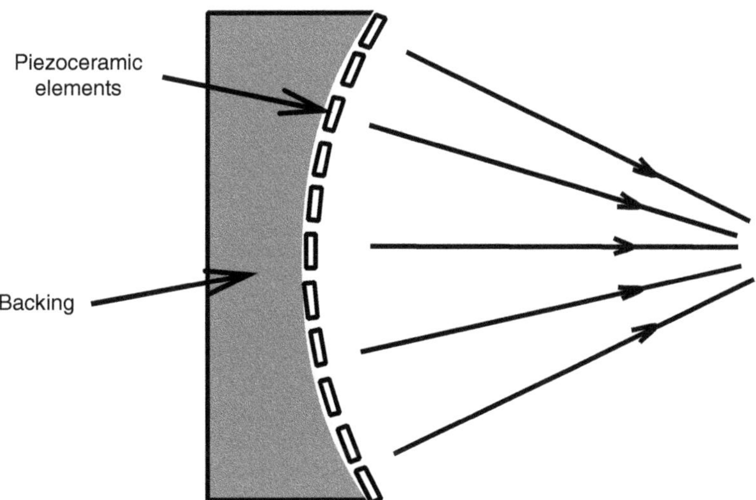

Figure 18.4 Fundamental principles for a piezoelectric lithotripter. Piezoceramic elements are placed onto the surface of a sphere. The wave will focus to the center of the radius of curvature of that sphere. Source: Cleveland 2007 [6]. Reproduced with permission of PMPH- USA.

Factors influencing extracorporeal shock wave lithotripsy outcomes

Coupling

The efficiency of shock wave propagation through different media depends on their differences in impedance. As a sound wave is transmitted from one medium to the next, a portion of the wave continues forward and a portion of the wave is reflected back. The acoustic impedances of water and soft tissue are similar, meaning that the majority of the wave's energy will be transmitted from water into tissue. In contrast, the impedances of water and air are drastically different, resulting in virtually all of the wave's energy (99.9%) being reflected at the water–air interface [8,10].

Early lithotripters (HM3) employed a water bath as a coupling medium. The water bath is ideal for transmission of shock waves but the equipment is inconvenient because it is large and stationary [22]. As shock wave lithotripsy evolved, dry shock heads were introduced in order to make lithotripters more affordable, compact, and portable [7,22]. Dry lithotripters feature an energy source housed within a therapy head, which is filled with water and covered by an acoustically neutral membrane. Acoustic waves travel through the membrane and are coupled to the body wall of the patient using a gel or oil [9,27].

With the widespread use of dry head lithotripters, the importance of coupling quality must be emphasized. Important research has been done to determine methods for improved stone comminution through optimization of shock wave coupling. Pishchalnikov et al. found that an almost linear inverse relationship exists between the surface area of air pockets at the coupling interface and the efficiency of stone fragmentation. They reported a 20–40% decrease in stone breakage with as little as 2% of the coupling interface being occupied by air pockets [8]. Neucks et al. showed that the method of applying the coupling agent can have an impact on the number of air pockets and thus treatment success. Stone fragmentation was improved when coupling gel was applied to the therapy head as a bolus, compared to spreading the gel by hand [9]. Cartledge et al. evaluated various coupling media and indicated that ultrasonography jelly is probably the optimum coupling agent available for use [27]. Studies by Jain and Shah also support this recommendation [10].

Focal zone and peak pressure

All lithotripters have a focal point where the acoustic waves are focused. The high pressure area surrounding the focal point is termed the focal zone. The focal zone is the elliptical shaped volume within which the measured pressure is 50% or more of the maximum peak positive pressure. The dimensions of the focal zone and peak positive pressures vary considerably between lithotripters and are established by the manufacture's design [6,11,25].

In general, lithotripters with narrower focal zones generate higher peak pressures. Interestingly, *in vitro* studies using stationary stones reveal that electromagnetic and piezoelectric devices (narrower focal zone, higher peak pressures) are not better, and in some cases are worse at stone fragmentation compared to electrohydraulic lithotripters (broader focal zone, lower peak pressures) [28]. Great emphasis has been placed on achieving higher acoustic pressures to improve stone comminution. However, once the threshold of the calculus is overcome, further increases in peak positive pressure have minimal influence on stone breakage [7].

A narrow focal zone is also disadvantageous because the target (stone) frequently moves outside the focal zone with patient respiration, resulting in fewer shock waves being delivered to the stone and decreased fragmentation. Because higher peak pressures are associated with narrower focal zones, the shocks administered while the stone is outside the focal zone can cause increased damage to surrounding tissues [11,13]. Assessments of renal injury in a pig model show evidence of highly focused, full-thickness (from cortex to medulla), intense tissue disruption using a lithotripter with narrow focal width and high acoustic pressure [11,12]. Similar experiments in pigs using lithotripters with broad focal zones and low peak pressures resulted in far less tissue injury, consisting of scattered areas of diffuse interstitial hemorrhage in the cortex and medulla [25].

Rate of shock wave delivery

Recent trends in shock wave lithotripsy have favored increasing the rate of shock wave delivery in order to decrease procedure times. Unfortunately, numerous *in vitro* and *in vivo* studies have shown that faster shock wave administration rates result in decreased efficiency of stone fragmentation [14,15,16,17,18,19,20,21]. Paterson et al. implanted artificial stones into pig kidneys and applied shock waves at varying rates. Stones treated at 30 SW/min fragmented better than those treated at 120 SW/min [16]. A meta-analysis by Semins et al. found that patients treated at 60 SW/min had greater treatment success than patients treated at 120 SW/min [29]. Koo et al. reported greater stone-free rates and improved cost-effectiveness in patients treated at slower rates (70 SW/min) versus faster rates (100 SW/min). Decreased cost was mainly attributed to lower retreatment rates and the need for fewer additional procedures in the slow treatment group [14].

Although the exact mechanism underlying the observation of improved stone comminution at slower rates is uncertain, it is thought to be related to the growth of cavitation bubbles. When shocks are delivered rapidly, cavitation bubbles persist and accumulate around stone fragments. The air–water interface of bubbles is acoustically dense and may impede incoming shock waves [17,20,26].

Voltage/power and number of shocks delivered

Multiple experiments have demonstrated that the severity of renal injury from shock wave lithotripsy increases as voltage/power setting and the number of shocks are increased [11,16,30,31]. The term *power index* is often discussed in the literature and is equal to shock wave intensity × number of shocks. It should be noted that this equation does not account for the size of the focal zone. The concept of *effective energy dose* does address the width of the focal zone and may be a more accurate formula for comparison of different lithotripters [7]. In order to decrease tissue damage and renal functional impairment, it is recommended that treatment be limited to the lowest shock wave dosage necessary to achieve stone fragmentation [12].

Sequence of shock wave delivery

The technique used during shock wave lithotripsy can have significant impact on treatment success. Both *in vitro* and *in vivo* studies have supported the concept of pretreating the kidney (≤100 shocks) at a low power setting followed by a clinical dose of higher energy shock waves – a strategy known as "ramping." Ramping has been shown to improve stone comminution and also has a protective effect on the kidney. Improved stone breakage is thought to occur secondary to conditioning of the stone by the low power shocks which yields more efficient breakage during subsequent application of higher energy shocks. The reduced renal trauma observed in pretreated kidneys is presumably due to vasoconstriction [11,22,32].

Conclusion

Through intense research and decades of clinical application, great insight has been gained into techniques for improved efficiency and the characteristics of an ideal lithotripter. That being said, it is reasonable to ask, "Which lithotripter is the best?". Unfortunately, there is no convincing evidence that any of the current generators yield results comparable to those of the HM3 [9,10]. Despite the increased problems associated with newer generation lithotripters, the informed urologist can employ various techniques to maximize the efficiency of shock wave application [11,22]. Attention to a few simple, yet important details can significantly improve treatment success and patient safety.

Key points: techniques to improve shock wave efficiency

- Coupling – apply gel to therapy head as a bolus to minimize air pockets
- Rate – slower shock wave administration rates (60–70 SW/min) improve the efficiency of stone fragmentation
- Voltage/power and number of shocks – treatment should be limited to the lowest shock wave dosage necessary to achieve stone fragmentation
- Sequence of shock wave delivery – pretreat the kidney (≤100 shocks) at a low power setting followed by a clinical dose of higher energy shock waves

References

1. Matlaga BR, Lingeman JE. Surgical management of upper urinary tract calculi. In: Wein AJ, Kavoussi LR, Novick AC, et al., eds. *Campbell-Walsh Urology*, 10th edn. Philadelphia: W.B. Saunders, 2011, pp. 1357–410.
2. Kerbl K, Rehman J, Landman J, Lee D, Sundaram C, Clayman RV. Current management of urolithiasis: progress or regress? J Endourol 2002; 16(5): 281–8.
3. Lingeman JE. Extracorporeal shock wave lithotripsy. Development, instrumentation, and current status. Urol Clin North Am 1997; 24(1): 185–211.
4. Chaussy C, Brendel W, Schmiedt E. Extracorporeally induced destruction of kidney stones by shock waves. Lancet 1980; 2(8207): 1265–8.

5. Bhojani N, Lingeman JE. Shockwave lithotripsy – new concepts and optimizing treatment parameters. Urol Clin North Am 2013; 40(1): 59–66.
6. Cleveland RO, McAteer JA. The physics of shock wave lithotripsy. In: Smith AD, Badlani GH, Bagley DH, et al., eds. *Smith's Textbook of Endourology*. Hamilton, Ontario: BC Decker, Inc., 2007, pp. 317–32.
7. Rassweiler JJ, Knoll T, Kohrmann KU, et al. Shock wave technology and application: an update. Eur Urol 2011; 59(5): 784–96.
8. Pishchalnikov YA, Neucks JS, VonDerHaar RJ, Pishchalnikova IV, Williams JC Jr, McAteer JA. Air pockets trapped during routine coupling in dry head lithotripsy can significantly decrease the delivery of shock wave energy. J Urol 2006; 176: 2706–10.
9. Neucks JS, Pishchalnikov YA, Zancanaro AJ, VonDerHaar JN, Williams JC Jr, McAteer JA. Improved acoustic coupling for shock wave lithotripsy. Urol Res 2008; 36(1): 61–6.
10. Jain A, Shah TK. Effect of air bubbles in the coupling medium on efficacy of extracorporeal shock wave lithotripsy. Eur Urol 2007; 51(6): 1680–6; discussion 1686–7.
11. Connors BA, McAteer JA, Evan AP, et al. Evaluation of shock wave lithotripsy injury in the pig using a narrow focal zone lithotriptor. BJU Int 2012; 110: 1376–85.
12. Connors BA, Evan AP, Blomgren PM, et al. Reducing shock number dramatically decreases lesion size in a juvenile kidney model. J Endourol 2006; 20(9): 607–11.
13. Evan AP, Willis LR. Extracorporeal shock wave lithotripsy: complications. In: Smith AD, Badlani GH, Bagley DH, et al., eds. *Smith's Textbook of Endourology*. Hamilton, Ontario: BC Decker, Inc., 2007, pp. 353–66.
14. Koo V, Beattie I, Young M. Improved cost-effectiveness and efficiency with a slower shockwave delivery rate. BJU Int 2009; 105: 692–6.
15. Greenstein A, Matzkin H. Does the rate of extracorporeal shock wave delivery affect stone fragmentation? Urology 1999; 54: 430–2.
16. Paterson RF, Lifshitz DA, Lingeman JE, et al. Stone fragmentation during shock wave lithotripsy is improved by slowing the shock wave rate: studies with a new animal model. J Urol 2002; 168: 2211–15.
17. Pishchalnikov YA, McAteer JA, Williams JC Jr. Effect of firing rate on the performance of shock wave lithotriptors. BJU Int 2008; 102(11): 1681–6.
18. Yilmaz E, Batislam E, Basar M, Tuglu D, Mert C, Basar H. Optimal frequency in extracorporeal shock wave lithotripsy: prospective randomized study. Urology 2005; 66(6): 1160–4.
19. Madbouly K, El-Tiraifi AM, Seida M, El-Faqih SR, Atassi R, Talic RF. Slow versus fast shock wave lithotripsy rate for urolithiasis: a prospective randomized study. J Urol 2005; 173(1): 127–30.
20. Pace KT, Ghiculete D, Harju M, Honey RJ. Shock wave lithotripsy at 60 or 120 shocks per minute: a randomized, double-blind trial. J Urol 2005; 174(2): 595–9.
21. Wiksell H, Kinn AC. Implications of cavitation phenomena for shot intervals in extracorporeal shock wave lithotripsy. Br J Urol 1995; 75(6): 720–3.
22. Lingeman JE. Lithotripsy systems. In: Smith AD, Badlani GH, Bagley DH, et al., eds. *Smith's Textbook of Endourology*. Hamilton, Ontario: BC Decker, Inc., 2007, pp. 333–42.
23. Zhou Y, Cocks FH, Preminger GM, Zhong P. The effect of treatment strategy on stone comminution efficiency in shock wave lithotripsy. J Urol 2004; 172(1): 349–54.

24. Eisenmenger W. The mechanisms of stone fragmentation in ESWL. Ultrasound Med Biol 2001; 27(5): 683–93.
25. Evan AP, McAteer JA, Connors BA, et al. Independent assessment of a wide-focus, low-pressure electromagnetic lithotripter: absence of renal bioeffects in the pig. BJU Int 2008; 101(3): 382–8.
26. Eisenmenger W, Du XX, Tang C, et al. The first clinical results of "wide-focus and low-pressure" ESWL. Ultrasound Med Biol 2002; 28(6): 769–74.
27. Cartledge JJ, Cross WR, Lloyd SN, Joyce AD. The efficacy of a range of contact media as coupling agents in extracorporeal shock wave lithotripsy. BJU Int 2001; 88: 321.
28. Teichman JMH, Portis AJ, Cecconi PP, et al. In vitro comparison of shock wave lithotripsy machines. J Urol 2000; 164: 1259–64.
29. Semins MJ, Trock BJ, Matlaga BR. The effect of shock wave rate on the outcome of shock wave lithotripsy: a meta-analysis. J Urol 2008; 179(1): 194–7.
30. Willis LR, Evan AP, Connors BA, et al. Shockwave lithotripsy: dose-related effects on renal structure, hemodynamics, and tubular function. J Endourol 2005; 19(1): 90–101.
31. Connors BA, Evan AP, Willis LR, Blomgren PM, Lingeman JE, Fineberg NS. The effect of discharge voltage on renal injury and impairment caused by lithotripsy in the pig. J Am Soc Nephrol 2000; 11(2): 310–18.
32. Willis LR, Evan AP, Connors BA, Handa RK, Blomgren PM, Lingeman JE. Prevention of lithotripsy-induced renal injury by pretreating kidneys with low-energy shock waves. J Am Soc Nephrol 2006; 17(3): 663–73.

CHAPTER 19

Ureteroscopic Lithotripsy: Indications, Access Endoscopes, Accessories, and Lithotrites

Julien Letendre and Olivier Traxer

Tenon Hospital, Assistance Publique – Hôpitaux de Paris, Pierre et Marie Curie University, Paris, France

Do's and don'ts box

Do:

- set the proper indication for URS
- use a safety guidewire when necessary
- use a ureteral access sheath when appropriate
- visualize your laser fiber when doing lithotripsy.

Don't:

- apply excessive force
- use the same laser settings for every case
- pull hard when using a stone basket in the ureter
- prestent everyone
- place a stent after every URS.

Introduction

Stones remain one of the most common urological problems and an important part of the urologist's practice. Advances in technology, mainly with flexible ureteroscopes, have allowed stone surgery for better outcomes and less morbidity. In this chapter, we review the indications, surgical aspects, and instruments and accessories of ureteroscopy (URS).

Indications

Indications for URS depend largely on stone size and location (see Figure 19.1).

Urinary Stones: Medical and Surgical Management, First Edition. Edited by Michael Grasso and David S. Goldfarb.

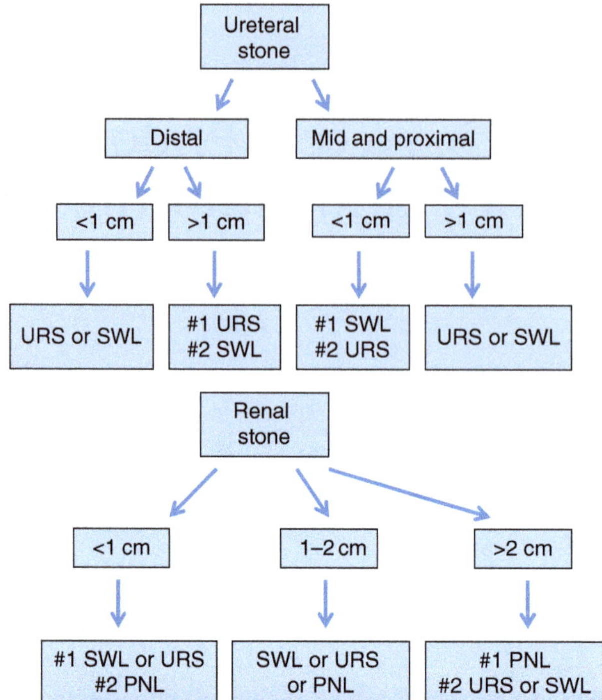

Figure 19.1 Indications of URS for the treatment of upper tract stones according to size and location.

Ureteral stones smaller than 1 cm can usually be observed with periodic evaluation until spontaneous expulsion. URS is therefore indicated after a failed period of observation of 1 month [1].

Contraindications to observation include the presence of:

- persistent obstruction
- acute renal insufficiency (renal failure, bilateral obstruction, solitary kidney)
- flank pain refractory to adequate pain medication
- fever.

The probabilities of expulsion for a stone larger than 1 cm are quite minimal and intervention can be planned either electively or semi-urgently.

Ureteroscopy can be safely performed in the urgent setting for stones smaller then 1 cm. However, it must be performed very carefully and should be interrupted in favor of a double J stent as soon as difficulties are encountered [2].

Ureteroscopy is usually recommended for distal ureteral stones independently of size, as it is associated with high success rates and low complication rates. For proximal stones, shock wave lithotripsy (SWL) has a higher stone-free rate (SFR) for stones less than 1 cm and URS for stones larger than 1 cm, but both approaches are feasible. URS is also appropriate following failed treatment with SWL. Flexible URS has improved the SFR for proximal stones significantly [1,3].

For renal stones, URS now shares the same indications as SWL as first-line treatment for stones less than 2 cm and is the preferred option for lower pole stones. Indications for retrograde intrarenal surgery are expanding with stones larger than 2 cm being treated with success [4,5].

Selection of the treatment modality also depends on stone composition. Stones presenting characteristics suggesting resistance to SWL (cystine, calcium monohydrate, >1000 Hounsfield units [HU], impacted) are more appropriately treated with URS. Patients presenting contraindications to SWL (coagulopathy, pregnancy, obesity, skeletal malformation, aneurysm, distal obstruction) are also usually better candidates for URS. In fact, URS is the most appropriate treatment modality in patients with bleeding disorders [6].

Ureteroscopy is obviously contraindicated in the context of sepsis. Urgent decompression should be obtained and definitive treatment for the stone delayed.

For a complete overview of stone management, see Chapter 13.

Setting up for surgery

To perform a URS adequately for a ureteral stone, suitable instrumentation and accessories must be available [7].

- Fluoroscopy
- Endourology-video unit
- Irrigation
- Guidewires
- Ureteral dilators or balloons
- Endoscopes (semi-rigid or flexible)
- Endocorporeal lithotripter including a holmium:YAG laser
- Stone retrieval devices
- Stents

General principles of ureteroscopy

Whether URS is performed with a semi-rigid or a flexible ureteroscope, it should be done following general principles. No manoevers should be attempted blindly. It should be done under visual or fluoroscopic guidance. Antegrade or retrograde progression should be done carefully.

Radiation safety

Minimizing radiation exposure for both the patient and surgeon is important and should follow the ALARA guidelines [8].

- Minimize time
  - Fluoroscopy controlled by the surgeon (foot pedal)
  - Pulsed fluoroscopy (15–30 frames per second)
  - Last image hold

- Maximize distance
- Maximize shielding
  - Glasses, thyroid shields, chest and pelvic aprons

Other suggestions include:
- place the source below the patient and the intensifier above and as close as possible to the patient
- use lead collimators to restrict exposure.

Gaining access to the ureter

Guidewire

Guidewires are the key accessories for gaining access to the ureter. Placement of a guidewire with a rigid cystoscope under fluoroscopy in the renal cavities is usually the first step of stone surgery. Insertion of a guidewire in the ureteral orifice is sometimes difficult due to a large median lobe or a cystocele. Emptying the bladder, using a flexible cystoscope, or placement with a semi-rigid ureteroscope can be helpful. If the wire does not advance easily or if adequate placement of the guidewire is doubtful, exchanging the guidewire for an open-ended ureteral catheter or a dual-lumen catheter allows performance of a pyelogram to assess the anatomy [9].

It is usually preferable to perform URS with a safety guidewire placed in the renal cavities, but this is left to the surgeon's preference [1]. Guidewires maintain continuity of the urinary tract, help straighten a tortuous path, serve as damage control when complications (perforation) occur, and facilitate multiple entry/re-entry in the upper tract.

Many different guidewires exist and each presents various characteristics. Guidewires can be compared according to their resistance, composition, and tip. More resistant (stiff) wires are ideal to maintain rigidity and to allow for the passage of instruments, such as dilators. However, since they are more resistant to bending, they are more prone to perforation of the ureter when they encounter an obstructing stone. Hydrophilic wires are more expensive but allow for easier placement of a guidewire past an obstructive ureteral stone. Because of their nature, they offer less friction, making them more likely to be accidentally pulled out. Hybrid guidewires combine the advantages of a stiffer body with a softer hydrophilic tip [7].

Guidewires may be:
- regular or stiff
- hydrophilic or non-hydrophilic
- straight or with an angled tip.

The standard guidewire used is a floppy-tipped PTFE, but we recommend using a stiff hydrophilic wire.

For flexible URS, two guidewires are usually necessary to allow placement of a safety wire beside a ureteral access sheath (UAS). When a flexible ureteroscope is placed over a guidewire to access the upper tract, the wire used should have a floppy tip on the distal end to prevent any damage.

Bypassing an impacted or obstructive stone is sometimes challenging.

- Changing for a softer hydrophilic guidewire is the first step. Manipulation of this wire is difficult, so passing it within an open-ended ureteral catheter placed just distally to the stone is helpful.
- Using an angled hydrophilic catheter is helpful.
- The next step could be to carefully try passing the guidewire under direct visualization with an ureteroscope.
- In case of failure, antegrade access could be attempted or a nephrostomy installed for 2 weeks for decompression.

Ureteral dilators

Routine ureteral dilation is unnecessary. Because of their progressive size, most semi-rigid ureteroscopes act as autodilators. However, if the ureteroscope or the UAS will not advance due to a ureteral stricture, spasm, or tight ureteral orifice, progressive co-axial dilators or balloon dilation can be used.

Balloon dilators are inflated under fluoroscopic guidance at 20 atm of pressure and dilate 4–10 cm in length at a size from 12 to 30 F (12–15 F for the ureter). Co-axial dilators are sequentially inserted from 6 F to 18 F under fluoroscopy ideally on a stiff guidewire (usually up to 12 F is sufficient) [10].

If multiple areas of the ureter appear narrow, placing a double J stent and deferring the procedure for 1 week to wait for passive dilation is a valid and safe option [11].

Ureteral access sheath

Ureteral access sheaths are now widely accepted. They consist of a two-piece hydrophilic device: the sheath and an internal dilator. The UAS is inserted under fluoroscopic guidance. We recommend not placing the UAS directly in the ureteropelvic junction (UPJ) since it limits deflection and may disrupt the fragile UPJ.

Various sizes exist to accommodate different flexible endoscopes. UAS size 12/14 F (inner channel 12 F/outer diameter 14 F) is currently the universal size since all flexible ureteroscopes can be placed inside. However, the large diameter prevents primary ureteral placement in about 20% of cases compared to 5% for 10/12 F [12]. Various lengths exist (20–55 cm) with 35 cm being the standard size.

The advantages of a UAS include:

- dilatation of the ureter
- easy multiple re-entry
- good irrigation by facilitating drainage
- maintain a low-pressure system

- easier stone extraction
- protect the ureteroscopes
- decreased operative time.

Recently, a new UAS has been developed, the ReTrace (Coloplast). It presents a unique characteristic consisting of the guidewire being able to exit on the side of the internal dilator just before the sheath. By pulling out the internal sheath, the guidewire is forced out of a side slit and becomes the safety wire (Figure 19.2). This feature eliminates the need for multiple manipulations in order to place a safety wire [12].

Two myths exist regarding the diameters of UASs. First of all, a wider UAS allows for more flow. This is not true. It has been determined that backflow and intrarenal pressure are the same whatever the size of the sheath [13]. Secondly, a larger sheath allows for the passage of bigger stone fragments. This is partly true, but the difference in diameter of a 10/12 F sheath compared to 12/14 F is 0.7 mm, which is of small clinical significance. Size of UAS should then be decided according to prestenting, ureteral orifice appearance on cystoscopy and available ureteroscopes, bearing in mind that the normal ureter size is 10 F.

Using UASs can induce ureteral wall injury. In fact, up to 50% of patients have some degree of ureteral wall injury, which translates into 4% ureteral

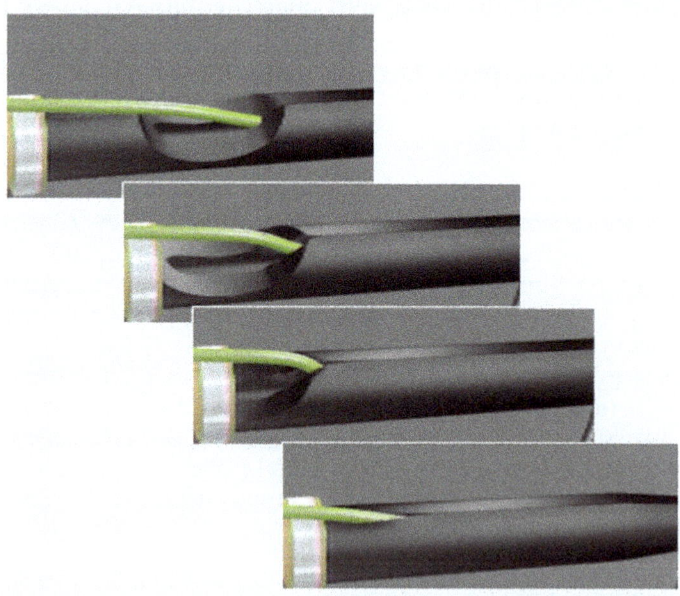

Figure 19.2 The ReTrace (Coloplast); the unique side slit in the internal sheath allows easy placement of a safety wire.

stenosis at 1 year [14]. It is important first of all to place UASs without too much force and also to evaluate the ureter at the end of surgery to assess for any damage.

Irrigation

Proper irrigation, with saline, is key to good visibility and adequate realization of URS, since endoscopes are long and working channels are small, which are obstacles to flow and optimal visibility. In fact, both irrigation and instruments are passed through the same channel, reducing flow. Stone dusting also reduces visibility. Various devices are helpful in maintaining constant and controlled irrigation to allow good visibility, short operative time, and better outcomes [15]. With a UAS in place, intrarenal pressure of less than 30 cmH_2O can be maintained with systems pressurized up to 200 cmH_2O. Keeping low intrarenal pressures prevents intrarenal reflux and the risk of sepsis.

Devices to maintain irrigation pressure include (can be used in combination) Figure 19.3:

- pressurized irrigation bag (not recommended because of inconsistent pressure)
- automated systems
- hand-held syringe or bulb device
- foot-controlled device.

Endoscopes

Semi-rigid

Semi-rigid ureteroscopes remain the most common instrument to access the ureter. The main improvement over the years has been the arrival of thinner ureteroscopes (7.5 versus 10 F) allowing for higher rates of achieved

(a)

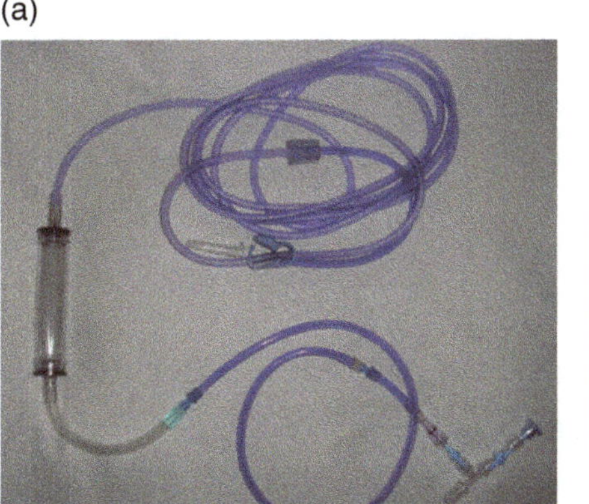

(b)

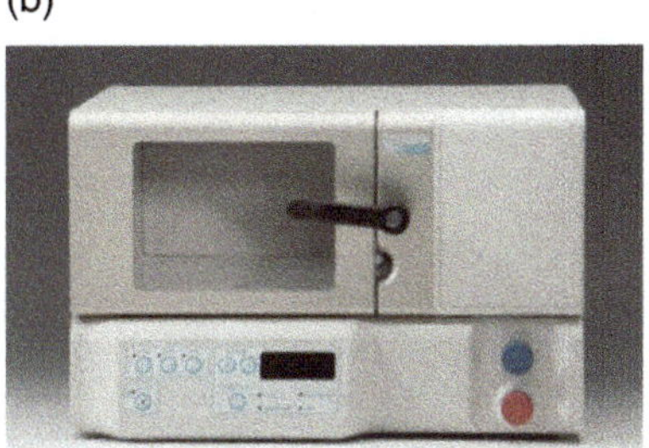

Figure 19.3 (a) Hand-held bulb pump irrgiation device (Traxer Flow, Rocamed). (b) Automated pressure and temperature system.

access, more efficiency, and less iatrogenic trauma and stricture [16]. Currently, tip diameters range from 4.5 to 9.0F and proximal diameter from 6.5 to 15.0F. Most semi-rigid ureteroscopes have one working channel, but some have two. Their size varies from 3.0 to 6.0F but most are 5.0F. At the time of writing, only one digital semi-rigid ureteroscope exists. Transition to digital imagery is less appealing than for flexible scopes since the image provided is already of good quality due to the high density of fiberoptic bundles already incorporated.

Semi-rigid ureteroscopes present several advantages. They are easier to manipulate and have wide working channels, allowing for a good irrigation flow and the use of larger instruments. They offer good visibility and are more durable. They are also easier to clean and sterilize. However, they are of limited use above the iliac vessels, mainly in the urgent setting or in first intention without prestenting, and are useless for calyceal stones.

Flexible

Flexible ureteroscopes revolutionized endourology and the treatment of urolithiasis [17]. Small size (tip size: 5.4–9F) and increased deflection (180–275°) have allowed urologists to reach any stone (Figures 19.4, 19.5) [7]. However, the added value of digital imagery is undeniable (Figure 19.6). Placing the chip on the end of the scope and taking out the fibers allows for a clearer and bigger image without pixels. Better visibility translates into faster stone fragmentation rate and up to 25% less operative time [18].

Working channels of the majority of flexible ureteroscopes are 3.6F in diameter, which allows for the use of instruments up to 3.2F. When placed in the working channel, instruments tend to reduce primary deflection and irrigation [19].

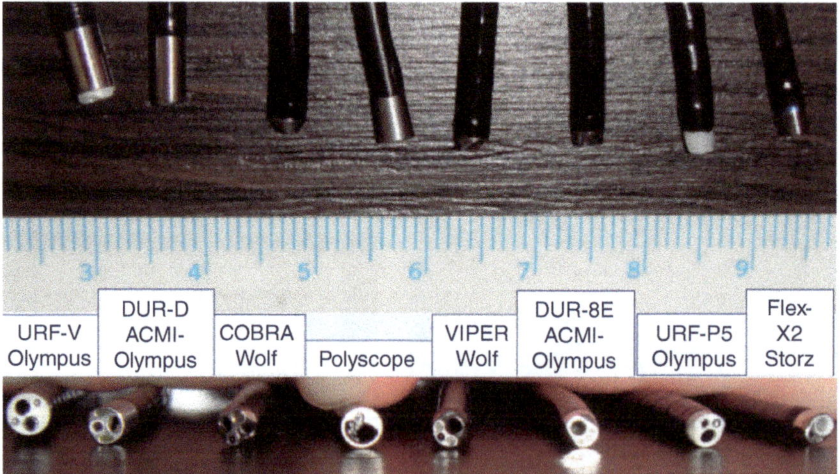

Figure 19.4 Various types of flexible ureteroscopes. URF-V and DUR-D are digital flexible ureteroscopes. Absent from this picture is the Storz Flex XC digital scope.

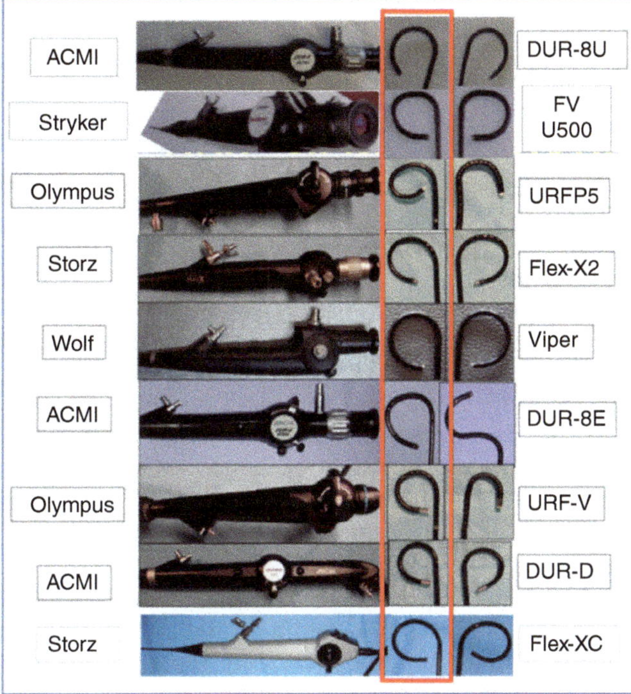

Figure 19.5 Fiberoptic and digital (*bottom three*) flexible ureteroscopes.

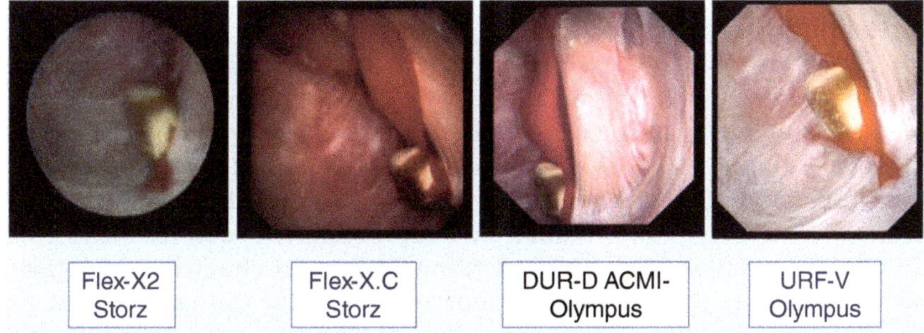

Figure 19.6 Comparison of the quality of a fiberoptic image (Storz Flex X2) with three digital flexible ureteroscopes.

One of the issues with digital ureteroscopes is the fact that the camera is not pendular, making orientation confusing. Referring to the position of air bubbles in the cavities helps to identify anterior from posterior.

Two main inter-related concerns arise from the use of ureteroscopes: cost and durability. Cost of flexible ureteroscopes and cost of repairs are very high, even more so for digital scopes. These costs are overemphasized by ureteroscopes needing repair every few cases and having a life expectancy of approximately 50 cases [20]. The need for more durable scopes is pressing.

Stone fragmentation and retrieval

Lithotripters

Ultrasonic lithotripsy

Ultrasonic lithotripsy results from the generation of vibrational energy transmitted through a probe, which breaks stones by direct contact, like drilling. The probes are rigid and vary from 4.5 to 12 F, the bigger ones combining a suctioning channel. The main disadvantages of ultrasonic lithotripsy are the rigid probes, the lack of efficiency on very hard stones, and the excessive heat generation. Even though they can be used for semi-rigid URS, their mainstay application remains for PCNL.

Ballistic lithotripsy

Energy developed by compressed air is transmitted to a probe, which in turn fragments stones like a "jack-hammer." Ballisitc lithotripsy has many advantages over ultrasonic. Fisrt, probes are reusable and come in both rigid (2.4–9.6 F) and flexible (2.4–2.7 F) forms. Second, they generate very little heat and are safer in regard to ureteral trauma [21]. However, the flexible probes allow for only 30° of flexibility when used with flexible ureteroscopes and are associated with high retropulsion rates.

Laser lithotripsy

Since their introduction, lasers have been used for various tasks in urology, but their main role is still for lithotripsy [22]. Many types of lasers have been tried, including alexandrite, pulsed-dye, and neodymium:YAG lasers. However, holmium:YAG lasers are most often employed for stone surgery. Laser energy is transmitted to the fiber tip, producing photothermal damage upon direct contact and a cavitation bubble, which results in efficient fragmentation of all types of stone. The main characteristic of this wavelength that makes it convenient to use in the urinary tract is its absorption in liquid at a distance smaller than 1 mm, thus minimizing the risk of damage to the urinary tract [23].

Fibers also come in various sizes (150–1000 μm) that allow their use in flexible ureteroscopes. However, misfires or improper use may result in significant and costly damages to the ureteroscope.

Tips to prevent ureteroscope damage include:

- test reusable fibers for leakage before use
- use small fibers in flexible ureteroscopes (150–273 μm)
- insert the fibers while the flexible ureteroscope is straight
- make sure the tip of the fiber is visible at all times during use (Figure 19.7)

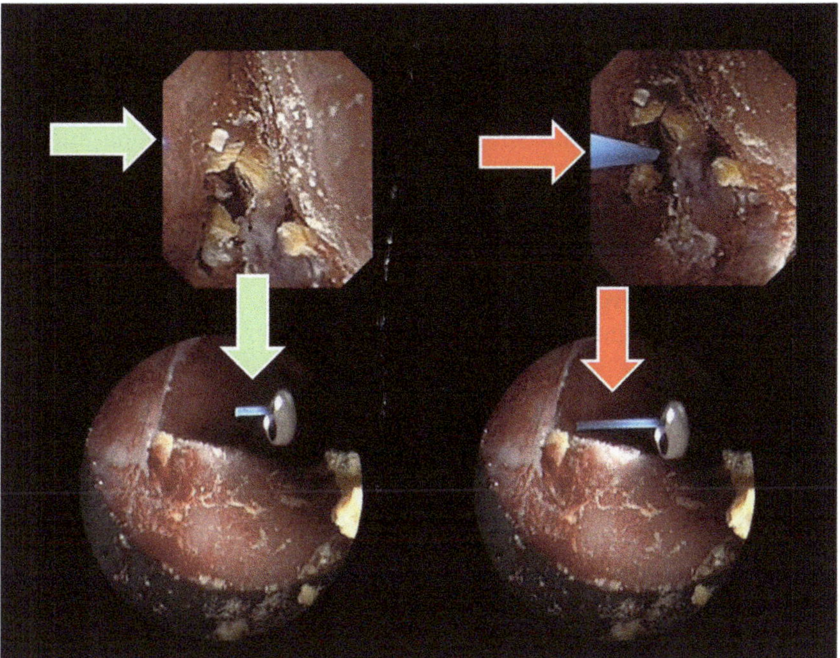

Figure 19.7 View from a nephroscope of a laser fiber exiting from a flexible ureteroscope. When the fiber is barely visible on the ureteroscope view (*top green arrow*), the fiber has already safely the working channel exited (*bottom green arrow*). Visualizing the laser fiber well ensures a safe distance from the ureteroscope (*red arrows*).

- relocate stones from lower pole to upper pole before lithotripsy
- lower power when firing with the scope highly deflected.

When using a holmium laser to fragment a ureteral stone, we suggest starting with the center of the stone and then moving laterally in order to prevent ureteral damage. Either dusting or fragmenting settings can be used. For renal stones, we prefer dusting the stone from the surface to the center to minimize the number of fragments to remove.

Laser settings for these procedures:

- Fragmentation: high energy (1–2 joules) and low frequency (4–5 Hz)
- Dusting: low energy (0.2–0.5 joules) and high frequency (15–20 Hz)
- Cutting: high energy (1.2–1.5 joules) and high frequency (10–14 Hz).

Large stones can produce a significant number of fragments, making stone removal long and hazardous. If we consider a stone as a cube, fragmenting a 1 cm stone in fragments of 5 mm produces eight pieces. Fragmenting a 9 mm stone into 3 mm fragments to allow removal into a UAS produces 27 fragments. UAS size has little effect on the number of fragments needed in this model. In order to reduce going in and out of the ureter for stone removal, dusting is sometimes preferable followed by removal of the larger residual fragments.

Holmium lasers in stone surgery also allow concomitant application of adjunct intervention. Endoscopic treatment of UPJ obstruction, ureteral stenosis, infundibular stenosis, and calyceal diverticulum can be performed using a holmium laser.

Antiretropulsion devices

Retropulsion is a significant issue in ureteral lithotripsy. It is responsible for more complicated intervention, longer operative times, and lower stone-free rates. To prevent retropulsion, various strategies may be used. The first step is to reduce the flow and pressure of irrigation to prevent proximal migration. A recent study from our center (to be published) demonstrated that using a smaller fiber produces less retropulsion for the same laser parameters. Also retropulsion is reduced by aiming at the edges of the stone instead of its center. Various devices have also been designed to help with this problem. They have been shown to be equally effective in blocking fragment migration as small as 1.5 mm [24].

A new product is also available, the Backstop (Boston Scientific). This is a gel applied proximally to the stone with a ureteral catheter that temporarily occludes the ureter [25]. The gel dissolves afterward in 2 h. However, laser lithotripsy of a fragment stuck inside the gel is difficult and the gel is not radiopaque and is transparent.

Stone retrieval devices

After lithotripsy, retrieval of the significant fragments takes place. For semi-rigid URS, metallic Alligator forceps allow adequate prehension under direct vision and allow for easy release in case of an obstruction. Otherwise Nitinol stone baskets are frequently employed since they can be used in both semi-rigid and flexible ureteroscopes owing to their small diameter and great flexibility. Extraction of stones with a basket should be done under direct visualization and excessive force should be prohibited because of the risk of ureteral avulsion.

If a stone becomes stuck in the ureter while being removed with a basket, the urologist can try to:

- readjust the angle of the stone by releasing the grasp and increasing irrigation
- release the stone from the basket
- pass a small laser fiber alongside the basket and fragment the stone in the basket
- disengage the basket from the handle.

Retrieval of small stone fragments is sometimes difficult because they are hard to immobilize in baskets. Some baskets are designed for grabbing small fragments (1 mm), like the N-Compass (Cook). For stone fragments in the kidney, injecting 5–10 cc of the patient 's blood into the calyces and waiting 10 min for the clots to entrap the small fragments allows for easier retrieval with a basket [26].

After stone extraction

Post-URS stent

At the end of the intervention, the ureter should be visualized to assess for ureteral damage.

Routine double J placement after URS is unnecessary [27]. No ureteral drainage is needed if the stone was removed rapidly and easily *in toto*. A ureteral catheter can be left in place for 24–48 h after lithotripsy of a small non-impacted stone without residual fragments >2 mm [28]. A double J catheter should probably be left in place for 8–10 days for other cases and for 4–6 weeks in case of ureteral trauma [28].

Indications for ureteral stenting post URS include [29]:

- perforation
- dilation (co-axial or balloon)
- significant edema
- deferring procedure due to a narrow ureter
- infected system
- large stone burden
- solitary kidney.

Double J stents are composed of either polyurethane or silicone. The senior author prefers silicone because it is less prone to encrustration and better tolerated by patients [30]. However, it needs to be installed over a stiff hydrophilic guidewire since it does not glide well on PTFE wires. The lock-in system facilitates safe placement in the cavities.

Placement of a stent of the appropriate length helps to minimize the patient's urinary problems and pain. α-Blockers, ketorolac or oxybutinin have also been shown to improve tolerability of double J stents [31].

Conclusion

Advances in the technology available for endoscopes and instruments have allowed urologists to extend the indications for ureteroscopic stone surgery. Miniaturization of endoscopes and laser fibers has allowed us to reach stones previously untreatable by endoscopy. However, URS is still not risk free and care taken by the urologist is still key. Adequate indications, proper preparation of the patient, selection of the right instruments, and knowing the limits are important principles to prevent any complication.

Key points

- Ureteroscopy is a first-line treatment option for distal ureteral stones, proximal ureteral stones >1 cm, and renal stones less than 2 cm.
- Making sure all the appropriate instruments and accessories are available before a case is mandatory.
- Hydrophilic stiff guidewires and hybrid wires offer the benefits of being less traumatic and facilitate bypassing an obstruction while rendering instrument passing possible.
- While a UAS presents several advantages in performing a flexible URS, including easy re-entry and exits, good irrigation drainage and low-pressure system, its use can be associated with ureteral wall injury, so careful use is necessary.
- Holmium laser lithotripsy is the main modality due to its versatility (semi-rigid and flexible), various uses (e.g. endopyelotomy), and safety. Different settings obtain different effects: fragmenting, dusting, and cutting.
- Various devices and techniques of stone retrieval and prevention of retropulsion help to obtain a stone-free status.

References

1. Türk C, Knoll T, Petrik A, Sarica K, Straub M, Sietz C. *Guidelines on Urolithiasis*. Arnhem: European Association of Urology, 2012, pp. 21–65.
2. Osorio L, Lima E, Soares J, et al. Emergency ureteroscopic management of ureteral stones: why not? Urology 2007; 69(1): 27–31; discussion 333.
3. Preminger GM, Tiselius H-G, Assimos DG, et al. 2007 Guideline for the management of ureteral calculi: diagnosis and treatment recommendation. EAU/AUA Nephrolithiasis Guideline Panel. Arnhem: European Association of Urology, 2007, pp. 31–7.
4. Aboumarzouk OM, Monga M, Kata SG, Traxer O, Somani BK. Flexible ureteroscopy and laser lithotripsy for stones >2 cm: a systematic review and meta-analysis. J Endourol 2012; 26(10): 1257–63.
5. Grasso M, Conlin M, Bagley D. Retrograde ureteropyeloscopic treatment of 2 cm. or greater upper urinary tract and minor Staghorn calculi. J Urol 1998; 160(2): 346–51.
6. Klingler HC, Kramer G, Lodde M, Dorfinger K, Hofbauer J, Marberger M. Stone treatment and coagulopathy. Eur Urol 2003; 43(1): 75–9.
7. Borofsky MS, Shah O. Advances in ureteroscopy. Urol Clin North Am 2013; 40(1): 67–78.
8. Mancini JG. How to protect patients and personnel from radiation. In: Smith AD, Preminger GM, Kavoussi LR, eds. *Smith's Textbook of Endourology*, 3rd edn. Oxford: Blackwell, 2012, pp. 10–18.
9. Geavlete P. Ureteroscopy complications. In: Smith AD, Preminger GM, Kavoussi LR, eds. *Smith's Texbook of Endourology*, 3rd edn. Oxford: Blackwell, 2012
10. Delvechhio FC. Access to the ureter: rigid ureteroscopy. In: Smith AD, Preminger GM, Kavoussi LR, eds. *Smith's Textbook of Endourology*, 3rd edn. Oxford: Blackwell, 2012.
11. Hubert KC, Palmer JS. Passive dilation by ureteral stenting before ureteroscopy: eliminating the need for active dilation. J Urol 2005; 174(3): 1079–80; discussion 1080.

12. Doizi S, Knoll T, Scoffone CM, et al. First clinical evaluation of a new, innovative ureteral access sheath (Re-Trace): a multicenter study. World J Urol 2013; May 3 (epub ahead of print).
13. Ng YH, Somani BK, Dennison A, Kata SG, Nabi G, Brown S. Irrigant flow and intrarenal pressure during flexible ureteroscopy: the effect of different access sheaths, working channel instruments, and hydrostatic pressure. J Endourol 2010; 24(12): 1915–20.
14. Traxer O, Thomas A. Prospective evaluation and classification of ureteral wall injuries resulting from insertion of a ureteral access sheath during retrograde intrarenal surgery. J Urol 2013; 189(2): 580–4.
15. Lechevallier E, Luciani M, Nahon O, Lay F, Coulange C. Transurethral ureterorenolithotripsy using new automated irrigation/suction system controlling pressure and flow compared with standard irrigation: a randomized pilot study. J Endourol 2003; 17(2): 97–101.
16. Yaycioglu O, Guvel S, Kilinc F, Egilmez T, Ozkardes H. Results with 7.5 F versus 10 F rigid ureteroscopes in treatment of ureteral calculi. Urology 2004; 64(4): 643–6; discussion 646–7.
17. Grasso M, Bagley D. Small diameter, actively deflectable, flexible ureteropyeloscopy. J Urol 1998; 160(5): 1648–53; discussion 1653–4.
18. Somani BK, Al-Qahtani SM, Gil de Medina SD, Traxer O. Outcomes of flexible ureterorenoscopy and laser fragmentation for renal stones: comparison between digital and conventional ureteroscope. Urology. 2013 Aug 31. PubMed PMID: 24001703.
19. Michel MS, Knoll T, Ptaschnyk T, Kohrmann KU, Alken P. Flexible ureterorenoscopy for the treatment of lower pole calyx stones: influence of different lithotripsy probes and stone extraction tools on scope deflection and irrigation flow. Eur Urol 2002; 41(3): 312–16; discussion 316–17.
20. Traxer O, Dubosq F, Jamali K, Gattegno B, Thibault P. New-generation flexible ureterorenoscopes are more durable than previous ones. Urology 2006; 68(2): 276–9; discussion 280–1.
21. Aridogan IA, Zeren S, Bayazit Y, Soyupak B, Doran S. Complications of pneumatic ureterolithotripsy in the early postoperative period. J Endourol 2005; 19(1): 50–3.
22. Denstedt JD, Razvi HA, Sales JL, Eberwein PM. Preliminary experience with holmium: YAG laser lithotripsy. J Endourol 1995; 9(3): 255–8.
23. Lee J, Gianduzzo TR. Advances in laser technology in urology. Urol Clin North Am 2009; 36(2): 189–98, viii.
24. Ahmed M, Pedro RN, Kieley S, Akornor JW, Durfee WK, Monga M. Systematic evaluation of ureteral occlusion devices: insertion, deployment, stone migration, and extraction. Urology 2009; 73(5): 976–80.
25. Sacco D, McDougal WS, Schwarz A. Preventing migration of stones during fragmentation with thermosensitive polymer. J Endourol 2007; 21(5): 504–7.
26. Patel A. Lower calyceal occlusion by autologous blood clot to prevent stone fragment reaccumulation after retrograde intra-renal surgery for lower calyceal stones: first experience of a new technique. J Endourol 2008; 22(11): 2501–6.
27. Nabi G, Cook J, N'Dow J, McClinton S. Outcomes of stenting after uncomplicated ureteroscopy: systematic review and meta-analysis. BMJ 2007; 334(7593): 572.
28. Djaladat H, Tajik P, Payandemehr P, Alehashemi S. Ureteral catheterization in uncomplicated ureterolithotripsy: a randomized, controlled trial. Eur Urol 2007; 52(3): 836–41.

29. Chew BH, Denstedt JD. Ureteroscopy and retrograde ureteral access. In: Wein AJ, Kavoussi LR, eds. *Campbell-Walsh Urology*, 9th edn. Philadelphia: Saunders Elsevier, 2007, pp. 1516–17.
30. Denstedt JD, Wollin TA, Reid G. Biomaterials used in urology: current issues of biocompatibility, infection, and encrustation. J Endourol 1998; 12(6): 493–500.
31. Chew B, Paterson R. Ureteroscopy: ureteral stents and postoperative care. In: Smith AD, Badlani GH, Preminger GM, Kavoussi LR, eds. *Smith's Textbook of Endourology*. Oxford: Blackwell, 2012, pp. 495–505.

CHAPTER 20

Ureteropyeloscopic Management of Upper Urinary Tract Calculi

Michael Grasso[1], Andrew I. Fishman[1], and Bobby Alexander[2]

[1]New York Medical College, Valhalla, NY, USA

[2]Lenox Hill Hospital, New York, NY, USA

Introduction

Ureteroscopic lithotripsy has progressed since the first reported cases employing rigid rod lens endoscopes in the late 1970s [1,2]. The application of fiberoptics allowed for endoscope miniaturization and also facilitated the application of steerable, deflectable ureteroscopes [3,4]. Over the last 30 years there has been a general trend toward smaller, actively deflectable, flexible endoscopes which are easier to place into the upper urinary tract, and when combined with powerful and precise lithotrites facilitate not only clearance of the average ureteral calculus, but also treatment of large complex intrarenal stone burdens [4,5,6,7,8,9].

Technological advances which improve the efficiency of ureteroscopic lithotripsy include the small diameter flexible ureteroscopes, holmium laser lithotrite, and a variety of Nitinol-based endoscopic retrieval devices. In the preceding chapter the currently available endoscopes and accessories were presented. With these instruments, a variety of surgical techniques have been developed to facilitate efficient clearance of upper urinary tract calculi. Variables including stone burden, calculus location, upper urinary tract obstruction, intrarenal anatomical variants, and stone composition all must be assessed when developing an endoscopic treatment plan. The only relative contraindication to proceeding with ureteroscopic lithotripsy is an active infection. Otherwise, with current instrumentation and the described techniques, most stones can be cleared in this minimally invasive, retrograde endoscopic fashion.

Ureteroscopic lithotripsy: general principles

The endoscopic suite where retrograde ureteroscopic lithotripsy is performed should be familiar to the urologist and assisting staff. A radiolucent operating table and real-time fluoroscopy are essential. Most ureteroscopic

Urinary Stones: Medical and Surgical Management, First Edition. Edited by Michael Grasso and David S. Goldfarb.

procedures are performed under general or, less frequently, regional anesthesia. The adage "one is none" is important when describing instrumentation available to the urologist in this setting. A variety of semi-rigid and flexible endoscopes, as well as a complete array of accessory instruments, should be readily at hand as necessary based on the clinical parameters encountered intraoperatively.

Choosing an endoscope

There are two basic classes of ureteroscopes: semi-rigid and actively deflectable flexible (Figure 20.1). These endoscopes are employed in different clinical settings and have complementary roles. Semi-rigid endoscopes are essential in treating intramural and distal ureteral lesions, but can be employed proximally in dilated systems. They are particularly useful in assessing the obstructed distal ureter when retrograde attempts at obtaining guidewire or catheter access have been unsuccessful. All other upper urinary tract stones are best treated with the actively deflectable, flexible ureteroscope. The steerability of these endoscopes allows the endoscopist to treat calculi throughout the calyceal system, without concerns about stone migration.

Semi-rigid ureteroscopes

The fiberoptic-based semi-rigid ureteroscopes replaced the rod lens rigid endoscopes over 20 years ago [10]. The application of fiberoptic bundles for illumination and visualization in a bendable metal cylinder facilitated miniaturization, which in turn allowed for easier ureteral access while maintaining a clear round endoscopic field of view even when the instrument was gently flexed [11,12,13]. This was remarkably different from the half moon optical defect that was common when the rod lens rigid ureteroscopes were torqued even minimally in the ureter.

The outer metal sheath of the semi-rigid ureteroscope is graduated in size. For example, a semi-rigid endoscope with a tip diameter of 7.5 F will have a shaft diameter of over 10 F at the base, and when passed into the ureter will facilitate intramural dilation under direct vision. This is particularly useful when other intramural dilation techniques are unsatisfactory. Direct ureteroscopic assessment can define intramural pathology prohibiting intramural dilation (e.g. stricture, hidden calculus, false passage of guidewire) and also dilate this segment when other fluoroscopically placed accessories have failed.

Semi-rigid ureteroscopes have two basic tip designs. The triangular or oval flush tip is found on two-channel endoscopes. These ureteroscopes have two dedicated working channels and are designed to employ two accessories simultaneously. The two dedicated channels allow for two working accessories to be fixed in space relative to each other. The application of a stone retrieval device or basket to immobilize a migrating calculus,

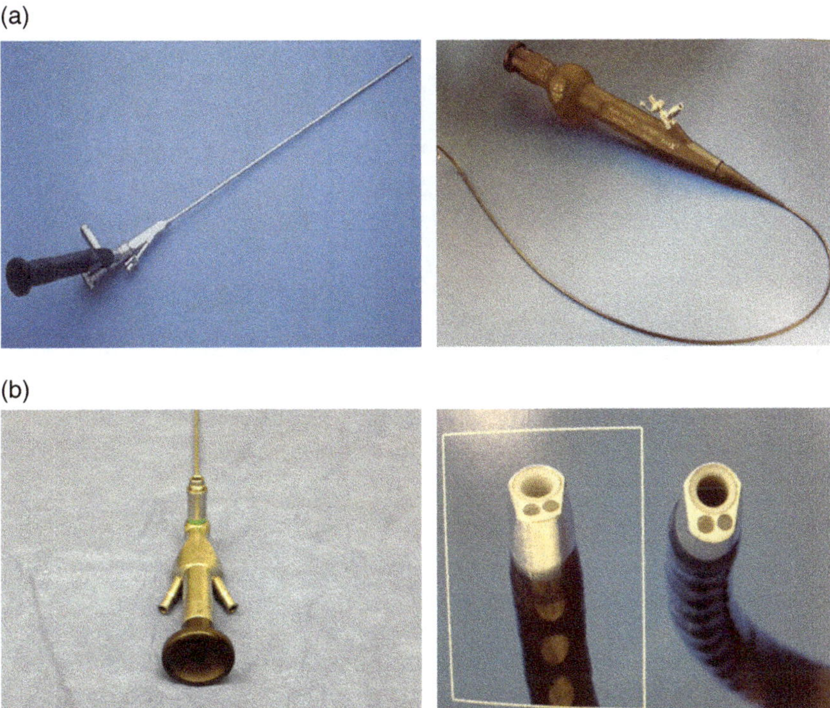

Figure 20.1 (a) Semi-rigid ureteroscopes (single channel and dual channel). (b) Flexible ureteroscope. Source: Grasso M. 2006 [16]. Reproduced with permission of Karl Storz.

for example, combined with a lithotrite like the holmium laser allows for efficient treatment of a mobile ureteral stone (Figure 20.2a). Rotation of the endoscope places the laser fiber circumferentially on the calculus, sculpting it to an extractable core. The beaked or bulbous single working channel semi-rigid endoscope has a larger working channel and better irrigant flow, but lacks the precise control of two simultaneously placed accessories as compared to the two-channel design.

Actively deflectable, flexible ureteroscopes

The actively deflectable, flexible ureteroscope has evolved with improved optics and mechanical advancements that facilitate universal retrograde intrarenal therapies. From an optics perspective, smaller diameter fiberoptic quartz bundles became commercially available in early 1990, and as such these endoscopes downsized from over 10 F in diameter to a standard 8 F tip and shaft [3,4,5,14]. This, more than any other advancement, facilitated flexible ureteroscope access. Subsequently, digital CMOS-based chips have replaced fiberoptics with a more detailed image, but initially

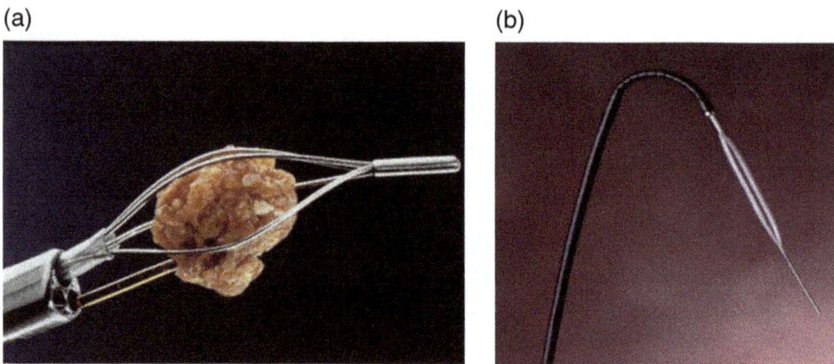

Figure 20.2 (a) Simultaneous placement of laser and basket through a two-channel semi-rigid endoscope. (b) Placement of an accessory device (Passport balloon) into a lower pole system using a flexible ureteroscope

requiring a larger overall endoscope diameter. Fortunately, the newest of the digital endoscopes are based on the smallest available digital chips and have similar diameter specifications as their fiberoptic predecessors [15].

Steerability and deflectability are key attributes of the flexible ureteroscope. Primary endoscope deflection refers to the ability to deflect the endoscope tip by depressing a lever in the handle. There are a variety of current flexible ureteroscope designs available. Attractive flexible ureteroscope features which improve treatment efficiency include two-way active tip deflection, large radius of deflection, a relatively stiff torquable distal shaft, and a passive deflecting segment approximately 3 from the active deflecting mechanism. It is this passive deflecting segment that is particularly useful in placing accessories through the endoscope's working channel into a dependent lower pole calyx [5] (Figure 20.2b).

Irrigation: clearing the optical field of view

The judicial administration of irrigation applied through the endoscope's working channel during ureteroscopy is essential to facilitate clear visualization. Sterile saline irrigant is the primary agent, which can be applied via a mechanical pump or piston syringe. The key is to deliver just enough irrigant to clear the optical field but not overdistend the collecting system, which can lead to obscuring hematuria.

A simple and straightforward system employs two 60 cc syringes of normal saline irrigant, connected through a three-way stopcock to Luer-Lock extension (i.e. arterial line) tubing (Figure 20.3). This delivery system offers the assistant precise control of pressure and flow to clear the visual field, especially when the endoscope's working channel is shared with a grasper or laser fiber [16]. Benefits of this simple system include continuous irrigation with minimal lapse in flow with syringe refill, and the ability to

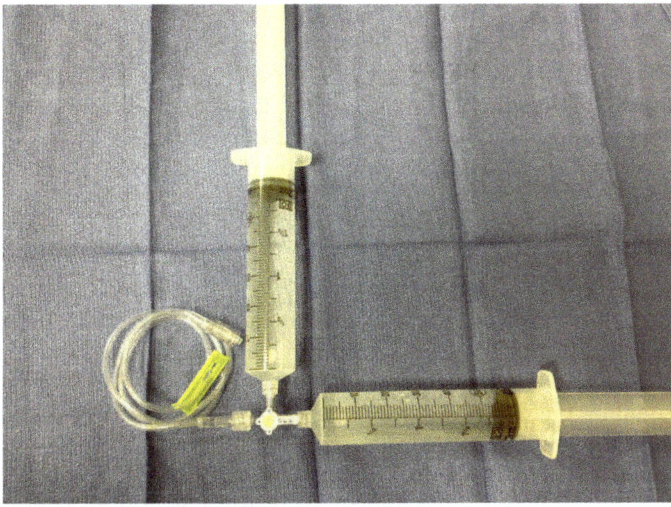

Figure 20.3 Two 60 cc syringes of normal saline irrigant, connected through a three-way stopcock to Luer-Lock extension (i.e. arterial line) tubing.

increase or decrease pressure as necessary when accessories of various diameter partially obstruct the delivery of saline through the endoscope's working channel.

Essential accessories

Guidewires, catheters, sheaths, and ureteral stents

A variety of guidewires are employed for both ureteral access, directing the endoscope into the upper urinary tract, and as a safety mechanism during complex ureteroscopic interventions. Basic components of guidewires include a core (i.e. mandrill) composed of stiff stainless steel or flexible Nitinol, with outer wraps composed of steel, Teflon, or a plastic polymer. Ureteral access catheters are either stiff and braided, employed to circumvent a stone and traverse an obstruction, or softer with multiple shaft perforations facilitating maximum drainage. In general, the combination of a lubriciously coated angled tipped Nitinol guidewire with a 5 F angiographic catheter is employed to traverse an obstructed segment secondary to an impacted ureteral calculus. Contrast material is instilled liberally through the catheter to define tip location and ureteral anatomy. In the setting of a particularly tortuous or kinked ureter, the steerable 5 F hockeystick-shaped Kumpe or broad-angled Cobra catheter can be employed. These catheters are particularly useful in exchanging from an access guidewire to one that will either straighten the ureter and/or facilitate endoscope placement.

Ureteral stents are commonly employed in conjunction with ureteroscopic lithotripsy. These internal double pigtail catheters serve two purposes: to help ensure upper urinary tract and to facilitate passive dilation of the ureter improving clearance of stone debris and drainage in general [9]. These catheters are of various lengths and diameters, and are composed of a variety of polymers. The larger diameter catheters facilitate improved drainage. Silicone ureteral stents appear to have the least tissue reaction, but the softness of the material can make placement challenging.

Examples of clinical challenges addressed with various guidewires and catheters are listed below.

- **Impacted ureteral stone**: the angled tip, lubriciously coated nickel titanium glidewire is the premier ureteral access wire, most often able to traverse ureteral obstructions including impacted stones or strictures caused by disease. This torquable and flexible guidewire, stabilized with a 5 F braided angiographic catheter, can be navigated through the most difficult obstructions under fluoroscopic guidance.
- **Flexible ureteroscopic access over a guidewire**: the angle tip, Teflon-jacketed Nitinol-based Zebra guidewire (Boston Scientific, Natick, Mass.) has many positive attributes that make it a superior delivery guidewire for the flexible ureteroscope. It is nickel titanium based and so virtually non-kinkable, it has a relatively stiff shaft which can straighten ureteral tortuosities, and the outer jacket is composed of a similar Teflon as the lining of the flexible ureteroscope working channel, allowing for a low coefficient of friction while having a waxy feel such that the assistant can properly place appropriate traction to facilitate endoscope placement.
- **Straightening the tortuous ureter**: stiff guidewires are necessary when attempting to minimize ureteral tortuosity and allow for a straight ureteral pathway for the endoscope. Nickel titanium and stainless steel combination guidewires like the Sensor (Boston Scientific, Natick, Mass.) and Roadrunner (Cook Urological, Spenser, Ind.) are densely radiopaque with a soft flexible tip that helps prevent ureteral perforation while maintaining a stiff shaft for straightening the ureter. They both can be employed as a flexible ureteroscope placement guidewire, but have a larger role in straightening the ureter for access and also as safety wires in complex presentations.
- **The ultimate safety guidewire**: the Amplatz super stiff guidewire offers maximal rigidity. It should never be placed directly into the ureter. Rather, an angiographic catheter should be directed into the collecting system first with the aid of a softer steerable guidewire, and once the catheter tip's position is verified with contrast under fluoroscopic guidance, it is exchanged for the super stiff wire. In addition, this wire should never be used as a flexible ureteroscope placement guidewire. It is kinkable, which can be frustrating, and the stiff shaft often has a sharp distal end that will play havoc with the endoscope's delicate working channel. That all being said, it is the premier safety wire and will temporarily fix in space a hypermobile kidney. It is also particularly useful in placing large-caliber (8–10Fr) and soft silicone-based double pigtail ureteral stents.

Stone movers and extractors

Historically, basket extractors were employed either under fluoroscopic guidance or with the assistance of a ureteroscope. Currently fluoroscopic-assisted stone basketing, termed "blind basketing," is prohibited by two guideline panel reports [17]. Extraction of smaller stones can be performed ureteroscopically, but with current endoscopic lithotrites like the holmium laser, it is preferred that stones which are too large to pass are rendered into smaller fragments with a lithotrite, and then those fragments are either extracted or allowed to pass spontaneously.

What has increased the safety margin of basket extractors is the application of pliable, non-kinkable Nitinol instead of stainless steel for the extractor wires. Tiny Nitinol wires are now available, with the smallest diameter basket currently employed only 1.7 F in sheath diameter, so small that it does not inhibit the active delectability of the flexible ureteroscope and can be easily placed into the lower pole collecting system. Other applications of small-diameter Nitinol wires include extractors that allow for grasping and dropping stone fragments. The 1.7 F N-gauge and 1.9 F Graspit are two varied designs on this theme. These accessories are particularly useful in relocating intrarenal calculi to more cephalad locations where larger diameter laser fibers can be employed, increasing the efficiency of stone fragmentation (Figure 20.4) [18].

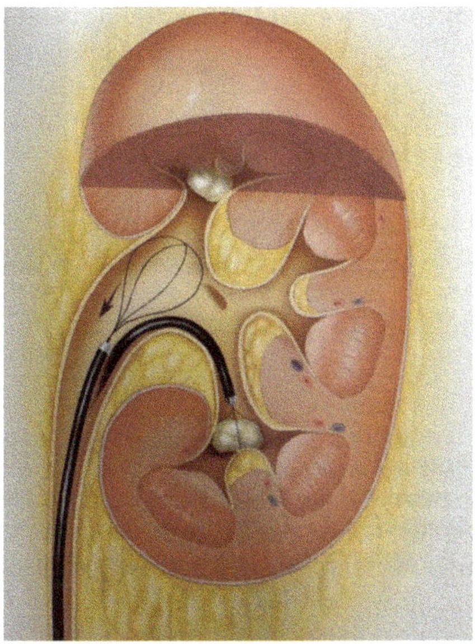

Figure 20.4 Relocation of lower pole intrarenal calculi to more cephalad location where larger diameter laser fibers can be employed, increasing the efficiency of stone. Source: Grasso M. 2006 [16]. Reproduced with permission of Karl Storz.

Endoscopic lithotrites

As described in the previous chapter, there are many energy sources and lithotrites available for stone fragmentation. Electrohydraulic lithotrites, commonly employed 20 years ago but rarely seen in contemporary endoscopy suites, were powerful but delivered energy imprecisely and were too often associated with ureteral wall trauma [19,20,21,22]. Since the first publication describing the holmium:yttrium-aluminum-garnet (Ho:YAG) laser as a powerful and precise endoscopic lithotrite in 1996, this energy source has become the primary ureteroscopic lithotripter employed worldwide [23]. Low water density quartz fibers of various diameters are employed to deliver pulsatile light energy, fragmenting stones of all compositions with both direct thermal and photoacoustic effects. Larger diameter 365 micron fibers have a proportionately larger fiber tip water vaporization bubble and more expeditiously fragment stone compared to the smaller, more flexible 200 micron variety, employed almost exclusively for lower pole calculi [24]. A variety of fragmentation schemes have been developed to efficiently treat upper urinary tract calculi with this laser energy, varying total energy in joules and frequency of pulsation in hertz to obtain the desired effect. Stone composition, density and fragility, location in the collecting system, and stone volume are all key variables when choosing laser settings. Representative clinical scenarios are described below.

- **Stone sculpting**: for large, hard, calcium oxalate and cystine-based stones, high-energy (1.0–1.5 J) and relatively low frequency (5–10 Hz) settings are used to core out the center of the stone, followed by reducing crescents and peripheral pieces into multiple smaller passable fragments. Reducing the settings will help in dividing the mobile fragments in half and then in half again, until they are rendered into the desired diameter (approximately 2–3 mm).
- **Stone dusting**: for large, soft, uric acid and calcium oxalate dihydrate-based stones, low-energy (0.6–0.8 J) and high-frequency (10–30 Hz) settings are used to dust the stone into fine sand. Starting from the periphery, the laser tip is gently passed back and forth at a set distance. This technique should leave no sizeable fragments and only fine passable debris at completion.

Ureteral access sheath

The ureteral access sheath, a combined dilator and hollow tube that facilitates easier placement of the ureteroscope directly into the ureter, has been available as an adjunct to standard ureteroscope technique since the 1980s. Positive attributes include helping to maintain lower collecting system pressure and easier endoscope placement when multiple passes of the endoscope are required, particularly when many small stone fragments are being meticulously extracted [25,26,27]. Historically, these catheters kinked and could trap an endoscope, inhibiting removal, but with newer material this has been less of a problem. One major issue is the relatively large outer diameter of these cylinders and the effect of this sustained dilation through an operative procedure on the ureter itself [28].

In a recent report by Traxer and Thomas, 359 consecutive patients undergoing retrograde intrarenal surgery using an ureteral access sheath were prospectively evaluated for ureteral wall injury. Ureteral trauma with wall damage was found in 167 patients, with high-grade full-thickness injury identified in 48 (13.3%). The most significant predictor of severe ureteral injury was lack of presenting prior to sheath placement ($p = 0.0001$). Presenting decreased the risk of ureteral injury seven-fold [29].

As a general rule, operative sheaths can be a useful adjunct during complex ureteroscopic procedures, but should be employed with caution in non-dilated systems.

Surgical technique

Obtaining retrograde access to the ureter and kidney

Upper urinary tract endoscopy begins with a systematic evaluation of the bladder. Meticulous cystoscopic assessment with either a rigid or flexible endoscope begins the evaluation. Contrast-based fluoroscopic imaging of the upper urinary tract is performed next. A retrograde pyelogram is performed with either a 5 F open-ended angiographic or 6 F cone-tipped catheter and dilute radiopaque contrast material. This is performed with real-time fluoroscopy, only injecting sufficient contrast material to opacify but not overdistend the collecting system. This produces a radiographic road map of the collecting system, helping to localize ureteral or renal stones, as well as defining obstructive lesions and anatomical variants (e.g. infundibular and ureteral strictures, duplications, ureteral tortuosity, etc.).

The techniques employed to access the ureter and place the ureteroscope proximally to the level of a calculus have evolved based in large part on endoscope miniaturization. When the ureteroscope outer diameter was in excess of 10 F, intramural dilation was routinely required to place the instrument into the ureteral lumen. With greater ureteral dilation, there is an increased risk of ureteral perforation and thus one or two guidewires were simultaneously employed, one acting as a safety wire to maintain access. If, for example, ureteroscopic interventions became difficult and the procedure required conversion to placement of an ureteral stent to maintain patency and drainage, the safety guidewire was available to facilitate placement of this internal catheter. As ureteroscopes have become smaller in outer profile, intramural dilation for access is less commonly required and frequently the endoscope can be placed into the ureter to the level of a stone under direct vision without the aid of a guidewire.

Techniques employed to achieve ureteroscopic access to the ureter and intrarenal collecting system: specific clinical presentations

The impacted intramural ureteral calculus

This clinical presentation can be one of the most challenging for the endourologist. Often the ureteral orifice is completely covered with edema and may be difficult to localize with a standard cystoscopic technique. If a guidewire cannot be placed with combined cystoscopic and fluoroscopic guidance, the next step is to try to intubate the orifice directly with a smallest diameter semi-rigid ureteroscope. Often the crowning stone will be noted and the tip of the endoscope employed to gently move the stone back into the dilated ureter, allowing for a guidewire to be passed proximally through the working channel under direct vision. Laser energy can also be employed to retropulse the stone, but *in situ* fragmentation should proceed with caution to minimize fragment perforation and create submucosal stone debris.

The obstructing distal ureteral calculus – the two-guidewire technique (Figure 20.5)

When a guidewire can be passed proximal to an obstructing distal ureteral calculus but the intramural ureter is tight or edematous, the two-wire access technique is often helpful. In this setting a small-caliber, two-channel semi-rigid ureteroscope is passed just to the ureteral orifice beside the safety guidewire. A second guidewire is passed proximally under direct endoscopic and fluoroscopic guidance. Irrigation is passed through the second endoscopic working channel to clear the optical field and the endoscope rotated, placing its tip between the two guidewires. The semi-rigid ureteroscope is then gently passed proximally between the two wires, compressing the edema and gently dilating the distal segment until the calculus is encountered. Once at the level of the calculus, the second wire is removed and lithotripsy can commence.

Passing the flexible ureteroscope through a tight distal ureter

Intramural ureteral dilation for endoscope access is used sparingly in the era of the small-diameter ureteroscope. When the intramural ureter is particularly narrow, often encountered in young muscular male patients or those with an intrusive prostate, intramural dilation is frequently required. Graduated 6–12 F Nottingham dilators are passed under fluoroscopic guidance over a pre-placed safety guidewire. If this is insufficient, a low-caliber 12 F dilation balloon is employed. Lastly, if the flexible ureteroscope still fails to pass, a small-caliber semi-rigid ureteroscope is employed to assess the ureter under direct vision. A submucosal or kinked guidewire can be determined promptly and changed, while the actual proximal passage of this endoscope with its graduated shaft will dilate the intramural tunnel to 12 F (i.e. dilation under direct vision).

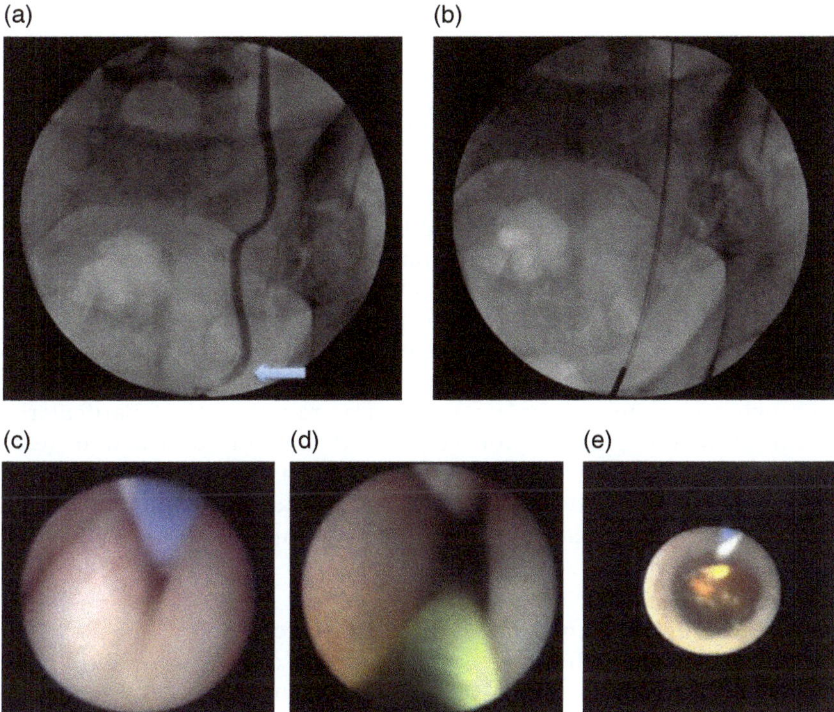

Figure 20.5 The obstructing distal ureteral calculus – the two-guidewire technique. (a) Fluoroscopic illustration of impacted distal ureteral stone. (b) Fluoroscopic illustration of two-wire technique. (c) Ureteroscopic view of Zebra wire. (d) Ureteroscopic view of two-wire technique. (e) Ureteroscopic view of impacted ureteral stone ready for lithotripsy.

No-touch flexible ureteroscopic access

Directing the actively deflectable, flexible ureteroscope into the ureter under direct vision without the aid of a guidewire or sheath was first described for mapping the upper urinary tract in treating malignant urothelial lesions. What was found is that often, the endoscope can be placed to the level of an obstructing calculus without a guidewire in a particularly atraumatic manner. There are some obvious limitations and when unsuccessful, more standard ureteroscopic access techniques should be promptly employed. The attractiveness of this technique, however, is that it allows for a virtually atraumatic placement of the endoscope under direct vision [30]. One limitation is when a calculus is located in the most distal ureter. The secondary deflecting segment of the flexible ureteroscope may lead to shaft buckling in the bladder, inhibiting precise steerability and laser fiber placement in this location. For these reasons, the semi-rigid endoscope is a more efficient platform for lithotripsy in the most distal ureter.

To intubate the ureteral orifice under direct vision with the actively deflectable flexible ureteroscope, the distal deflecting end should be straightened to be in line with the intramural ureter, as if a straight angiographic catheter was being passed into the orifice. If the orifice has a flap-like configuration, a standard stainless steel guidewire can be passed through the working channel, just intubating the orifice to hold it open for endoscope passage. Once the endoscope enters the ureter, it is directed proximal by turning up and lateral, following the natural turns of the distal-most ureter. It is essential to advance the shaft beyond the deflecting components to gain steerability from the handle and to prevent shaft buckling. Once the endoscope has progressed beyond the distal-most 5 cm of the ureter, it will pass more easily under direct vision to the level of the stone in question and treatment begins. This no-wire no-touch technique minimizes guidewire trauma and is particularly useful in defining causes for concurrent ureteral obstruction (e.g. stricture, edema, iatrogenic false passage, etc.) in a clear endoscopic field of view [30]. Obviously, this technique is not feasible in many clinical settings but as endoscopic miniaturization continues, its applicability will continue to grow.

Access through the tortuous proximal ureter

Passing the actively deflectable flexible ureteroscope proximal through a ureteral kink or narrowing can be a frustrating endeavor. It is essential to remember that the most proximal ureter has minimal surrounding support with the thinnest ureteral wall structure, and thus vigorous maneuvers in this segment can be calamitous. Radiopaque contrast can be instilled through the working channel of the endoscope to help define the more proximal ureter fluoroscopically, creating a road map. If the endoscope cannot be passed under direct vision through a serpiginous ureter, the placement of a guidewire through the working channel and beyond one tortuous segment is often helpful. Just as a catheter and angle tipped Nitinol wire is used to traverse tortuous segments in a stepwise fashion, the endoscope in this setting is analogous to the catheter. The angle tipped Teflon-jacketed Nitinol-based Zebra guidewire is particularly useful in this setting.

It s very important to remember that overdilation of the proximal ureter, with either a balloon or graduated dilator, will thin the ureter and increase the risk of perforation or avulsion. When the ureteropelvic junction (UPJ) of the proximal ureter is narrowed from either edema or fibrosis, and dilation is required for retrograde endoscope passage, the act of dilation should be minimal in diameter (i.e. 10–12 F) with the least traumatic device. In this setting a low-pressure 12 F dilation balloon can either be passed through the working channel of the endoscope (Passport balloon, Boston Scientific or Bagley Balloon, Cook Urological) or over a safety guidewire. Ultimately if the endoscope does not pass easily through a segment, placement of an internal stent and staging the procedure, allowing for a period of passage dilation with catheter drainage, is optimal.

Intrarenal lower pole calyceal access

Directing the flexible ureteroscope into the lower pole calyceal system requires an understanding of the construction of the distal end of the ureteroscope shaft and intrarenal collecting system anatomy. The lower pole calyceal system can have a variety of configurations. The most challenging for endoscope placement is a lower pole infundibulum that is parallel to the ureter and is longer than 3 cm. The standard flexible ureteroscope should have at least 270° two-way active tip deflection, a deflecting radius that will allow intubation of the lower pole infundibulum, and a proximal shaft secondary passive deflecting segment. Just intubating the lower pole infundibilum is often insufficient for stone therapy. The endoscope tip must be placed into the peripheral calyceal system, ideally with an endoscopic lithotrite or grasper passed through the endoscope's working channel, onto a calculus [5,18].

To facilitate lower pole access, one must understand that the endoscope has both the actively deflecting segment and also a passively deflecting portion of the shaft. By widening the space between the endoscope articulating vertebrae just beyond the actively deflecting segment, a buckling or passive secondary deflecting segment designed for lower pole access can be obtained. By maximally deflecting the distal end by depressing the lever and then advancing the endoscope, the shaft will buckle when contacting the renal pelvis or upper pole infundibulum, and the tip will roll into the most dependent portion of the lower pole calyceal system. To place an accessory into the lower pole requires its passage just to the tip of a straight endoscope, and then performing the aforementioned steps. Once in the lower pole calyceal system, the accessory can be advanced from the tip position onto a stone. If, however, one attempts to place a stiff sharp laser fiber into the lower pole after the endoscope is maximally deflected, all too often this results in working channel perforation and damage to the instrument.

Traversing the obstructed or strictured infundibulum

When attempting to place the flexible ureteroscope beyond an infundibular stricture or through a narrow calyceal diverticular neck, the endoscopist first assesses the intrarenal collecting system directly, and then with radiopaque contrast and real-time fluoroscopy. Small-caliber catheters (Luminator Guide Wire, Boston Scientific, Natick, Mass.) can be placed through the working channel of the endoscope to inject contrast into a groove or pit to verify that this is indeed the aperture. Opening the aperture can be performed by either incising or dilating. Balloon dilation is preferred if the diverticular neck is long or tortuous. The small-caliber dilating balloons (e.g. Passport and Bagley balloons) described previously which can be placed through the endoscope's working channel are useful in this setting (see Figure 20.2b). These are low-pressure balloons and should be filled precisely with a Levine insufflator to only a few atmospheres of pressure. These balloons can rupture easily if overinflated. If this occurs, the endoscope and balloon should be removed as a unit, thus insuring the balloon does not disengage from the delivering catheter. It is often technically difficult to place these stiff shaft balloons into the most dependent segments of the collecting system. It is here, and with short-necked obstructing segments, that direct ureteroscopic incision is useful.

Ureteroscopic incision of a calyceal diverticular neck or infundibular stricture can be performed with either a small-caliber electrode (e.g. 2F Bugbee) or small-diameter 200 micron laser fiber and holmium laser energy. Understanding that often large-caliber vessels lie just below these infundibulae should give pause to any deep incisions. The infundibulotomy should be performed superficially at first, in a telegraphed manner, through the thinnest segment. Pure cutting current at a low setting for electrocautery, with holmium laser energy of 1.0–1.4J and high-frequency pulsation of 20Hz, is a good place to begin, with subtle adjustments on delivered power based on the density of the tissue encountered. After the superficial initial incision, the energy source is then used to connect the serrated perforations, connecting them into the peripheral obstructed segment while allowing the irrigant to hydro-distend the underlying tissue and thus protect adjacent vasculature.

The efficient application of the laser lithotripter

Since its introduction in the early 1990s, the holmium laser has been the primary endoscopic lithotrite employed worldwide [23,24,31]. The foundation of its success is the combination of a flexible fiberoptic delivery system, compatible with both semi-rigid and actively deflectable flexible ureteroscopes, and a solid state laser delivering 2150nm of light which when employed in a water-based medium creates a vaporization bubble able to fragment even the most dense calculi. Holmium laser energy fragments calculi in two ways: direct thermal vaporization and delivering the light energy in a pulsatile fashion, creating a photoacoustic effect. By varying the delivered energy in joules and the frequency of pulsation in hertz, the efficiency of stone fragmentation can be maximized.

Endoscopic fragmentation parameters are varied based on the composition, and thus density, of the offending calculus. An endoscopic assessment will commonly differentiate stone composition, directing the surgeon to employ different laser parameters. Dense, smooth black calcium oxalate monohydrate and cystine, for example, require higher energy settings (1.0–1.4J) and relatively low frequency of pulsation to prevent stone migration. Pinning smaller mobile fragments and lowering the frequency of pulsation will minimize migration and help to efficiently reduce the calculus to small debris. The opposite settings are useful for relatively soft crystalline calcium oxalate dihydrate and uric acid calculi. Lower energy and higher frequency of pulsation allow the endoscopist to powder the stone into fine dust by directing the laser fiber tip back and forth, painting the surface with laser energy.

Ureteropyeloscopic lithotripsy: techniques based on stone location

Distal ureteral calculi

Stone location in part dictates the technique employed for endoscopic lithotripsy. Distal ureteral stones are efficiently treated with the semi-rigid endoscope, often employing a basket extractor to prevent stone migration and laser energy for fragmentation. Two-channel endoscopes are useful in this setting in that the two accessories can be precisely employed relative to each other. For example, once engaged in a basket, the calculus can be efficiently fragmented with laser energy by rotating the endoscope, thus placing the fiber tip circumferentially as necessary to smooth the stone to an extractable core.

Middle third and proximal ureteral calculi

Middle third and proximal ureteral calculi are often mobile and will easily migrate into the intrarenal collecting system. By positioning the patient in Trendelenburg and raising the ipsilateral side, the stone will migrate into a more easily accessible cephalad calyx where efficient fragmentation can be performed. Even though in some patients semi-rigid endoscopes can be employed in the proximal ureter, the actively deflectable flexible ureteroscope allows the endoscopist to follow and treat a migrating calculus and thus is preferred in this setting.

Intrarenal calculi

Lower pole calculi can be the most difficult to access and treat with the actively deflectable flexible endoscope. Employing the small-diameter 200 micron laser fibers allows for greater tip deflection, but its proportionally smaller vaporization bubble fragments stone significantly slower than the larger core fibers. As treatment progresses, the cooling irrigant will hydrodistend the collecting system, making access to the lower pole more challenging. For large lower pole calculi, fragmentation is performed not to dust the calculus but rather to create moveable fragments which are repositioned with a smaller caliber endoscopic grasper to a more easily accessible cephalad calyx. Endoscopic lithotripsy can then be performed more efficiently in the upper pole calyx, employing a stiffer but larger diameter 365 micron laser fiber.

Ureteropyelosocpic treatment of large upper urinary tract calculi

Ureteroscopic treatment of large upper urinary tract calculi was first described in 1998, where patients with co-morbidities prohibiting percutaneous nephrostolithotomy were treated with retrograde endoscopic techniques [32]. Over the next 14 years some 10 centers presented their experience with excellent stone-free rates and minimal morbidity (Table 20.1). The most recent series was based on 145 patients with 164 stone burdens in excess of 2 cm in diameter, including 36

Table 20.1 Ureteroscopic management of upper urinary tract calculi >2 cm

Study	Date	Number of patients	Mean stone diameter (mm)	Mean number of procedures	Stone free (%)	Complications number (%)
Grasso et al. [32]	1998	51	24.9	1.3	93	3 (3)
El-Anany et al. [33]	2001	30	>20	1	77	3 (10)
Mariani [34]	2007	16	33	2.4	88	4 (10)
Ricchiuti et al. [35]	2007	23	30.9	1.4	74	0 (0)
Breda et al. [36]	2008	15	22	2.3	93	3 (9)
Wheat et al. [37]	2009	9	38	2.3	33	0 (0)
Riley et al. [38]	2009	22	30	1.8	91	4 (10)
Hyams et al. [39]	2010	120	24	1.2	83	8 (6)
Bader et al. [40]	2010	24	29.8	1.7	92	5 (12)
Takazawa et al. [41]	2011	20	31	1.4	90	3 (5)
Cohen et al. [9]	2012	145	29	1.6	87	5 (2)

partial staghorn calculi with a mean diameter of 37 mm. Stone-free rate at 3 months was 87%, with an average of 1.6 procedures per patient (Figure 20.6). There were only five minor complication noted in this large patient population.

A tenet of retrograde ureteropyeloscopic treatment of large upper urinary tract calculi is a sterile preoperative urine culture. Patients with infectious struvite calculi are poor candidates for this treatment in that there is a higher risk of perioperative infectious complications, and residual infectious stone debris may act as a nidus for stone regrowth and future infections. In cases of uncorrectable bleeding diathesis, or with renal ectopy where a nephrostomy cannot be placed safely due to the proximity of adjacent structures, retrograde ureteroscopic lithotripsy could be employed for struvite calculi, albeit with higher risk.

From a technical perspective, this procedure begins in a similar fashion to any flexible ureteropyeloscopic procedure. The flexible ureteroscope and laser lithotripter are employed to fragment the calculus into fine dust and small residual passable debris. To help maintain lower pressure in the collecting system, a small diameter (e.g. 14 F) Foley catheter is placed transurethrally beside the flexible ureteroscope to maintain continuous bladder drainage during the procedure, with sterile saline as the optimum irrigant. The application of the ureteral access sheath has been described in this setting as well, but in general there is concern about pressure necrosis of the ureteral wall when employing these large-diameter cylinders for lengthy procedures. Ureteroscopic fragmentation continues until the endoscopic field of view is obscured by dust and debris, with 90 min as an arbitrary operative stop time. All patients are counseled that second-stage

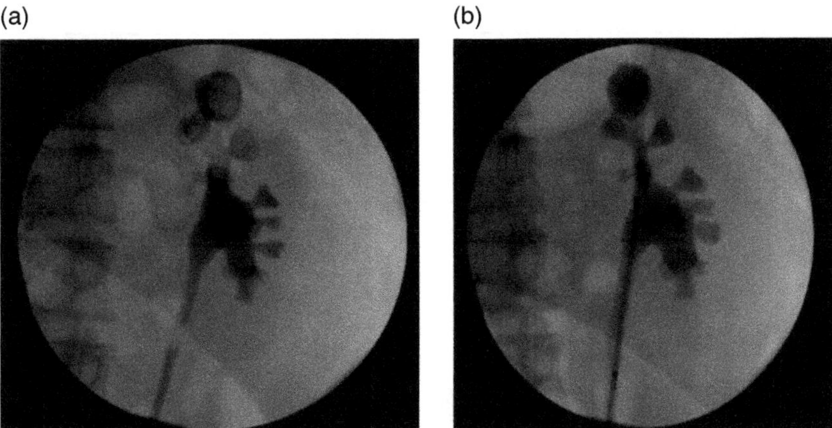

Figure 20.6 (a) Large upper pole partial staghorn calculus in cystinuric patient. (b) Completion retrograde pyelogram post staged ureteroscopic treatment.

ureteroscopy may be required. In those patients with the largest stone burdens, it is often difficult to determine whether the entire stone burden has been completely treated since the intrarenal collecting system is often coated with stone dust, potentially obscuring sizeable residua. For this reason, staged second-look endoscopy is planned from the onset in those with the largest stone burdens (>3 cm) and is essential in ensuring complete fragmentation.

Ureteroscopic lithotripsy is concluded when the stone burden is converted into fine dust and small fragments <3 mm, or when visualization is impeded by stone debris. Holmium laser settings are adjusted based on stone density and volume. Higher settings are employed to convert a large central stone burden into fine dust. Lower settings minimize the kinetic effects of the laser, and are employed to systematically reduce mobile stones into passable debris. At the conclusion of endoscopic lithotripsy, large-caliber ureteral stents (8–10 F) are employed to maximize drainage and passively dilate the ureter over time, which will ultimately help clear stone debris.

Staged ureteropyeloscopic lithotripsy and retrograde intrarenal irrigation

Patients with a sizeable residual stone burden after ureteroscopic lithotripsy that require staged therapy are either treated with an interval of internal ureteral stenting as an outpatient, or with a short course of retrograde intrarenal irrigation employed to clear stone dust and debris. Alkalinizing retrograde intrarenal irrigation is particularly useful in clearing cystine and uric acid stone debris, but in general stone dust of all compositions can be irrigated from the collecting system in this fashion (Table 20.2). In general, a two-catheter system is employed. A 5 F Cobra catheter positioned with

Table 20.2 Irrigant choice for intrarenal irrigation

Stone type	Irrigant choice
Cystine	THAM-E and Mucomyst*
Uric acid	THAM-E
Calcium-based	Normal saline and gentamicin

*THAM-E is pH 10 tromethamine tris-hydroxymethyl aminomethane; Mucomyst is N-acetylcysteine

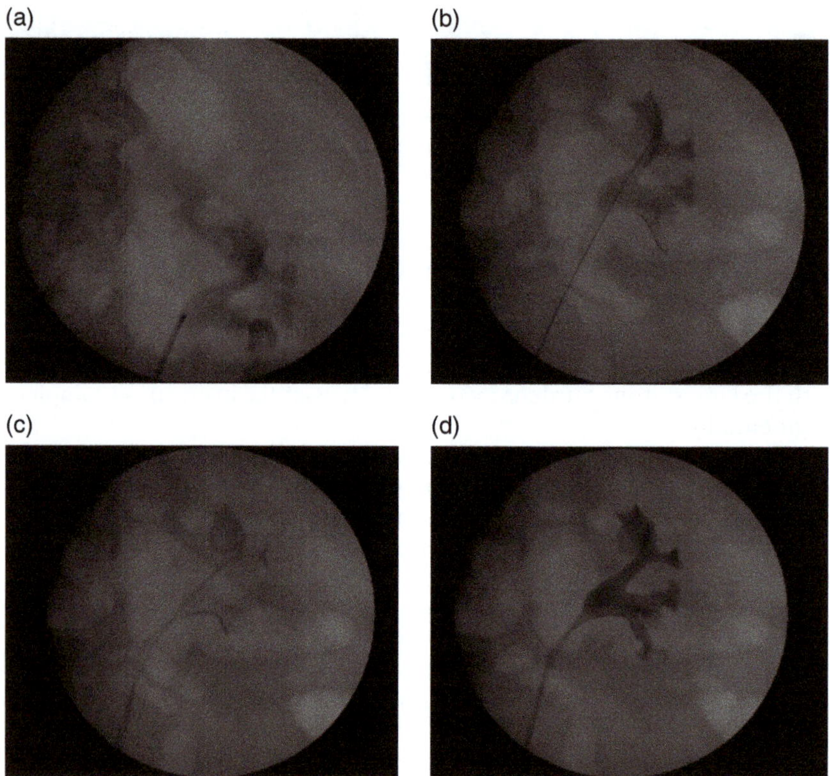

Figure 20.7 (a) Large obstructing lower pole uric acid stone. (b) Placement of two wires. (c) 5 F Cobra catheter positioned with its tip in the lower pole employed for irrigant inflow, and a single pigtail stent (e.g. 6 or 8 F in diameter) positioned centrally used for outflow drainage. (d) Fluoroscopic view of irrigation system.

its tip either in the lower pole or beside the majority of stone debris is employed for irrigant inflow, and a single pigtail stent (e.g. 6 or 8 F in diameter) positioned centrally is used for outflow drainage (Figure 20.7). The irrigation catheters are secured to a bladder Foley catheter, and their position in the intrarenal collecting system is verified with radiopaque contrast and fluoroscopic imaging.

Intrarenal irrigation is performed for 36–72 h to help clear stone dust and debris and to allow for more effective second-stage ureteroscopic lithotripsy. Irrigation commences at a rate of 50 mL per hour, and is gradually increased to 100 mL per hour as tolerated. The irrigation is immediately halted with clinical symptoms of high intrarenal pressure: flank pain, nausea and emesis, and/or fever. The catheters are hand irrigated to remove any obstructing debris and set to gravity drainage, with intrarenal irrigation only restarted when the clinical parameters improve.

Operative success when treating large intrarenal calculi with staged ureteroscopic lithotripsy is often defined on plain radiography as a smudge outline of the collecting system, reflecting tiny stone fragments and dust filling a calyx. Sonography immediately postoperative will define bright stone dust filling a calyx, which is echobright but shadow minimally. Over time this debris will systematically clear through the now dilated ureter, with overall stone-free rates at 3 months of 87%, and with stone regrowth only noted in those with uncorrectable hypermetabolic states (e.g. primary hyperoxalosis, uncorrectable cystinuria, hypervitaminosis D, malignant secondary hypercalcemia, etc.) [9].

References

1. Cockett WS, Cockett AT. The Hopkins rod-lens system and the Storz cold light illumination system. Urology 1998; 51(suppl 5A): 1–2.
2. Gow JG. Harold Hopkins and optical systems for urology – an appreciation. Urology 1998; 52: 152–7.
3. Bagley DH. Intrarenal access with flexible ureteropyeloscope: effects of active and passive tip deflection. J Endourol 1993; 7: 221.
4. Grasso M, Bagley DH. A 7.5/8.2 F actively deflectable, flexible ureteroscope: a new device for both diagnostic and therapeutic upper urinary tract endoscopy. Urology 1994; 43: 435–41.
5. Johnson GB, Grasso M. Exaggerated primary endoscope deflection: initial clinical experience with prototypic flexible ureteroscopes: the first 115 procedures. Br J Urol 2004; 93: 109–14.
6. Lam JS, Greene TD, Gupta, M. Treatment of proximal ureteral calculi: holmium:YAG laser ureterolithotripsy versus extracorporeal shock wave lithotripsy. J Urol 2002; 167: 1972–6.
7. Erhard M, Salwen J, Bagley DH. Ureteroscopic removal of mid and proximal ureteral calculi. J Urol 1996; 155: 38.
8. Graff J, Pastor J, Funke PJ, et al. Extracorporeal shock wave lithotripsy for ureteral stones: a retrospective analysis of 417 cases. J Urol 1988; 139: 513.
9. Cohen J, Cohen S, Grasso M. Ureteropyeloscopic treatment of large, complex intrarenal and proximal ureteral calculi. BJU Int 2013; 111: E127–31.
10. Grasso M. Intracorporeal lithotripsy: ultrasonic, electrohydraulic, laser, and electromechanical. In: Marshall FF, ed. *Textbook of Operative Urology*. Philadelphia: Saunders, 1996.

11. Stoller ML, Wolf JS, Hofmann R, Marc B. Ureteroscopy without routine balloon dilation: an outcome assessment. J Urol 1992; 147: 1238.
12. Abdel-Razzak OM, Bagley DH. The 6.9 F semi-rigid ureteroscope in clinical use. Urology 1993; 41: 45.
13. Bagley DH. Ureteroscopic stone retrieval: rigid versus flexible endoscopes. Semin Urol 1994; 12: 31.
14. Grasso M. Ureteropyeloscopic treatment of ureteral and intrarenal calculi. Urol Clin North Am 2000; 27: 623–31.
15. Binbay M, Yuruk E, Akman T, et al. Is there a difference in outcomes between digital and fiberoptic flexible ureterorenoscopy procedures? J Endourol 2010; 24(12): 1929–34.
16. Grasso M, Bagley DH. Flexible Ureteroscopy with the Flex-X2 Ureteroscope. Storz Manual. Tuttlingen, Germany: Endo-Press, 2006.
17. Segura JW, Preminger GM, Assimos DG, et al. Ureteral Stones Clinical Gudelines Panel summary report on the management of ureteral calculi. The American Urological Association. J Urol 1997; 158(5): 1915–21.
18. Grasso M, Ficazzola M. Retrograde ureteropyeloscopy for lower pole caliceal calculi. J Urol 1999; 162: 1904–8.
19. Raney AM. Electrohydraulic lithotripsy: experimental study and case reports with the stone disintegrator. J Urol 1975; 113(3): 345–7.
20. Raney AM. Electrohydraulic cystolithotripsy. Urology 1976; 7(4): 379–81.
21. Purohit GS, Pham D, Raney AM, Bogaev JH. Electrohydraulic ureterolithotripsy. An experimental study. Invest Urol 1980; 17(6): 462–4.
22. Denstedt JD, Clayman RV. Electrohydraulic lithotripsy of renal and ureteral calculi. J Urol 1990; 143: 13.
23. Grasso M. Experience with the holmium laser as an endoscopic lithotrite. Urology 1996; 48(2): 199–206.
24. Johnson DE, Cromeens DM, Price RE. Use of the holmium:YAG laser in urology. Lasers Surg Med 1992; 12(4): 353–63.
25. Kourambas J, Byrne RR, Preminger GM. Does a ureteral access sheath facilitate ureteroscopy? J Urol 2001; 165: 789–93.
26. Rehman J, Monga M, Landman J, et al. Characterization of intrapelvic pressure during ureteropyeloscopy with ureteral access sheaths. Urology 2003; 61: 713–18.
27. Auge BK, Pietrow PK, Lallas CD, et al. Ureteral access sheath provides protection against elevated renal pressures during routine flexible ureteroscopic stone manipulation. J Endourol 2004; 18: 33–6.
28. Delvecchio FC, Auge BK, Brizuela RM, et al. Assessment of stricture formation with the ureteral access sheath. Urology 2003; 61: 518–22.
29. Traxer O, Thomas A. Prospective evaluation and classification of ureteral wall injuries resulting from insertion of a ureteral access sheath during retrograde intrarenal surgery. J Urol 2013; 189(2): 580–4.
30. Johnson GB, Portela D, Grasso M. Advanced ureteroscopy: wireless and sheathless. J Endourol 2006; 20(8): 552–5.
31. Scarpa RM, de Lisa A, Porru D, et al. Holmium:YAG laser ureterolithotripsy. Eur Urol 1999; 35: 233–8.
32. Grasso M, Conlin M, Bagley DH. Retrograde ureteropyeloscopic treatment of 2 cm or greater upper urinary tract and minor staghorn calculi. J Urol 1998; 160(2): 346–51.
33. El-Anany FG, Hammouda HM, Maghraby HA, Elakkad MA. Retrograde ureteropyeloscopic holmium laser lithotripsy for large renal calculi. BJU Int 2001; 88: 850–3.

34. Mariani AJ. Combined electrohydraulic and holmium:YAG laser ureteroscopic nephrolithotripsy of large (greater than 4 cm) renal calculi. J Urol 2007; 177: 168–73.
35. Ricchiuti DJ, Smaldone MC, Jacobs BL, Maldone AM, Jackman SV, Averch TD. Staged retrograde endoscopic lithotripsy as alternative to PCNL in select patients with large renal calculi. J Endourol 2007; 21: 1421–4.
36. Breda A, Ogunyemi O, Leppert JT, Lam JS, Schulam PG . Flexible ureteroscopy and laser lithotripsy for single intrarental stones 2 cm or greater – is this the new frontier? J Urol 2008; 179: 981–4.
37. Wheat JC, Roberts WW, Wolf JS. Multisession retrograde endoscopic lithotripsy of large renal calculi in obese patients. Can J Urol 2009; 16: 4915–20.
38. Riley JM, Stearman L, Troxel S. Retrograde ureteroscopy for renal stones larger than 2.5 cm. J Endourol 2009; 23: 1395–8.
39. Hyams ES, Munver R, Bird VG, Ueroi J, Shah O. Flexible ureterorenoscopy and holmium laser lithotripsy for the management of renal stone burdens that measure 2 to 3 cm: a multiinstitutional experience. J Endourol 2010; 24: 1583–8.
40. Bader MJ, Gratzke C, Walther S, et al. Efficacy of retrograde ureteropyeloscopic holmium laser lithotripsy for intrarenal calculi > 2 cm. Urol Res 2010; 38: 397–402.
41. Takazawa R, Kitayama S, Tsujii T. Successful outcome of flexible ureteroscopy with holmium laser lithotripsy for renal stones 2 cm or greater. Int J Urol 2012; 19: 264–7.

CHAPTER 21

Percutaneous Nephrolithomy: Access and Instrumentation

Arvind P. Ganpule, Sachin Abrol, Abhishek Laddha, and Mahesh R. Desai
Muljibhai Patel Urological Hospital, Nadiad, Gujarat, India

Introduction

The definition of correct access in a percutaneous nephrolithomy (PCNL) is a short straight tract from the skin and subcutaneous tissue, through the cup of the calyx into the desired calyx [1]. Proper access forms the "cornerstone" for successful completion of the percutaneous procedure. The prerequisites for gaining perfect access are proper instrumentation, equipment, and appropriate preoperative imaging. The well-described methods for gaining adequate access are ultrasound and fluoroscopy, computed tomography guided and endoscopy guided. Recently, the use of "see through needles," iPad-guided access and computed tomography-guided access have been described [2,3]. The choice of access is a matter of surgeon preference. The factors which decide the calyx of choice are the location of the calyx, location of the stone in relation to the pelvicalyceal system, and the lie of the kidney.

In this chapter, we outline the various approaches to accessing the pelvicalyceal system, explaining the pros and cons of each, and discuss the relevant literature. We also cover the instrumentation for percutaneous nephrolithotomy and the instruments used during access and stone removal.

Planning access preoperatively

Access is challenging in situations such as a non-dilated system, large stone burden, aberrant anatomy and in obese patients and those with history of previous surgery [4]. The desired calyx is selected after evaluation of preoperative imaging studies. The factors which decide the most appropriate calyx are: stone location, relation and position of stone in the pelvicalyceal system, and function of the kidney.

Urinary Stones: Medical and Surgical Management, First Edition. Edited by Michael Grasso and David S. Goldfarb.

Role of computed tomographic urography (CTU) in planning access

Optimal access is key to the success of PCNL. CTU provides more accurate stone morphometry data for standard PCNL [5]. The entry calyx for PCNL should be the optimal calyx chosen, keeping in view the relation of ribs and adjoining viscera, that could clear the maximum stone burden. Success of PCNL depends upon the stone burden and its distribution in the collecting system. It has been shown by Mishra and colleagues that staghorn morphometry predicts the chance of stone clearance [6]. An unfavorable calyx was defined as one that had an acute angle with the entry calyx and infundibular width of less than 8 mm. A favorable calyx, in contrast, has an obtuse angle with the entry calyx and infundibular width of more than 8 mm. Three-dimensional CTU with stone morphometry can calculate the total stone volume and the percentile volume in various calyces and also delineates the relative anatomy of various calyces very accurately and easily. In this way, CTU can be of tremendous help in choosing the optimal entry calyx and thus clearing the stone burden with the minimal number of tracts and staged procedures. It also helps in discussing the outcome with patients.

Positioning for access

Prone position

Prone is the most common position employed for gaining percutaneous renal access. The position of the bolsters varies from surgeon to surgeon. We prefer to place the bolsters below the chest while another bolster is placed below the hip. This allows the abdomen and panus to fall down away from the line of puncture. The problem with this position is the potential difficulty in maintaining the airway. This is of significance in patients with cardiorespiratory compromise. The obvious disadvantages of prone position for PCNL are the need for repositioning and the theoretical chance of limb and nerve injuries.

Supine position

The obvious advantages of supine positioning for access are no need to change position, ability to simultaneously access ureter if required, easier airway control, theoretical chance of lower intrapelvic pressures, and lesser chance of colonic injury. There are a few modifications of supine PCNL, including the flank position and Valdevia position [7].

Access techniques

Ultrasound-guided access

The advantages of ultrasound-guided access are that it offers straight-line access from the skin to the cup of the desired calyx, traversing a minimum number of vessels, it is more precise as it offers continuous "real-time" control of puncture with the needle remaining in the puncture plane and visualization of the needle puncturing the renal pelvicalyceal system, and it is potentially associated with less blood loss and intraoperative complications compared to fluoroscopy-guided access. Reduction in fluoroscopy time is an added advantage. Ultrasound-guided access is superior in delineating the 3D anatomy of the pelvicalyceal system, particularly the posterior calyx. It is the method of choice in pregnant women and anomalous kidneys such as pelvic ectopic kidneys. It also has the potential to visualize the intervening structures [8,9]. Ultrasound-guided access also has potential advantages in the pediatric population [1].

The limitations of this approach are its operator dependence, difficulty in visualization of the needle due to rib shadows and other artifacts during needle advancement, which is augmented in obese patients.

Technique

Preferably, access is gained with a ultrasound probe using a puncture guide. Once inserted in the needle guide, the needle traverses a path marked by a dotted line seen on the ultrasound screen.The ultrasound probe frequency ranges from 3.5 MHz to 5 MHz. The color Doppler mode helps to determine the access tract, avoiding vascular structures [10]. The Echotip™ needle helps ultrasound-guided puncture. A useful tip for seeing the trajectory of the needle is to place the bevel of the needle facing the ultrasound probe.

Access can be gained in supine, lateral or prone position. In prone position, the ultrasound scan is done starting posterior and proceeding anteriorly. The first calyx to be seen is the posterior calyx .The ultrasound scanner should be positioned in such a way that the calyx infundibulum and the pelvis are seen in a straight line. The position of the needle on the screen is ascertained by a "jiggling" movement of the needle. The patient is asked to hold the breath if the procedure is being performed under local anesthesia or the anesthetist holds respiration in expiration (Figure 21.1).

The needle can be seen positioned in the pelvicalyceal system; this is confirmed by return of fluid and a contrast study. If the contrast fills up the pelvis first followed by the calyces, it indicates a proper puncture.

In a recent randomized study comparing the outcome in fluoroscopy-guided versus ultrasound-guided punctures, the authors found that the mean time to successful puncture, mean radiation exposure, and mean number of attempts for successful puncture were less in patients in whom access was gained using the ultrasound approach. The stone-free rates were comparable in both groups. They concluded that ultrasound-guided puncture in PCNL helps to increase the accuracy of puncture and decrease radiation exposure for both patients and the surgical team [8].

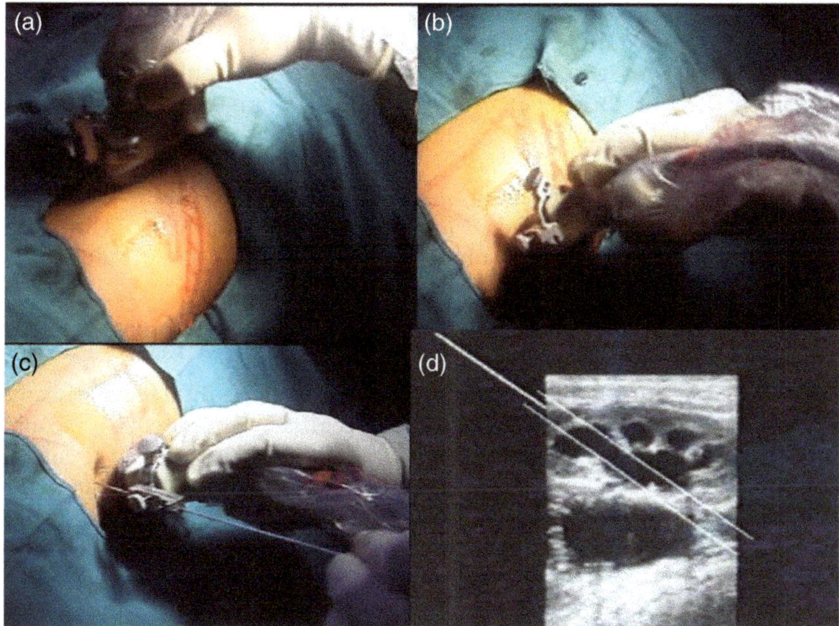

Figure 21.1 (a) The ultrasound scan starts posteriorly.The surface marking helps to orient the scanned portion in relation to the surrounding structure. (b) The probe is scanned anteriorly. The first calyx to be seen is the posterior calyx. (c) The ultrasound-guided puncture can be done either with or without a puncture guide. (d) The optimal needle path should follow the dotted line traversing along the cup of the calyx, the infundibulum and thereafter into the renal pelvis.

Fluoroscopy-guided puncture

One advantage of the fluoroscopic approach is its technical simplicity. However, it is a known fact that radiation hazard is directly proportional to radiation exposure. A dose as low as 0.15 Gy can lead to temporary oligospermia, while permanent sterility can be induced with doses of 5–6 Gy. This is of much significance in prepubertal females [11]. Thus it is important to reduce the amount of radiation the patient and surgeon receive during the procedure. The strategy to be followed is that of ALARA (as low as reasonably achievable). Opinion is divided about the person who gains the access. The ultrasound-guided puncture should be popularized by structured training programs and orientation courses in ultrasound.

Fluoroscopic access can be gained by injecting approximately 2–3 cc air in the pelvicalyceal system through a ureteric catheter. As air is light, the bubble is easily seen and helps in gaining access [8].

Technique

Fluoroscopy-guided percutaneous access technique is more commonly used by urologists, because intrarenal collecting system anatomy and pathology are better delineated and all the steps of the procedure can be precisely monitored under fluoroscopy (Figure 21.2).

Two fluoroscopy-guided percutaneous access techniques are well described: eye of the needle technique and triangulation technique. There is no clear advantage of one over the other and both have their proponents.

First, a plain fluoroscopic film is taken to note the radiopaque pathology and then the contrast is injected through a retrograde device. Once the collecting system is opacified, some retrograde air is injected to delineate the posterior calyces as air rises up them.

Eye of the needle technique

A fluoroscopic film is taken from above the patient directed vertically downward and the desired entry calyx is identified. Then the fluoroscopic unit is rotated 30° or a little more towards the operator so that it comes more or less in line with the posterior calyces. Now mark a site directly over the desired calyx and make a small skin incision to accept the needle and dilators. Place the tip of the needle in the incision and, keeping the tip of the needle steady, move the shaft of the needle and bring it in line with the axis of the fluoroscopic unit. By doing so, the hub of the needle will appear as a circle and the shaft will appear as a dot, thus forming a bull's eye appearance. In fluoroscopy, it seems like the surgeon is looking through the needle into the calyx. Now the needle is advanced, maintaining the bull's eye, and a "pop" is felt when the renal capsule is punctured. Now rotate the fluoroscopy unit back to vertical or 10–15° more away and the needle is seen as a straight line. Adjust the depth of the needle, keeping the mediolateral and cephalocaudal axis of the needle steady, to get into the desired calyx. Aspiration of urine confirms the entry. To minimize radiation exposure to the surgeon's hand, hold the needle with a hemostat or a purpose-built needle holder (Figure 21.2a,b).

Triangulation technique

In this technique, a fluoroscopic view is taken from above the patient vertically downward and the desired entry calyx is selected. The needle is placed in an approximate position for the desired angle of entry. Now the fluoroscopy unit is moved lateral and cephalad. From this fluoroscopic view, the needle is moved in a mediolateral direction, keeping the needle tip fixed, so that it points towards the entry calyx. The top of the fluoroscopy unit is now moved medially 45° and from this axis, the needle is moved in a craniocaudal direction, keeping the mediolateral orientation fixed, until it again targets the entry calyx. In both these positions, the needle should point towards the entry calyx. If the needle is advanced and the position of the needle is maintained in both craniocaudal and mediolateral planes, the desired calyx is contacted. The depth of the needle is continuously monitored in both planes (Figure 21.2c).

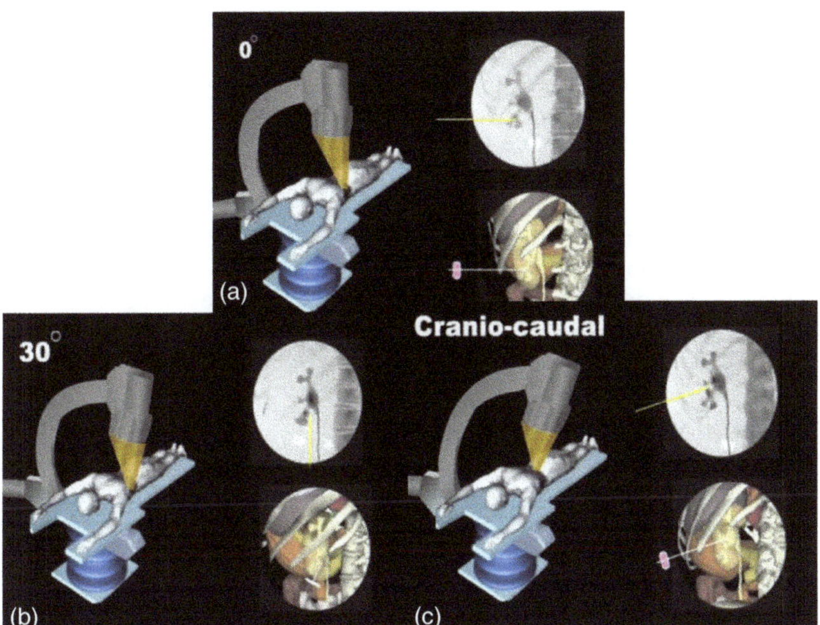

Figure 21.2 The patient is in prone position. The position of the needle is confirmed on zero position of the C-arm and thereafter in 30° and craniocaudal position of the C-arm.

Endoscopy-guided percutaneous access

The basis for endoscopy-guided access can be considered in the original Hawkins-Hunter and Lawson techniques, in which access was gained "inside-out" using deflectable guidewires and ureteral catheters. Successful access could be gained in over 85% of cases. The drawback of this method is difficulty in gaining access in impacted ureteric calculus. In addition, the tract is not necessarily straight or the shortest one [12].

The first description of endoscopy-guided access was done by Grasso et al. [13]. Endoscopy-guided access can be either under flexible ureteroscopy vision or using the microperc optics. This access is gained using the flexible ureteroscope for ascertaining that the puncture is done in an appropriate calyx. Thereafter the tract is dilated under vision, ascertaining that the needle is in the proper position. The obvious disadvantage of this approach is the need for two sets of equipment and two operators both well versed in endoscopic techniques. The added instrumentation is likely to add to the procedural time and the subsequent cost.

Technique

A 0.035 inch floppy tip glidewire is passed retrograde into the ureter, introduced using a flexible ureteroscope. An access sheath is passed retrograde;

the length of the access sheath is 55 cm in males and 35 cm in females. A contrast study is done to map the pelvicalyceal system. Direct access to the desired calyx is obtained using an18 gauge needle, which is advanced under fluoroscopy control. If the infundibular stone is obstructing the calyx and preventing direct vision of needle entry, the stone is fragmented and thereafter the ureteroscope is advanced into the pelvicalyceal system.

Bader et al. demonstrated the feasibility of the flexible endoscope for ensuring the proper position of the needle for gaining access. The instrumentation included a "see-through needle" which gave an idea about the adequacy of the access. Later Desai et al. modified the microperc technique for completion of the procedure [14].

iPad-guided access

Any navigated surgery involves preoperative imaging, planning of the operation, intraoperative imaging, and tracking. In the iPad-guided approach, first multi-slice CT is performed in exactly the same position as required during PCNL (prone position on PCNL cushion). Five colored radiopaque markers are placed around the target organ for percutaneous access and the images are taken in end-inspiratory phase. The radio markers are removed and marked with waterproof pen. On the operating table, the patient is placed in exactly the same position as during preoperative CT. The back-facing camera of the iPad captures the images of the access site and sends them to the nearby server (a standard computer). The server in turn runs the algorithm to analyze the position of markers in relation to the iPad and computer registration of video image and CT, and thus creates the augmented reality-enhanced image and sends it back to the iPad. This is a continuous process and depends upon the actual position of the iPad.

The 3D display of the kidney and the collecting system on the iPad guides the puncture site, followed by short fluoroscopic orientation of the needle. The desired calyx is entered, checked by fluoroscopy. The glidewire is passed and the tract is dilated under fluoroscopic control [3].

Instruments

Access needles

The access needle helps in gaining optimal access and also acts as a conduit for passage of guidewires into the pelvicalyceal system. The access needle has two parts, a shaft and a hub. Traditionally they are classified as two-part and three-part needles (Figure 21.3).

Initial puncture needle: three-part bevel tip

This is the first instrument used for gaining access. A 0.035 inch guidewire is used with it. The initial puncture needle is 18 gauge and 20 cm in length,

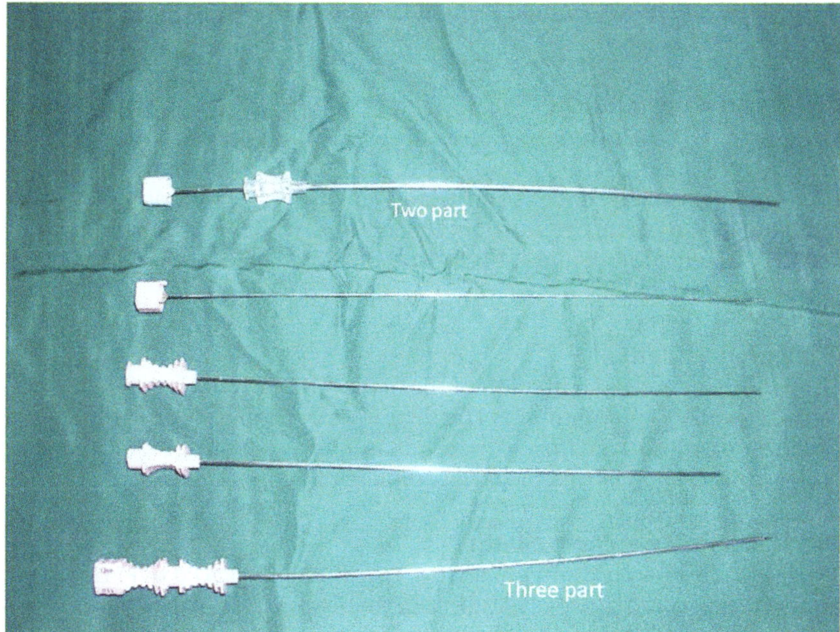

Figure 21.3 Access needles, two part and three part.

with a three-part bevel.The bevel helps entry of the guidewire into the pelvicalyceal system.The bevel tip should be facing the crystals in the ultrasound dilator for acoustic visualization of the needle.

Initial puncture needle: two-part trocar tip

The needle is 20 cm in length and 18 gauge, with a two-part trocar tip.

Chiba needle: two-part bevel tip

This 22 gauge, two-part 22 cm needle is also called a skinny needle and is used for opacification of the pelvicalyceal system. It is inserted paraspinally and the inner needle is removed. The outer skinny needle helps in contrast insertion. The pelvicalyceal system is thus opacified and helps in gaining access.

TLA introducer needle

Used for placement of a 0.038 inch guidewire. The radiopaque sheath allows better visualization and the trocar point aids easy introduction. It is made up of a 5 F sheath, it weighs 19 g and is 20 cm in length.

Percutaneous nephrolithotomy tract dilators

These dilators are used for formation of the PCNL tract, dictated by the size of stone and the degree of hydronephrosis. The type of dilator is a matter of surgeon preference. Single step and serial dilators (Amplatz and serial metallic) may be used.

Amplatz renal dilator set

These sets, which include radiopaque dilators and sheaths, are used for progressive dilation of the nephrostomy tract prior to percutaneous kidney stone removal. They have a short tapered tip with a smooth surface to reduce tissue trauma.The introducer catheter, which is 30 cm in length, acts as a guide for dilators 14–30 F and allows safety wire placement (Figure 21.4b).

Plastic serial dilators

These are used for serial dilation of the access tract after access is achieved. The sizes range from 6 F to 18 F. The dilators are cheap but their use is associated with more bleeding as each dilator is used once, removed and replaced with a larger dilator until complete dilation is achieved.

Metallic serial telescopic dilators

These are placed over a stiff guidewire. One dilator is placed over the other as the tract gets progressively larger and finally a 32 F sheath is placed over a 30 F dilator and then all are removed as one over the wire. They are cheap and reliable and allow dilation all the way up to the stone-bearing entry calyx. The dilators are made from stainless steel, reusable and cost effective. There are nine serial dilators and the first one may be rigid or flexible; it is braided and has a ball at the distal end which prevents the rest of dilators from advancing beyond the first. The assembly resembles a folded radio antenna (Figure 21.4a).

Balloon dilators

These are placed over a stiff guidewire. The distal end of the balloon is placed as close to the stone-bearing calyx as possible and the balloon is inflated. Finally an Amplatz sheath is placed over the balloon and the balloon is removed (Figure 21.4b). Dilation is rapidly achieved and they are easy to use. The disadvantage is that the balloon has a tapered end so dilation up to the stone-bearing calyx may not be complete. Balloon dilators are not recommended with staghorn calculi, cast calculi, and calyceal diverticulae (Figure 21.4c,d).

One-step dilators

Single-step dilators when compared to metal dilators have less radiation exposure with comparable success and complication rates. Some studies have shown that although they reduce radiation access and work rapidly, they may cause more damage to renal tissue than serial metallic dilation, the clinical significance of which is not known at present [15].

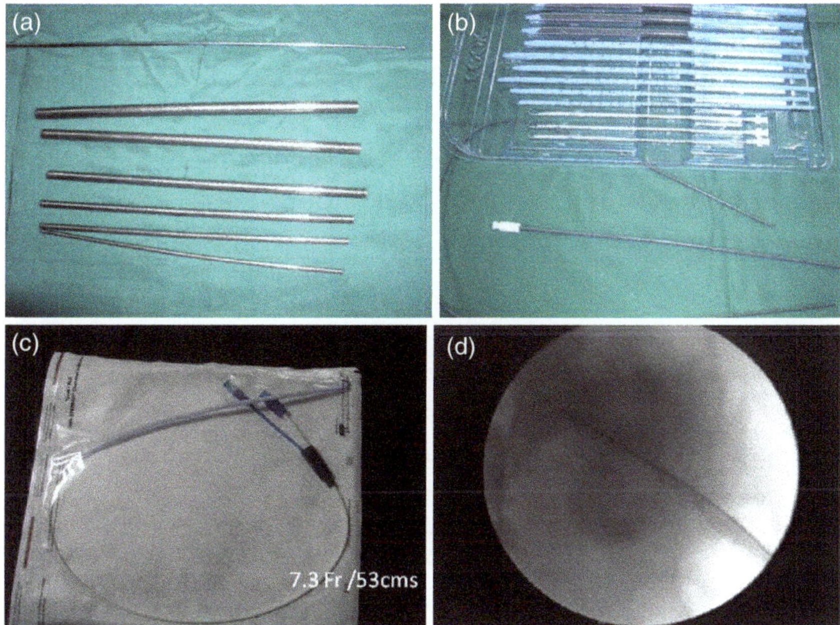

Figure 21.4 (a) Metal serial dilator. These are available from 9 F to 24 F. The assembly resembles a collapsed radio antenna. The rod is 6 F and the knob is 9 F. (b) Amplatz dilators are available up to 30 F. The assembly includes a plastic cannula and a Cobra catheter. (c) The balloon dilators are 53 cm in length and 7.3 F in diameter. (d) The fully inflated dilator.

Amplatz sheath

This is used for mantainenence of an already created nephrostomy tract. The size varies from 12 to 34 F, the length varies from 16 to 30 cm. It is used during renal dilation to provide an atraumatic working tract after removal of the dilator. It is made from radiopaque material for verification of position during fluoroscopy. The specially engineered polymer provides high resistance to abrasion. The preferred method of sterilization is with ethylene oxide. The beveled end of the sheath helps atraumatic entry in the calyx [16].

Guidewires and glidewires

BiWire®Nitinol core wire guide

This provides two options for urethral access: straight and angled ends, with flexible tips. The hydrophilic coating allows smooth and easy advancement.The BiWire has been designed to provide two options for ureteral access. Diameter 0.028 to 0.038 inch, length 150 cm and tip length 3 cm.

HiWire®Nitinol core wire guide

Used for access to the ureter in routine or demanding cases which require precise control. Instruments can be changed over the wire once in position. Available in standard and stiff shaft, so can be used in difficult cases and with tortuous ureters. One-to-one torque control allows placement in difficult and challenging anatomy with precise control. It has flexible tapered tip and hydrophilic coating for smooth and easy advancement. Diameter 0.028 to 0.038 inch, length 150 cm and tip length 3 cm (straight or angled).

Roadrunner® PC wire guide

Used to place and exchange catheters when the ureter is kinked or tortuous or with large ureteric stones. The Nitinol core allows maximum deflection without kinking and the radiopaque tip of platinum aids use with fluoroscopy. A microthin layer of hydrophilic polymer (AQ® coating) holds and attracts water to the wire when activated, allowing placement with low resistance and friction. Diameter 0.035 to 0.038 inch, length 145 cm , tip configuration 3 cm/7 cm/8 cm/16 cm, straight and angled tips.

Roadrunner® PC wire guide, double flexible

A double flexible tipped design that allows safe entrance into the body and protects against damage while being introduced. The other features are the same as those above. It has a diameter of 0.035 to 0.038 inch, length 145 cm, double flexible tip. It has marking increments at 5 cm.

Amplatz fixed core wire guide

Made of stainless steel, this has straight and flexible tip designs. It is mainly used for ureteral access, percutaneous access, and replacement and exchange of devices during endourological procedures. The diameter is 0.035 to 0.038 inch with a length of 145 cm, with a 5 cm double flexible tip.

Fixed core wire guide

Made of stainless steel, this has straight and flexible tip designs. It is used for ureteral access, percutaneous access, and replacement and exchange of devices during endourological procedures. Diameter 0.028 to 0.038 inch, length 145 cm, tip configuration 1 cm/3 cm/15 cm flexible tip.

Movable core wire guide

Made of stainless steel. Urinary tract access via the moveable core design allows the surgeon greater versatility by varying the length of the flexible portion [17].

Nephroscopes

With the advent of percutaneous stone removal, various forms of nephroscopes, flexible and rigid, are now available, and proper selection is vital for each particular case.

Dresden percutaneous universal nephroscope

Used for diagnostic and therapeutic renal procedures, also for ultrasound litholapaxy or electrohydraulic lithotripsy, this nephroscope has a small sheath of 20.8 F with a large working channel of 14 F and axillary instruments up to 3.5 mm can be used with it [18].

Lahme miniature nephroscope 15/18Fr

Very useful for stones in the renal pelvis and staghorn calculi, this nephroscope can be used in children and adults. It is made of titanium and stainless steel to decrease the weight [18].

Invisio® Smith digital percutaneous nephroscope

An advanced scope, much lighter than traditional versions (470 g versus 935 g), decreasing fatigue during long procedures. Its light weight allows the surgeon to use the non-dominant hand to hold the scope and the dominant hand to manipulate instruments [19].

Nephrostomy tubes

The nephrostomy tube helps to drain the kidney after the procedure, acts as a conduit to remove residual stones after a PCNL if they are detected on postoperative film, and helps to tamponade any bleeding.

Available nephrostomy tubes include the following.

- **Councilman catheter**: this is a modified Foley catheter, with a end-on hole. This type of nephrostomy drainage is useful if the nephrostomy tube requires frequent changes.
- **Kays tamponade balloon**: originally this catheter was designed to arrest post-PCNL bleeding. The tamponade is provided by the balloon and the central channel provides drainage.
- **Nelaton catheter**: ranging in size from 12 F to 28 F. This is the preferred method of drainage after PCNL.

Graspers and baskets (Figure 21.5)

- **Nitinol basket**: the memory of this basket helps in retrieval of stones in awkward calyces. The basket cannot be used with a laser as this leads to a barbed wire effect.
- **Triflange, biflange grasper**: the choice between these two varieties is decided by the size of the stone and the size of the calyx. Larger stones in compact calyces are removed with a biflange, while capacious calyx calculi are dealt with using a triflange.

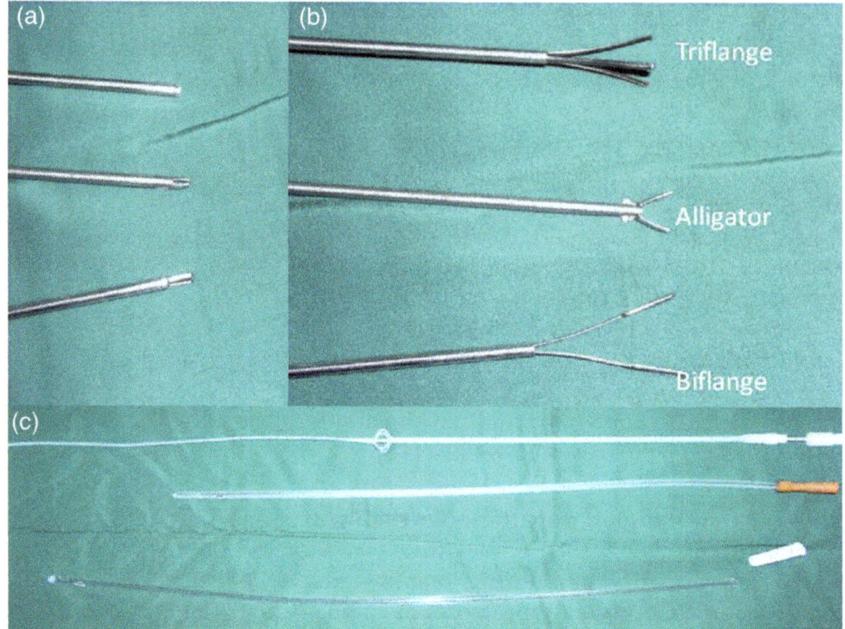

Figure 21.5 (a,b) The three varieties of graspers: triflange, biflange and alligator. (c) The nephrostomy catheters include re-entry catheter, Nelaton catheter and Council tip Foley catheter.

References

1. Desai M. Ultrasonography guided punctures – with and without puncture guide. J Endourol 2009; 23: 1641–3.
2. Desai MR, Sharma R, Mishra S, Sabnis RB, Stief C, Bader M. Single step percutaneous nephrolithotomy (microperc): the initial clinical report. J Urol 2011; 186(1): 140–5.
3. Rassweiller J. iPad assisted percutaneous access to the kidney using marker based navigation: initial clinical experience. Eur Urol 2012; 61: 627–31.
4. Sountoulides PG, Kaufmann OG, Louie MK, et al. Endoscopy guided percutaneous nephrostolithotomy: benefits of ureteroscopic access and therapy. J Endourol 2009; 23(10): 1649–54.
5. Olcott EW, Sommer FG, Napel S. Accuracy of detection and measurement of renal calculi: in vitro comparison of three dimensional spiral CT, radiography and nephrotomography. Radiology 1997; 20: 419–25.
6. Mishra S, Sabnis RB, Desai M. Staghorn morphometry: a new tool for clinical classification and prediction model for percutaneous nephrolithotomy monotherapy. J Endourol 2012; 26(1): 6–14.
7. Karami H, Rezaei A, Mohamaddahosseni M, Javanmard B, Mazloomfard M, Lofti B. Ultrasonography guided percutaneous nephrolithomy in the flank position versus fluoroscopy guided percutaneous nephrolithotomy in the prone position: a comparative study. J Endourol 2010; 24(8): 1357–61.

8. Agrawal MS, Jaiiswal A, Kumar D, Yadav H, Lavania P. Safety and efficacy of ultrasonography as an adjunct to fluoroscopy for renal access in percutaneous nephrolithotomy (PCNL). BJU Int 2011; 108: 1346–9.
9. Desai MR, Jasani A. Percutaneous nephrolithotripsy in ectopic kidneys. J Endourol 2000; 14(3): 289–92.
10. Xu Y, Wu Z, Yu J, et al. Doppler ultrasound guided percutaneous nephrolithomy with two step tract dilation for management of complex renal stones. Urology 2012; 79: 1247–51.
11. Castenada WR, Espenan GD. How to protect yourself and others from radiation. In: Smith AD, Badlani G, Bagley D, eds. *Smith's Textbook of Endourology*. St Louis: Quality Medical, 1996, pp. 21–8.
12. Kahn F, Borin JF, Pearle MS, Mcdougall EM, Clayman RV. Endoscopically guided percutaneous renal access: "seeing is believing". J Endourol 2006; 20(7): 451–5.
13. Grasso M, Lang G, Taylor FC. Flexible ureteroscopically assisted percutaneous renal access. Tech Urol 1995; 1: 39–43.
14. Desai MR, Sharma R, Mishra S, Sabnis RB, Stief C, Bader M. Single-step percutaneous nephrolithotomy (microperc): the initial clinical report. J Urol 2011b; 186(1): 140–5.
15. Aminsharifi A, Alavi M, Sadeghi G, Shakeri S, Afsar F. Renal parenchymal damage after percutaneous nephrolithotomy with one-stage tract dilation technique: a randomized clinical trial. J Endourol 2011; 25(6): 927–31.
16. Cook Medical: www.cookmedical.com/uro/dataSheet.do?id=1941
17. Cook Medical: www.cookmedical.com/uro/familyListingAction.do?family=Wire+Guides
18. Richard Wolf Medical Systems: www.richard-wolf.com/en/human-medicine/urology.html
19. Gyrus Acmi Medical Systems: www.gyrusacmi.com/acmi/user/display.cfm?display=product&pid=9849&catid=76&maincat=Urology&catname=Percutaneous%20Nephroscopes

CHAPTER 22

Percutaneous Management of Intrarenal Calculi

Michael Degen and Majid Eshghi
Westchester Medical Center *and* New York Medical College, Valhalla, NY, USA

Introduction

The first reported percutaneous stone extraction through a tract was performed in 1975 [1]. The procedure gained wide acceptance in the early 1980s and is currently the gold standard for large intrarenal calculi [2]. The number of percutaneous nephrolithotomies (PCNL) being performed in the US has decreased since the arrival of extracorporeal shock wave lithotripsy (SWL) in the 1980s, as well as constantly improving ureteroscopic and laser technology. As a result, patients who undergo PCNL usually fall into one of several catagories.

- Failed SWL.
- Unsuccessful ureteroscopy or failed passage of stone or fragments.
- Anatomical abnormalities such as ureteropelvic junction (UPJ) obstruction, infundibular stenosis or long narrow infundibula, and calyceal diverticula in which SWL and ureteroscopic methods would either fail or have very poor outcomes.
- Large-volume and staghorn calculi.
- Patients with urinary diversions including continent urinary reservoirs, augmentation and ureteral reimplant that prevent access to the ureteral orifice and the upper tract.
- Retained or forgotten stents with both proximal/distal encrustation and proximal stone ball formation.
- Narrow ureteral lumens or significant retroperitoneal fibrosis resulting in hydronephrosis.
- Other congenital or postsurgical anatomical variations such as horseshoe kidneys, pelvic kidneys, cross-fused ectopia, and transureteroureterostomy.

The only absolute contraindication for PCNL is an uncorrected bleeding diathesis [3].

Urinary Stones: Medical and Surgical Management, First Edition. Edited by Michael Grasso and David S. Goldfarb.

Preoperative antimicrobial prophylaxis

While there is not enough evidence to support a clinical guideline for preoperative antibiotics, the AUA has issued a best practice policy statement. Based on this analysis, it is suggested to prescribe prophylactic antimicrobials for all patients undergoing percutaneous renal surgery. This is based on two studies. In the first, 35% of patients with negative preoperative urine cultures who underwent PCNLs suffered from postoperative urinary tract infections (UTI) [4]. In the second, patients receiving preoperative intravenous, versus oral versus no antibiotics developed postoperative urinary tract infections in 0%, 17%, and 40% respectively [5]. The AUA suggest a first- or second-generation cephalosporin or aminoglycoside + metronidazole or clindamycin as the antimicrobials of choice. Alternative antimicrobials that are commonly used include aminoglycoside/sulbactam or fluoroquinolone [6].

Access

While percutaneous access is beyond the scope of this chapter and is discussed elsewhere in this text, we will briefly describe our approach to obtaining access. Bilateral sequential compression devices (Covidien, Dublin, Ireland) are placed at the beginning of the case unless contraindicated. Once general anesthesia has been administered, we begin with flexible cystoscopy on the stretcher with the patient in a supine position. A 5 or 6F open-ended catheter (Cook Medical, Bloomington, IN) is placed in the ipsilateral collecting system of the stone. This allows us to perform a retrograde pyelogram to outline the collecting system once in the prone position. The open-ended catheter also allows us access to place a "through-and-through" wire in a retrograde fashion for safety once access has been established. The open-ended catheter is then secured to the Foley catheter prior to placing the patient in the prone position. We routinely leave the guide wire inside the ureteral catheter for readjustment under flueroscopy after the patient is in prone position. We typically use a narrow strip of anesthesia tape with split ends to allow easy removal when the patient is in the prone position. Silk ties should not be used to avoid dislodging the silk tie into the bladder during catheter manipulation.

The patient is then positioned on the endourology table in the prone position, about 20–30° up on the side of surgery. Chest rolls and face protection are placed. Axillary supports are placed to assure a physiologic alignment of shoulders, head, neck and upper extremities. Again proper cushioning is applied in all pressure areas. In a female patient, the breast should be placed medially and the chest adequately elevated to avoid excessive pressure. In a male patient, the penis and scrotum should be placed in a non-pressure location which is easily accessible for manipulation of the open-ended catheter. The genitals and flank should be prepped. The open-ended catheter is then placed over a half sheet before the final drape is placed. The final drape is then placed and a fenestration is created to access the open-ended catheter.

Using the open-ended catheter, a retrograde pyelogram of the kidney is performed with the C-arm angled about 10° forward. We routinely add 80 mg of gentamicin to the contrast material. In cases of chronic infection or indwelling foreign bodies, diflucan is also added. Based on stone size and location, access is initiated under fluoroscopic guidance by puncturing the appropriate calyx with an 18 G needle from the percutaneous entry set (Cook Medical). Entry into the calyx is confirmed by the aspiration of urine into a 10 cc syringe attached to the 18 G needle via intravenous (IV) extension tubing, as the needle is slowly withdrawn. Once in the collecting system, a 0.038 inch sensor guidewire with an angled tip (Boston Scientific, Natick, MA) is placed through the 18 G needle into the collecting system and ideally manipulated down into the ureter and the bladder under fluoroscopic guidance (Figure 22.1). If necessary, a Cobra or Kumpe access catheter (Cook Medical) can be used to direct the wire into the pelvis and down the ureter. An incision of the skin and fascia is performed with an 11-blade to help with dilation of the tract later in the case. A fascia incising needle which slides over the guide wire can also be used to make a cruciate incision of fascia. Under fluoroscopic guidance, the tract is then dilated up to 10 F with sequential teflon fascial dilators over the wire (Percutaneous Entry Set, Cook Medical). Dilation with a 30f Nephromax balloon (Boston Scientific) is performed and the working sheath is advanced into in position over the balloon. The balloon is removed while still inflated, the wire is left in place and stone clearance can begin after initial inspection of the collecting system. The inflated balloon should be saved and can be used as a dilator inside the sheath whenever the sheath is displaced out of the renal parenchyma and needs to be adjusted. Different commercial sets have smaller sheaths such as 20, 22, 24or 26 french incase the operator wants to use a smaller scope or a flexible cystoscope or even a rigid ureterscope. There are also single custom made sheaths in smaller sizes such as 16, 18 or 20 French usually

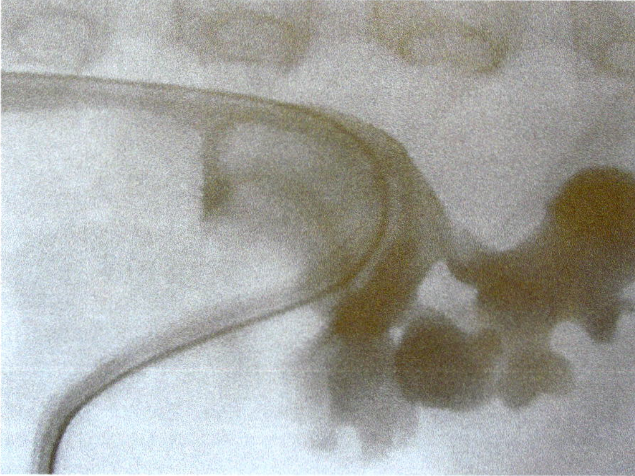

Figure 22.1 Percutaneous access through a lower pole calyx with the wire and a catheter manipulated down the ureter.

used for pediatric cases, follow up as nephrscopy or in transplant kidneys. For a right-handed surgeon, the nephroscope eyepiece and camera should be on the left side with the light cord and irrigation tubing coming in from the left as well. This will allow for a free excursion of the right hand to access the working channel. The first step is a general inspection of collecting system and accessing the tip of open ended catheter to retrieve the guide wire to be brought out through the sheath, thus creating a through and through access. To avoid inadvertent dislodgement a small clamp is placed at the tip of the wire on both sides.

Irrigation fluid

Our protocol is to use a standard 3 L saline bag with 80 mg of gentamicin in the first bag. In cases of chronically infected kidneys or indwelling foreign bodies, 400 mg of diflucan is also added. We hang the saline bags from a Level 1® fluid warmer (Smiths Medical, London) which allows us to adjust the height and temperature of the irrigant.

Stone clearance

The goal of PCNL is to clear all the stone burden and do it in an efficient and least traumatic manner. This can be performed in a variety of ways.

Mechanical clearance

In several cases, the size of the 30 F working sheath may allow for removal of the intrarenal calculi without the need for lithotripsy. A variety of forceps and baskets can be used for this purpose. Most commercial nephrosopes carry a variety of two or three prong forceps. One device that we frequently use is a large zero tip basket, with a hand spring action (Perc N Circle® Nitinol Tipless Stone Extractor, Cook Medical) that can be used for stone removal through the rigid nephroscope (Figure 22.2).

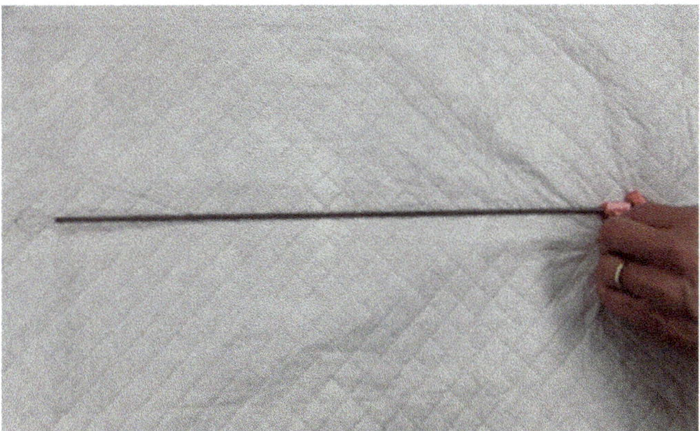

Figure 22.2 Perc N Circle® Nitinol Tipless Stone Extractor. Source: Cook Medical.

The atraumatic nature of this basket allows the removal of multiple stones up to 1–1.5 cm in size, depending on the shape with minimal damage to the collecting system. Flexible nephroscopy with a regular stone basket can also be used for calyces that are not accessible with a rigid scope.

Lithotripsy

There are several lithotripsy techniques and devices to fragment and clear intrarenal calculi.

- Electrohydraulic
- Ultrasonic
- Pneumatic
- Laser
- Combination devices

Electroydraulic lithotripsy (EHL) was first reported in Russia in 1955. The mechanism is an electrical current producing a spark gap that results in a cavitation bubble on contact with the stone, leading to fragmentation. One of the benefits of EHL is that its smaller probes are flexible and can be used in flexible scopes. It is also the cheapest of the lithotripters [7]. Unfortunately, it does have some disadvantages, the worst of which is its 2.9–17.6% risk of collecting system perforation [8]. Another drawback is its propensity to create multiple fragments with larger stone burdens, and unlike the ultrasonic lithotripter, it lacks the ability to evacuate small fragments. Overall, it has been proven safe and effective and one study showed it to have approximately a 90% fragmentation rate and 82% stone-free rate for ureteral and renal stones [9].

The trend of percutaneous intrarenal lithotripsy for many years has been ultrasonic lithotripsy. One of its main advantages is its ability to provide

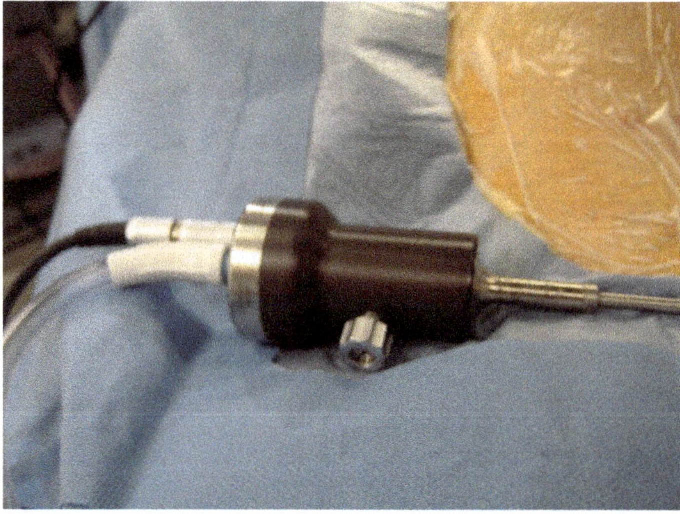

Figure 22.3 Ultrasonic lithotripter with suction attachment.

continuous suctioning during lithotripsy (Figure 22.3). This enables it to evacuate small pieces as the stone is being fragmented and also decreases repulsion of the stone during fragmentation. Another advantage is its low risk of collecting system injury and perforation as demonstrated in multiple animal trials [10,11]. Its main disadvantage is its rigidity. It must be used in a rigid scope, although for the percutaneous treatment of intrarenal stones, this is a minor issue. It has an overall success rate of approximately 80–100% [12,13,14,15] and it is relatively inexpensive [7].

Pneumatic lithotripsy requires direct contact to fragment stones and, similar to ultrasonic lithotripsy, has a low risk of collecting system perforation [10,16]. Most of the probes are rigid, although some of the smaller probes can be used in flexible endoscopy. One of its main advantages is its ability to effectively fragment harder stones [17], although its expense may make it a less desirable option [18]. The StoneBreaker pneumatic lithotripter (Cook Medical) is a compact hand-held device with various probe sizes that can be used in the kidney and ureter. It is relatively easy to use with minimal maintenance.

Each lithotripsy technique has its own advantages in different situations, but in general, the combination device that uses both pneumatic and ultrasonic lithotripsy has proven to be more efficient and possibly better at stone clearance [19,20,21]. It does so by combining the fragmentation capability of the pneumatic lithotripter with the suction capability of the ultrasound lithotripter.

Finally, there is the option to use laser lithotripsy. The holmium laser is the most widely used for this purpose in urology. The benefit of this modality is that it is flexible and can be used in flexible endoscopy. This gives the surgeon the advantage of accessing hard-to-reach calyces that the rigid nephroscope and the previously discussed modalities cannot reach. This helps to avoid performing multiple percutaneous accesses. In PCNL it has a success rate of approximately 61–89% [22,23,24]. Unfortunately, it has some drawbacks, including an inability to suck out fragments, and if one is not careful, the ability to perforate the collecting system.

Even with the best lithotripsy device, stone fragment migration into the ureter is always a concern. To combat this, we usually place a double-lumen catheter over the "through-and-through" wire in a retrograde fashion. This catheter has several advantages it dilates the distal ureter thus preventing UVJ obstruction by stone dust or small fragments. It allows for retrograde flushing of the ureter and UPJ area, to clear any stone fragments that may have migrated. Retrograde flushing also helps antegrade ureteroscopy by providing better visualization, especially in cases of impacted upper ureteral stones. Another advantage of this catheter is that it allows for the placement of a safety wire in an antegrade or retrograde fashion. Stone fragment migration can also be prevented by using specially designed catheters with balloons that block the UPJ.

Chemolysis

Chemolysis can be performed as a primary or secondary treatment for intrarenal stones. The main indications include patients who are not healthy enough for surgical intervention, patients who have undergone multiple procedures in the past, patients who are at high risk for recurrence, and those with residual fragments following a procedure for stones.

The general principles were set forth by Nemoy and Stamey [25] and include:

- an unobstructed efflux of irrigant and thus a low intrapelvic pressure (<20–25 cmH_2O)
- an intact urinary system (no evidence of extravasation)
- a sterile urinary tract prior to initiation of irrigant.

Irrigant installation can be performed via several methods which involve a combination of ureteral stents, open-ended catheters or nephrostomy tubes. The goal is to allow a significant amount of the irrigant to be in contact with the stone while keeping the intrapelvic pressure <20–25 cmH_2O [26,27]. This helps prevent irrigant absorption and parenchymal rupture [28]. If a nephrostomy tube is being used, one should wait 24–48 h after its insertion to start irrigant. This will give the tissue time to seal around the nephrostomy tube and decrease the risk of extravasation and absorption.

Prior to starting the irrigant, a contrast study is valuable to rule out extravasation and confirm adequate drainage. Once confirmed, normal saline should be used as the initial irrigant at a rate of 30–40 mL/h. If the intrapelvic pressure remains less than 25 cmH_2O, the rate can be increased by 10 mL/h until a maximum rate of 120 mL/h is reached. After approximately 24 h of normal saline at a maximal rate, the irrigant of choice can be started at 30–50 mL/h and titrated up to a maximum rate of 120 mL/h [29]. Irrigation is usually continued for 24–48 h after the last radiographic evidence of intrarenal stone is seen [29]. During the irrigation, the intrapelvic pressure must be monitored and the patient should remain on antibiotics. The patient and staff should be aware of key signs and symptoms suggesting obstruction or sepsis which include flank pain, fever, chills or irrigant leakage in which case, the irrigation should be immediately stopped.

Three stones that respond well to chemolysis are uric acid, cystine and struvite but stones are rarely homogeneous. Calcium and oxalate stones are typically not responsive to chemolysis.

Uric acid stones are usually treated with tromethamine (THAM, pH 8.6) with a goal of raising the pH to approximately 7.5 [30]. At this pH, rapid stone dissolution is seen without precipitation of other minerals. Sodium bicarbonate solution can also be used although studies show that THAM causes quicker stone dissolution [31].

Cystine stones' unique disulfide bonds are responsible for joining two cysteine molecules. It is these bonds that are targeted by chemolytic agents. These include D-penicillamine and α-mercaptopropionylglycine. Direct chemolysis alone would require a significant period of time to dissolve cystine stones [32] and therefore it is usually used as an adjunct to fragmentation procedures such as PCNL and SWL which will increase the surface area of the stone and thus the area for the chemolytic agent to work.

Struvite (magnesium ammonium phosphate) stone is the main component of staghorn calculi. These stones are most commonly secondary to recurrent

UTIs caused by urease-producing bacteria, in particular *Proteus* [33]. Chemolysis of these stones is usually accomplished with hemiacidrin [34], a solution which chemically interacts with the components of the struvite stone and at the same time increases the solubility of struvite by decreasing the pH below 5.5 [35]. It is important to note that use of this solution can lead to sepsis secondary to UTI and even death as the stone dissolves. Therefore patients must be carefully monitored for signs of infection during chemolysis and the irrigant must be stopped if infection is suspected.

During chemolysis, daily urine cultures must be performed and serum magnesium must be checked because magnesium is added as a mucosal protective agent in some chemolytic solutions.

Miniscope and Pediatric nephroscope

When the stone burden is small, a repeat or second-look procedure is required, we usually use a 12 F miniscope with two working sheaths up to 15 F. This requires minimal dilation and it is also ideal for surveillance follow-up of the collecting system after resection of tumor, intracavitary chemotherapy and in transplant kidneys (22.8). It can easily be used without a sheath for follow up endoscopy. It has a small working channel that allows for biopsy, basketing, pediatric ultrasound probe and laser lithotripsy. A dedicated 17 F pediatric nephroscope can be used in children and transplant kidneys as well. (Figure 22.4).

Exit strategy

Both before and during the procedure, the surgeon should be thinking about an exit strategy. Multiple factors come into play when deciding on

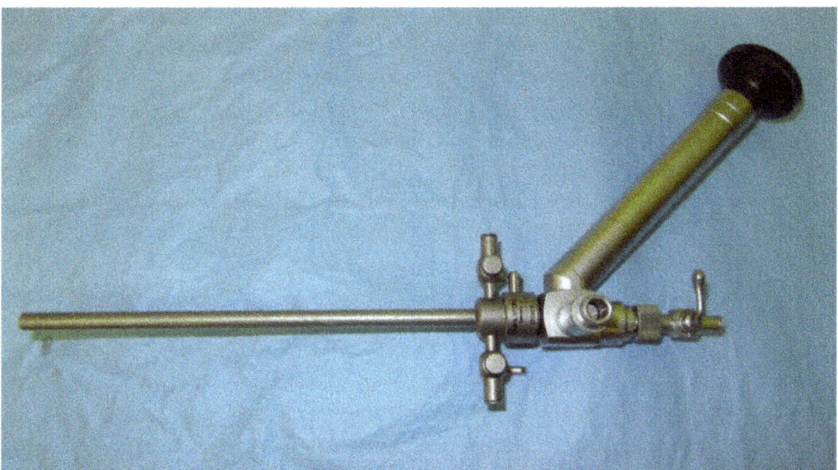

Figure 22.4 Pediatric nephroscope 17 F. Source: Karl Storz, Tuttlingen, Germany.

this step and unfortunately no one strategy is suitable for every scenario. Some of the key issues that will help the surgeon in determining this strategy include the degree of bleeding, any injury to the collecting system, evidence of an infected system, residual stone fragments, distal ureteral obstruction, and the possibility of a second look for a staged procedure. The shape and size of the collecting system plays and important role as well.

The classic teaching was to always leave a large-bore nephrostomy tube, but with the advent of "tubeless" percutaneous renal surgery [36], there are now several options. These include leaving a nephrostomy tube, leaving a ureteral stent without a PCN tube, and completely tubeless percutaneous renal surgery. We will discuss some of the situations that may suggest using one or another of these approaches, the risks and benefits, and our own opinions based on our experience.

For the majority of our cases, we leave an 18F or 20F silicone council catheter with a short open tip (Cook Medical). The benefits of using this type of catheter include adequate drainage of the kidney, access to perform a nephrostogram in the postoperative period, and the ability to tamponade bleeding from the tract in the immediate postoperative period if necessary. The drawback of this catheter is that it is not suitable for a small renal pelvis. Some believe that a smaller tube (<10F) may result in less postoperative pain, less analgesia, and less postoperative urine leakage [37,38], but current studies show this to be controversial. Malecot re-entry nephrostomy catheters (14–24F) or single pigtail nephrostomy tubes (10–16F) are also used, depending on the circumstances. In cases of injury or erosion near the ureteropelvic junction or upper ureter, a re-entry catheter is recommended. Alternatively, an indwelling double pigtail stent and a nephrostomy tube can be used.

There should always be some excursion length on the nephrostomy tube to avoid inadvertent dislodgment of the tube from the collecting system. Therefore the anchoring stich should be placed in a way that allows the nephrostomy tube to move in and out to accommodate the mobility of the kidney specially in overnight patients.

In an attempt to decrease patient discomfort, analgesic use and hospital stay, under certain circumstances, it is feasible to perform PCNL without leaving a percutaneous nephrostomy tube – "tubeless" PCNL. This includes two options: leaving only a stent as first described by Bellman [36] or totally tubeless as described by Karami [39]. The criteria we use for these exit strategies include:

- preferably for access below the 12th rib
- short operative time (indicating a lower stone burden or less complex stone/anatomy)
- minimal blood loss (decreased risk of clots that may cause obstruction postoperatively)
- no evidence of remaining stone (no need for second look)
- no evidence of collecting system perforation (decreased risk of urinary extravasation)

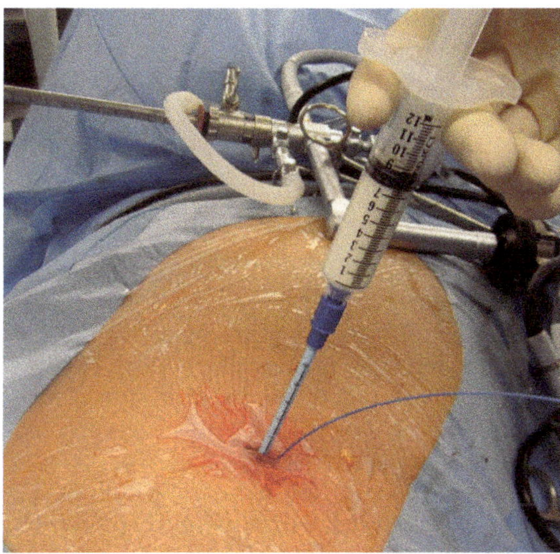

Figure 22.5 Installation of sealant at the conclusion of a "tubeless" percutaneous nephrolithotomy.

- no evidence of an infected system/stone (would require adequate drainage of infected system and avoid pleural complications when access is above 12th rib)
- a patulous ureter (decreased risk of postoperative obstruction).
- it is a good idea to observe the tract for bleeding for one to two minutes with only a guide wire in place to make sure there is no excessive bleeding before deciding on tubeless exit strategy.

One of the main concerns when one does not leave a percutaneous nephrostomy tube after PCNL is hemostasis of the access site. Several options exist to provide adequate hemostasis, including sealants and thermoablative techniques. We prefer to use a Gelatin sealant (e.g. FloSeal) injected into the access site with the applicator tip (Figure 22.5), the injection starts at the edge of parenchyma and is continued as the syringe is being withdrawn to the skin and occasionally we place a single absorbable suture over the incision site if superficial bleeding is encountered. In our experience, there has never been an issue with formation of a sealant clot within the collecting system when using a gelatinous sealant, but this complication has been reported by others [40,41].

Special anatomical considerations

Ureteropelvic junction obstruction

In cases of concominant UPJ obstruction, after the stone has been cleared, an antegrade endopyelotomy can be performed by incising the lateral to posterolateral aspect of the UPJ. We prefer a cold hook knife. An endopyelotomy stent with a large-diameter proximal end that tapers at the distal end (14 F/7 F or 10 F/7 F) can then be inserted with the larger portion traversing the incised UPJ region [42]. A Malecot Foley type nephrostomy is also placed for approximately 48 hours. A nephrostogram should be done prior to removal of their tube. Stent will be removed 4–6 weeks later.

Horseshoe kidneys

Stone formation is the most common urological disorder seen in horseshoe kidneys with an incidence of approximately 20% [43]. PCNL is the standard of care for stones >2 cm and failed SWL in horseshoe kidneys [43,44]. In relation to a kidney in normal anatomical position, there are several anatomical variations that one should be aware of when performing PCNL of horseshoe kidneys. These include a more overall caudal position, a more anterior position of the renal pelvis, a more posterior position of the calyces, a higher ureteral insertion, and a variable blood supply. These variations lead to a more medial puncture site, a longer tract which can require longer instruments [45], an increased risk of vessel injury with lower pole access [46], making a mid or upper pole access site more preferable (Figure 22.6), and impaired renal drainage, making it important to remove all stone fragments [47].

Even with these variations, the complication and success rates of PCNL in horseshoe kidneys are similar to anatomically normal kidneys. The success rate is approximately 70–100% but may require more than one procedure [47].

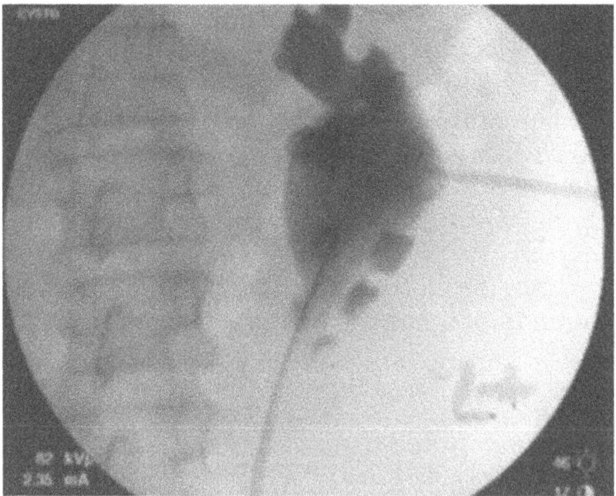

Figure 22.6 Horseshoe kidney with percutaneous nephrostomy tube in the left midpole calyx.

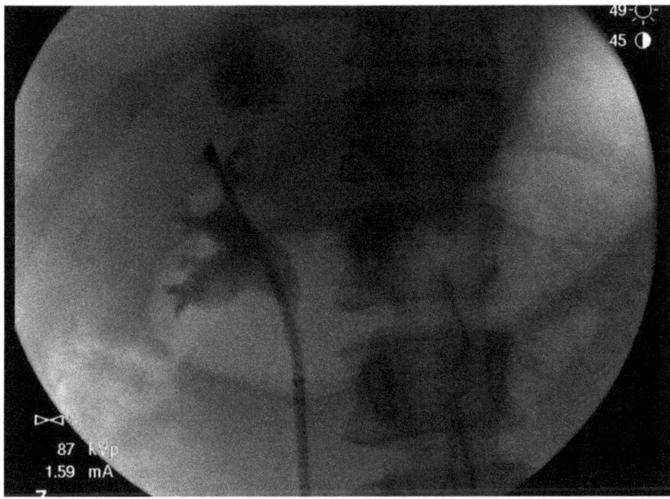

Figure 22.7 Right upper pole calyceal diverticulum seen on retrograde pyelogram.

Calyceal diverticulum/infundibular stenosis

Calyceal diverticula are very rare and are believed to be congenital smooth-walled, non-secretory cavities with a urothelium lining which communicates with the calyx, usually through a narrow diverticular neck or infundibulum (Figure 22.7). Most are less than 1 cm in size and asymptomatic, but stones can be seen in up to 40% of calyceal diverticula, leading to significant symptoms requiring treatment [48]. Current treatment options include SWL, PCNL, ureteroscopy, and laparoscopic surgery.

With PCNL, the goal is to gain access through the diverticulum and if possible advance the guidewire through the diverticular neck into the renal pelvis and down the ureter. If this is not possible secondary to the size or position of the neck, the guidewire can be coiled in the diverticula. The stone can then be cleared using the rigid nephroscope and the previously described techniques. Stone-free rates of 70–100% have been reported using this approach [48]. At the end of the procedure, the diverticular wall can be ablated with electrocautery laser and sometimes chemically with the goal of obliterating it [48]. Another approach calls for the dilation of the diverticular neck and placement of a stent creating a large enough neck to inhibit the stasis of urine within the diverticulum [49]. Both approaches have been successful, but we usually drain diverticulum unless it is a very large cavity.

Infundibular stenosis is defined by a dilated calyx, draining through a narrowed infundibulum into a non-distended renal pelvis [50]. Similar to calyceal diverticulum, stones can form proximal to stenotic infundibula. Treatment options include PCNL, ureteroscopy, and laparoscopic surgery.

In cases of true calyceal dilation with infundibular stenosis, after the stone has been removed, the goal is to dilate or incise the stenotic infundibulum, to relieve the obstruction and stasis of urine. An antegrade stent or a nephrostomy tube can then be placed so that it traverses the stenotic portion of the infundibulum. Unfortunately, there are limited data reported on outcomes. In our study, 14 patients underwent successful direct percutaneous infundibulotomies [51]. We found that direct puncture into the involved calyx provided the best access for stone removal and incision or dilation of the infundibular stenosis. We prefer a straight cold knife for the incision and leaving a nephrostomy tube such as the Cook 20F catheter with the balloon placed in the renal pelvis or a Malecot type re-entry nephrostomy and additional fenestrations created to be ideally positioned in the calyx proximal to the incision. These additional fenestrations provide adequate drainage of this region.

Transplant and true pelvic kidneys

Congenital or transplant pelvic kidneys can also present with renal stones with or without obstruction. The approach to transplant kidneys with renal stones is technically similar to native kidneys, except for the fact that the patient is in the supine position. The access, dilation, and lithotripsy are similar to native kidneys. In cases of small stone burden, a miniscope is ideal [52] (Figure 22.8).

In cases of true pelvic kidneys, a combination of retrograde puncture and laparoscopy can be performed to access the collecting system. Once a wire has been retrieved through the abdominal wall, the dilation and placement of the working sheath will be monitored with laparoscopy.

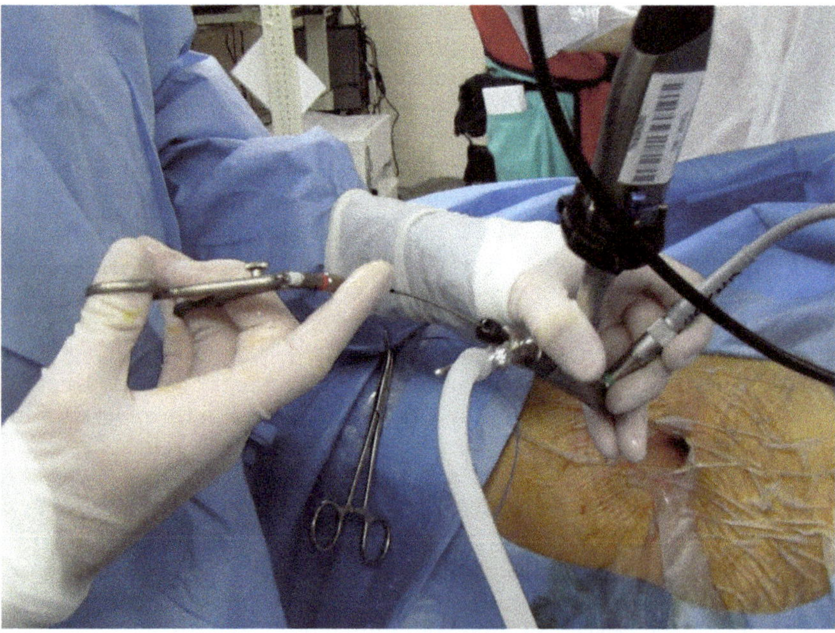

Figure 22.8 Miniscope. Source: Karl Storz, Tuttlingen, Germany.

Once the working sheath is in place, a nephroscope will be inserted with standard stone removal techniques. Adequate drainage of these kidneys during the postoperative period is extremely important to avoid intraperitoneal leakage [53].

Complications

As with most other surgeries, bleeding and infection are two complications of PCNL. The most frequent complications associated specifically with PCNL include:

- collecting system injury
- intra-abdominal organ injury
- pleural injury
- loss of access.
- variety of minor complications such as stone dislodgement into retroperitoneum, distal ureteral stone migration, secondary UPJ obstruction.

Bleeding is the most common complication of PCNL. Intraoperative bleeding from PCNL requires transfusion in 0.5–4% of cases [54]. If significant bleeding is encountered following removal of the access sheath, electrocautery or sealants can be used. We prefer placing a 20F Cook catheter, inflating the balloon with up to 10cc of sterile water, depending on the size of the renal pelvis, and applying pressure to the inciscion site while holding slight traction on the catheter. This is usually sufficient enough to tamponade parenchymal bleeding. The balloon is then partially deflated. It is not recommended to irrigate a bleeding nephrostomy tube since it disturbs the initial clotting that helps tamponade the bleeding. A balloon tamponade catheter is also commercially available but infrequently used.

Collecting system injury can occur while obtaining access or during the procedure. The majority of these injuries are detected intraoperatively, and the case should be aborted if the injury is extensive, at the discretion of the surgeon. Treatment requires adequate drainage of the system and healing usually occurs within 48h. If it is not detected intraoperatively, one should suspect possible perforation if the patient exhibits significant extravasation at the time of nephrostogram, or respiratory issues, abdominal distension, ileus or fever postoperatively [54].

While there have been reports of injury to the small bowel, biliary system, duodenum, spleen and liver, the most common intra-abdominal organ injury is to the colon. It is seen in <1% of cases, and the left side is twice as likely to be injured than the right [55]. The injury is usually extraperitoneal and can therefore be treated conservatively by converting the nephrostomy tube into a colostomy tube and then providing drainage of the kidney with either a new puncture and nephrostomy tube or a ureteral stent [55]. If the injury is intraperitoneal or if the patient's condition deteriorates with conservative management, a CT scan with contrast and or CT nephrostogram can help with diagnosis. One should strongly consider diagnostic laparoscopy for definitive diagnosis and possible repair. Open surgical repair is an option if laparoscopy is not feasible or successful.

One should exercise caution during access if the patient has known hepatomegaly or splenomegaly, or if supracostal access is being performed. These are the situations in which the liver and spleen are at most risk for injury. Injuries to the liver can usually be managed conservatively as there is a lower risk of significant bleeding [55]. Injuries to the spleen, however, have a much higher risk of bleeding and may require surgical intervention [56].

Pleural injury such as hydrothorax, hemothorax, and pneumothorax are rare unless access is being obtained above the 12th rib. Less than 0.5% of cases where access was below the ribs resulted in pleural injury [57]. We routinely scan with fluoroscopy to check the status of both lungs intraoperatively and at the end of each procedure. Special attention is given to this step when the access is above the 12th rib. We also instruct the anesthesia team to monitor the ipsilateral lung frequently during the procedure and to inform the surgical team if there is difficulty aerating the lungs, which can be an early sign of hydrothorax, hemothorax or pneumothorax. When the puncture is supracostal we place the nephrostomy tube through the sheath. Once this tube is in proper position we ask the anesthesiologist to give the patient a deep breath and hold while the sheath is removed and immediate pressure with dressing applied around the site. This maneuver decreases the risks of pneunothorax. When intraoperative fluoroscopic chest imaging was negative, a chest tube was never needed based on the postoperative chest X-ray (CXR) results [58]. We always obtain a portable CXR in the postanesthesia care unit (PACU) following our cases, but we find a negative intraoperative fluoroscopic chest image makes us confident that the patient is at minimal risk for discovering a pleural injury postoperatively. If the index of pleural injury or pneumothorax is high, a repeat CXR should be performed the next morning.

Infection is always a concern and all our patients have a preoperative urine culture and sensitivity. Positive cultures are treated accordingly and negative cultures receive the appropriate antibiotics based on the AUA best practice statement. Even with all these precautions, there is still a 1–2% chance of sepsis [59]. If "frank pus" is encountered upon access to the kidney, a percutaneous drain should be left and the procedure aborted [54]. The risk of pleural infection is high in such cases. It has also been suggested that a 2 step approach decreases the incidence of sepsis in infected kidneys and paraplegics.

Follow-up

Generally we obtain a nephrostogram approximately 24 to 48 h after PCNL to assess adequate drainage of the kidney, and ruling out collecting system extravasation and no evidence of residual stone fragments, prior to removing the nephrostomy tube. The exception is a perfect nephrostogram at the end of the procedure. In this case, the nephrostomy tube is removed 24–48h later without a repeat nephrostogram. If the nephrostogram is "negative," the nephrostomy tube is clamped for several hours. If the patient exhibits no signs of obstruction, and minimal residual when unclamped, the nephrostomy tube is removed. The patient will usually be followed up within 1–2 weeks. In cases of "tubeless" PCNL, an ultrasound can be performed prior to discharge if indicated, such as a patient with unusual pain, abdominal distension, respiratory issues or unexplained fever. The purpose is to rule out hydronephrosis, urinoma or perirenal collection.

We recommend postoperative antibiotics up to 1 week unless there is a strong history of infection or in cases of struvite stones. In such cases, we continue low-dose antibiotic treatment such as nitrofurantoin 100mg daily or a more specific antibiotic based on the sensitivity of the stone culture sent at the time of operation since the stone culture and urine culture are not always identical. This should be continued until the urine has been sterilized.

References

1. Fernstrom I, Johannson B. Percutaneous pyelolithotomy. A new extraction technique. Scand J Urol Nephrol 1976; 10: 257.
2. Kim S, Kuo R, Lingeman J. Percutaneous nephrolithotomy: an update. Curr Opin Urol 2003; 13: 235.
3. Segura J. Percutaneous nephrolithotomy: technique, indications, and complications. AUA Update Series 1993; 12: 154.
4. Charton M, Vallancien G, Veillon B. Urinary tract infection in percutaneous surgery for renal calculi. J Urol 1986; 135: 15.
5. Darenkov A, Derevianko I, Martov A. The prevention of infectious-inflammatory complications in the postoperative period in percutaneous surgical interventions in patients with urolithiasis. Urol Nephrol 1994; 2: 24.
6. Wolf J, Bennett C, Dmochowski R. Urologic Surgery Antimicrobial Prophylaxis Best Practice Policy Panel. J Urol 2008; 179: 1379.
7. Zheng W, Denstedt J. Intracorporeal lithotripsy. Update on technology. Urol Clin North Am 2000; 27: 301.
8. Hofbauer J, Hobarth K, Marberger M. Electrohydraulic versus pneumatic disintegration in the treatment of ureteral stones: a randomized, prospective trial. J Urol 1995; 153: 623.
9. Basar H, Ohta N, Kageyama S, et al. Treatment of ureteral and renal stones by electrohydraulic lithotripsy. Int Urol Nephrol 1997; 29: 275.
10. Piergiovanni M, Desgrandchamps F, Cochand-Priollet B, et al. Ureteral and bladder lesions after ballistic, ultrasonic, electrohydraulic, or laser lithotripsy. J Endourol 1994; 8: 293.
11. Howards S, Merrill E, Harris S, et al. Ultrasonic lithotripsy: laboratory evaluation. Invest Urol 1974; 11: 273.
12. Segura J, Patterson D, LeRoy A, et al. Percutaneous lithotripsy. J Urol 1983; 130: 1051.
13. Elder J, Gibbons R, Bush W, et al. Ultrasonic lithotripsy of a large staghorn calculus. J Urol 1984; 131: 1152.

14. Segura J, Patterson D, LeRoy A, et al. Percutaneous removal of kidney stones: review of 1000 cases. J Urol 1985; 134: 1077.
15. Servadio C, Winkler H, Neuman M, et al. Percutaneous nephrolithotomy. Isr J Med Sci 1986; 22: 541.
16. Santa-Cruz R, Leveillee R, Krongrad A. Ex vivo comparison of four lithotripters commonly used in the ureter: what does it take to perforate? J Endourol 1998; 12: 417.
17. Denstedt J. Use of Swiss Lithoclast for percutaneous nephrolithotripsy. J Endourol 1993; 7: 477.
18. Lasser M, Pareek G. Percutaneous lithotripsy and stone extraction. In: Smith A, Badlani G, Preminger G, Kavoussi L, eds. *Smith's Textbook of Endourology*, 3rd edn. Hoboken, NJ: Blackwell Publishing Ltd, 2012.
19. Hoffmann R, Weber A, Heidenreich Z, et al. Experimental studies and first clinical experience with a new Lithoclast and ultrasound combination for lithotripsy. Eur Urol 2002; 42: 376.
20. Pietrow P, Auge B, Zhong P, et al. Clinical efficacy of a combination pneumatic and ultrasonic lithotrite. J Urol 2003; 169: 1247.
21. Lehman D, Hruby G, Philips C, et al. Prospective randomized comparison of a combined ultrasonic and pneumatic lithotrite with a standard ultrasonic lithotrite for percutaneous nephrolithotomy. J Endourol 2008; 22: 285.
22. Jou Y, Shen C, Cheng M, et al. High-power holmium:yttrium-aluminum-garnet laser for percutaneous treatment of large renal stones. Urology 2007; 69: 22.
23. Hyams E, Shah O. Percutaneous nephrostolithotomy versus flexible ureteroscopy/holmium laser lithotripsy: cost and outcome analysis. J Urol 2009; 182: 1012.
24. Cuellar D, Averch T. Holmium laser percutaneous nephrolithotomy using a unique suction device. J Endourol 2004; 18:780.
25. Nemoy N, Stamey T. Surgical bacteriological, and biochemical management of "infection stones." JAMA 1971; 215: 1470.
26. Dretler S, Pfister R, Newhouse J. Renal stone dissolution via percutaneous nephrostomy. N Engl J Med 1979; 300: 341.
27. Blaivas J, Pais U, Spellman R. Chemolysis of residual stone fragments after extensive surgery for staghorn calculi. Urology 1975; 6: 680.
28. Mulvaney W. The hydrodynamics of renal irrigations: with reference to calculus solvents. J Urol 1963; 89:765.
29. Eshghi M, Smith A. Chemolysis of calculi: systemic and direct approaches. In: Smith A, Castaneda-Zuniga W, Bronson J, eds. *Endourology: Principles and Practice*. New York: Thieme Inc, 1986.
30. Rodman J, Vaughan ED. Chemolysis of urinary calculi. AUA Update Series 1992; 11: Lesson 1.
31. Sadi M, Saltzman N, Feria G, et al; Experimental observation on dissolution of uric acid calculi. J Urol 1985; 134: 575
32. Stark H, Savir A. Dissolution of cystine calculi by pelviocalyceal irrigation with D-penicillamine. J Urol 1980; 124: 895.
33. Silverman D, Stamey T. Management of infection stones: the Stanford experience. Medicine 1983; 62: 44.
34. Mulvaney W. A new solvent for certain urinary calculi. J Urol 1959; 82: 546.
35. Jacobs D, Heimbach D, Hesse A. A chemolysis of struvite stones by acidification of artificial urine – an in vitro study. Scand J Urol Nephrol 2001; 35: 345.
36. Bellman G, Davidoff R, Candela J, et al. Tubeless percutaneous renal surgery. J Urol 1997; 157: 1578.

37. Maheshwari P, Andankar M, Bansal M. Nephrostomy tube after percutaneous nephrolithotomy: large-bore or pigtail catheter? J Endourol 2000; 14: 735.
38. Pietrow P, Auge B, Lallas C, et al. Pain after percutaneous nephrolithotomy: impact of nephrostomy tube size. J Endourol 2003; 17: 411.
39. Karami H, Jabbari M, Arbab A. Tubeless percutaneous nephrolithotomy: 5 years of experience in 201 patients. J Endourol 2007; 21: 1411–13.
40. Uribe C, Eichel L, Khonsari S, et al. What happens to hemostatic agents in contact with urine? An in vitro study. J Endourol 2005; 19: 312.
41. Borin J, Sala L, Eichel L, et al. Tubeless percutaneous nephrolithotomy using hemostatic gelatin matrix. J Endourol 2005; 19: 614.
42. Badlani G, Eshghi M, Smith A. Percutaneous surgery for ureteropelvic junction obstruction (endopyelotomy): technique and early results. J Urol 1986; 135: 26.
43. Yohannes P, Smith A. The endourological management of complications associated with horseshoe kidney. J Urol 2002; 168: 5.
44. Clayman R, Surya V, Miller R, et al. Percutaneous nephrolithotomy: an approach to branched and staghorn renal calculi. JAMA 1983; 250: 73.
45. Stein R, Desai M. Management of urolithiasis in the congenitally abnormal kidney (horseshoe and ectopic). Curr Opin Urol 2007; 17: 125.
46. Horton A, Madigan R, Munneke G, et al. Nephrostomy – why, how and what to look for. Imaging 2008; 20: 29.
47. Skolarikos A, Murat B, Apostolos B, et al. Percutaneous nephrolithotomy in horseshoe kidneys: factors affecting stone-free rate. J Urol 2011; 186: 1894.
48. Monga M, Smith R, Ferral R, et al. Percutaneous ablation of caliceal diverticulum: long term followup. J Urol 2000; 163: 28.
49. Hulbert J, Reddy P, Hunter D, et al. Percutaneous techniques for the management of caliceal diverticula containing calculi. J Urol 1986; 135: 225.
50. Krambeck A, Lingeman J. Percutaneous treatment of calyceal diverticula, infundibular stenosis, and simple renal cysts. In: Smith A, Badlani G, Preminger G, Kavoussi L, eds. *Smith's Textbook of Endourology*, 3rd edn. Hoboken, NJ: Blackwell Publishing Ltd, 2012.
51. Eshghi M, William T, Fernandez R, et al. Percutaneous (endo) infundibulotomy. J Endourol 1987; 1:107.
52. Eshghi M, Smith A. Endourologic approach to transplant kidney. Urology 1986; 28: 504.
53. Eshghi M, Roth J, Smith A. Percutaneous transperitoneal approach to a pelvic kidney for endourological removal of a staghorn calculus. J Urol 1985; 134: 525.
54. Wolf J. Percutaneous approach to the upper urinary tract collecting system. In: Wein A, Kavoussi L, Novick A, Partin A, Peters C, eds. *Campbell-Walsh Urology*, 10th edn. Philadelphia: Elsevier Saunders, 2012.
55. El-Nahas A, Shokeir A, El-Assmy A, et al. Colonic perforation during percutaneous nephrolithotomy: study of risk factors. Urology 2006; 67: 937.
56. Kondas J, Szentgyorgyi E, Vaczi L, et al. Splenic injury: a rare complication of percutaneous nephrolithotomy. Int Urol Nephrol 1994; 26: 399.
57. Munver R, Delvecchio F, Newman G, et al. Critical analysis of supracostal access for percutaneous renal surgery. J Urol 2001; 166: 1242.
58. Ogan K, Corwin T, Smith T, et al. Sensitivity of chest fluoroscopy compared with chest CT and chest radiography for diagnosing hydropneumothorax in association with percutaneous nephrostolithotomy. Urology 2003; 62: 98.
59. Dogan H, Fuad G, Yesim S, et al. Importance of microbiological evaluation in management of infectious complications following percutaneous nephrolithotomy. Int Urol Nephrol 2007; 39: 737.

CHAPTER 23

Laparoscopic and Open Surgical Management of Urinary Calculi

Ahmed Alasker, Reza Ghavamian, and David Hoenig
Albert Einstein College of Medicine, Montefiore Medical Center, Bronx, NY, USA

Do's and don'ts box

Renal calculi

Pyelolithotomy

- Don't perform pyelolithotomy as first-line treatment for renal stone unless pyeloplasty or other anatomical repair is needed.
- Don't use fluid irrigation when using the flexible nephroscope to retrieve the stones because large amounts of fluid are hard to remove intraoperatively and may produce postoperative ileus and give the false impression of anastomotic leak.
- Do place indwelling stents and surgical drains to reduce urinary leak.
- Do close the collecting system in watertight fashion.

Anatrophic nephrolithotomy

- Do reserve anatrophic nephrolithotomy as an option for staghorn stones if other approaches are insufficient in the face of stone burden, instrumentation or anatomical abnormalities.
- Do cover the patient with broad-spectrum antibiotic therapy due to the risk of urosepsis related to struvite stones.
- Do use intraoperative imaging to confirm complete stone removal.

Calyceal diverticulectomy

- Do appropriately select the candidate for this approach based on preoperative images (typically anterior diverticula).
- Don't perform laparoscopic diverticulectomy for severely scarred diverticulum failing PNL approach.

Simple nephrectomy

- Do evaluate the renal function using nuclear renal scan after relieving the obstruction before proceeding to nephrectomy for renal stone.

Ureteric calculi

Ureterolithotomy

- Do reserve laparoscopic ureterolithotomy for very selected cases of proximal large ureteric stones when access to modern endourology is limited.

Urinary Stones: Medical and Surgical Management, First Edition. Edited by Michael Grasso and David S. Goldfarb.

- Don't leave the ureter without stenting or closure – at least one is required.
- Do place a periureteric drain not overlying the suture line.

Bladder calculi

Open cystolithotomy

- Do evaluate and manage the etiology of stones in case of bladder stones.
- Do evaluate stone burden by cystoscopy or preoperative images to select the appropriate approach.
- Do close the bladder with only absorbable sutures.

Introduction

Current advances in endourological procedures and extracorporeal shock wave lithotripsy (ESWL) have minimized the role of open stone surgery in the management of patients with urinary calculi [1]. Technological revolutions and improved surgical expertise have significantly diminished the number of patients needing open surgery [2]. Over 95% of urinary stone are performed by ESWL and/or endourological interventions such as percutaneous nephrolithotomy (PNL) and ureteroscopy (URS) [3]. However, open stone surgery has a role in very carefully chosen cases. The most common indication is complex stones with a high stone burden, especially in combination with anatomical variations [4].

Laparoscopic surgery has evolved in the last two decades and provides several advantages over open surgery, including less morbidity and faster recovery. It has been well accepted as a standard treatment for many benign and malignant urological disorders yet the number of studies on the role of laparoscopic management of renal stones is quite limited [5]. In this chapter, we will focus on the role of open and laparoscopic surgery to treat renal, ureteric, and bladder stones.

Renal calculi

Current guidelines from the American Urological Association reserve the option of open surgery as a last resort for treating staghorn stones, typically as anatrophic nephrolithotomy [6]. Side by side, the European Association of Urology guidelines limit open surgery for complex stone burden, treatment failure of ESWL and/or PNL, intrarenal anatomical abnormalities such as obstruction of the ureteropelvic junction (UPJ), infundibular stenosis, stone in the calyceal diverticulum (mainly in an anterior calyx), non-functioning lower pole (partial nephrectomy), and non-functioning kidney (nephrectomy) [7].

Laparoscopy is a method that reproduces the steps of open surgery and may be indicated as an alternative in cases of therapeutic failure using less invasive methods. Moreover, laparoscopic surgery is effective for complex renal stones and allows adjunctive procedures, such as pyeloplasty, ablation of calyceal diverticula, partial nephrectomy, and nephrectomy [7].

Pyelolithotomy with or without pyeloplasty

Laparoscopic pyelolithotomy (LP) can be an effective treatment modality for stone extraction, especially in the setting of UPJ repair where concomitant pyeloplasty needs to be performed (Table 23.1). It offers a high stone-free rate in a single operative session. A study of 19 patients who underwent laparoscopic pyelolithotomy with pyeloplasty demonstrated stone-free rates of 90%. Stone retrieval was achieved by guiding a flexible nephroscope into the renal pelvis through a laparoscopic port site. Indwelling stents and peritoneal drains usually are placed [8]. In a randomized and comparative study of 105 patients with solitary large renal pelvic stones who were divided into two groups, group 1 included 55 patients who were treated by LP performed retroperitoneally without pyeloplasty and group 2 included 50 patients who were treated by PNL. Mean estimated blood loss, mean hospital stay, mean time of postoperative analgesia, rate of postoperative blood transfusion, and stone-free rate (100% versus 96%) were similar. On the other hand, the mean operative time was significantly longer in the LP group (130.6 ± 38.7 min versus 108.5 ± 18.7 min; $p<0.05$), respectively [9].

In another study by Lee et al., 77 patients underwent LP as first-line treatment for large renal stones (≥15 mm). They classified their cases based on the complexity of renal stones. Overall stone-free rate was 81.8% after a single operative session. However, stone location, as well as total stone burden, was an important predictor of surgical outcome of LP in renal stone. For example, stone-free rate at 3 months for complete staghorn stone was 33% compared to 96% in stone located only in the renal pelvis [10].

Many technical innovations have facilitated such stone retrieval procedures, including the use of special laparoscopic graspers, flexible nephroscope with the use of carbon dioxide to insufflate the collecting system, and the use of an injected coagulum to retrieve all the stone fragments as one piece [11,12]. Moreover, robot-assisted surgery continues to expand its application for the management of large upper tract urinary stones, especially with simultaneous pyeloplasty. The results of early trials involving robot-assisted pyelolithotomy have revealed safe and efficacious outcomes. It offers superb visualization, by enhanced optics, facile dexterity and ergonomics by wristed instrumentation which makes complex reconstruction of the collecting system, including UPJ repair, much easier. However, larger studies are needed to explore this new technology in treating renal stones [13].

Anatrophic nephrolithotomy

Anatrophic nephrolithotomy was pioneered by Boyce and Elkins in 1974. They used renal anatomical and physiological principles and reconstructive surgical techniques to synthesize this operation. It was the preferred treatment for patients with staghorn calculi until the development of

Table 23.1 Summary of open and laparoscopic renal calculi surgeries

Surgery	Favorable approach	Indications	Reported complications	Technical tips
Pyelolithotomy	Lap	• Anatomical variations in location or shape of the kidney, i.e. pelvic kidney, horseshoe kidney, malrotated or ectopic kidney • Ureteropelvic junction obstruction that requires pyeloplasty • Failed PNL or ESWL • Morbid obesity	• Urinary leakage • Urinary tract infection • Stone migration • Peritonitis and abscess formation • Prolonged ileus	• Stone retrieval can be achieved by a laparoscopic grasper and/or a flexible nephroscope with stone basket • Carbon dioxide can be used to insufflate the collecting system • Colored fibrin sealant (with methylene blue) can be used with thrombin solution as a coagulum to retrieve all the stone fragments in one piece • Intraoperative fluoroscopy or ultrasound can be used to locate migrated stones
Anatrophic nephrolithotomy	Open	• Large-volume calculi and complex collecting system (>2500 mm^2) • Morbid obesity • Failed PNL	• Acute tubular necrosis • Hemorrhage • Vascular injuries and AV fistula • Urinoma	• The anatrophic plane is defined by occluding the posterior segmental artery and administering methylene blue intravenously • Doppler ultrasound can be used to facilitate identification of renal artery • The use of iced slush decreases ischemia effect on the kidney • Liberal use of hemostatic/sealant agents helps to reduce the risk of bleeding and leakage

(Continued)

Table 23.1 (continued)

Surgery	Favorable approach	Indications	Reported complications	Technical tips
Calyceal diverticulectomy	Lap	• Large stones within the calyceal diverticulum • An anterior calyx diverticulum with a long and narrow neck • Failed PNL, URS or ESWL	• Urinary leakage	• Retrograde injection of indigo carmine, methylene blue, fluoroscopy and/or ultrasound can help to locate the stone
Simple nephrectomy	Lap	• Symptomatic stones in non-functioning kidney	• Bowel perforation • Vascular injury • Open conversion	• Always control renal hilum before mobilizing the kidney laterally • Carry renal dissection outside Gerota's fascia in case of excessive adhesion

AV, arteriovenous; ESWL, extracorporeal shock wave lithotripsy; Lap, laparoscopic; PNL, percutaneous nephrolithotomy; URS, ureteroscopy.

percutaneous nephrolithotomy. It still remains a viable therapeutic alternative for a small number of patients harboring complex staghorn calculi (see Table 23.1) [14]. Lam et al. reported that when the stone surface area was greater than 2500 mm^2, the chance of attaining stone-free status with PNL at their center was only 50% [15]. In contrast, almost 90% of patients with staghorn calculi less than 2500 mm^2 were rendered stone free with PNL [14,15]. On the other hand, anatrophic nephrolithotomy offers high stone-free rate in a single operation exceeding 90% for large complex renal stones [1]. Other potential candidates for this procedure are those individuals with excessive morbid obesity (600 lb or greater) with large staghorn calculi as safe, effective percutaneous access may be difficult or impossible. However, the wider availability of long nephroscopes (22 cm versus 15 cm) makes PNL the first-line therapy for stones larger than 2 cm even in obese patients [1].

Technically, anatrophic nephrolithotomy requires a parenchymal incision made in an intersegmental plane (Brodel's white line), allowing removal of large renal calculi (Figure 23.1). Initially, the main renal artery is located and isolated and then the posterior segmental artery is identified and temporarily occluded. After that, methylene blue is administrated intravenously in order to define the anatrophic plane. By using iced slush, renal hypothermic ischemia is established, and then a nephrotomy is made through Brodel's white line. The stones are extracted, which may require incising stenotic infundibula to facilitate removal. In addition, radiography can be performed intraoperatively to confirm complete stone removal. Finally, the collecting system is reconstructed and then the renal capsule is closed with absorbable sutures after which the renal circulation is restored [14].

Laparoscopic anatrophic nephrolithotomy has been reported in a few series. Although it is technically demanding, it may be promising especially with the introduction of robotic-assisted laparoscopy. Among currently published series, the number of patients is extremely limited: the largest series included 11 patients. Stone-free rates varied between 60% and 90% and the mean warm ischemia time was 20–32 min [16,17,18,19]. Clearly, improvement in technique, instrumentation, outcomes, and experience will be required before a 60–90% result can be expected.

Calyceal diverticulectomy

Calyceal diverticula are non-secretory cystic intrarenal cavities that communicate with the collecting system by a narrow neck, and are typically located at a calyceal fornix or infundibulum (Figure 23.2) [20]. Although they are usually asymptomatic, such diverticula are prone to urinary stasis and may present clinically when infection and stones develop.

Urologists approach stones in calyceal diverticula by various strategies. Percutaneous nephrolithotomy directed toward the diverticulum with neck dilation and diverticular fulguration remains the main approach. Other potential therapeutic endourological modalities exist, such as extracorporeal shock wave lithotripsy and retrograde ureteroscopy. Similarly, laparoscopic management of calyceal diverticula is a feasible

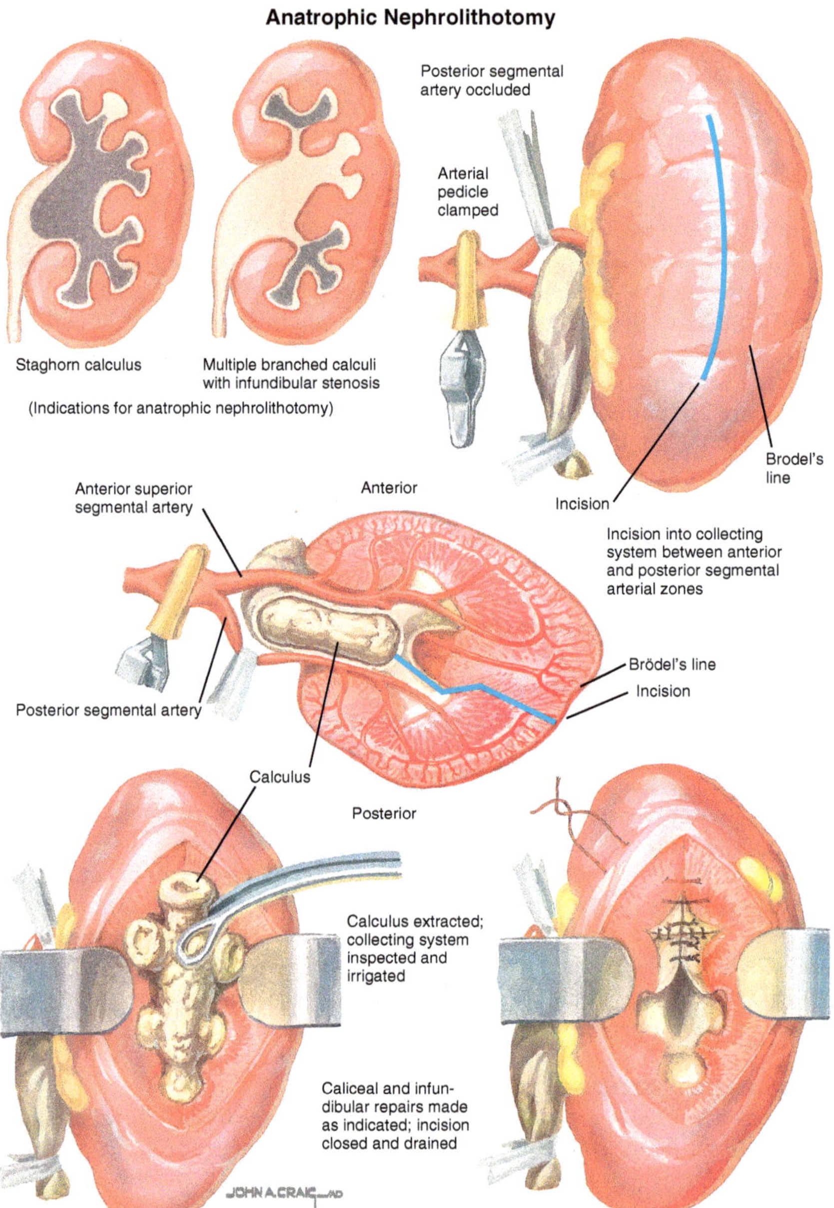

Figure 23.1 Anatrophic nephrolithotomy. Source: www.netterimages.com. Netter illustration used with permission of Elsevier, Inc. All rights reserved.

option mainly in symptomatic calyceal diverticula with thin overlying renal parenchyma, or for anterior diverticula inaccessible or unsuccessfully managed by endourological techniques. The overlying capsule and parenchyma are excised, stones are removed, and the cavity marsupialized.

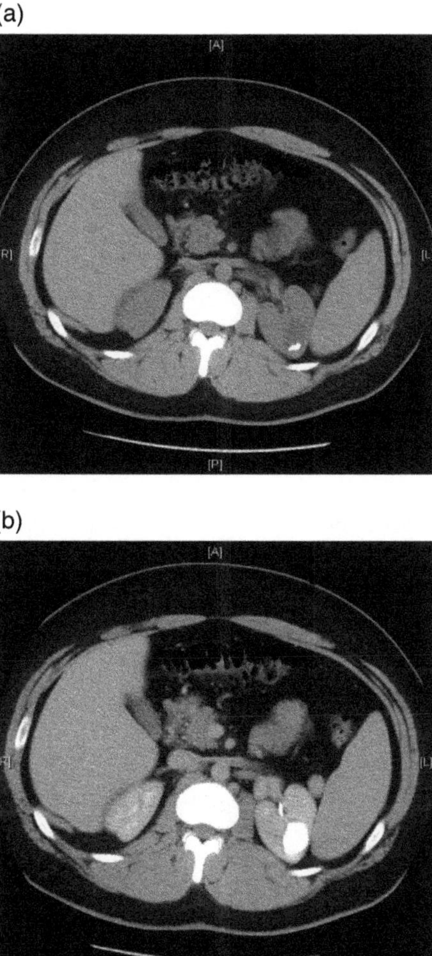

Figure 23.2 (a) Renal stone in a posterior calyceal diverticulum which makes a PNL approach more favorable. (b) The narrow diverticular neck is visualized by the contrast passively filling the diverticulum, precluding a retrograde access.

Techniques for intraoperative localization of the stone-bearing diverticulum include retrograde injection of indigo carmine, fluoroscopy and/or laparoscopic ultrasound (Figure 23.3) [21,22].

Several authors have demonstrated the success of the laparoscopic approach to a calyceal diverticulum with stone-free rates ranging between 92% and 100% [21,22,23]. These results were comparable with those using PNL approaches. The diverticulum was obliterated in between 92% and 100% of cases with a very high percentage of patients becoming symptom free [5]. However, most of these published series are limited by their small patient numbers and, again, more extensive studies are needed.

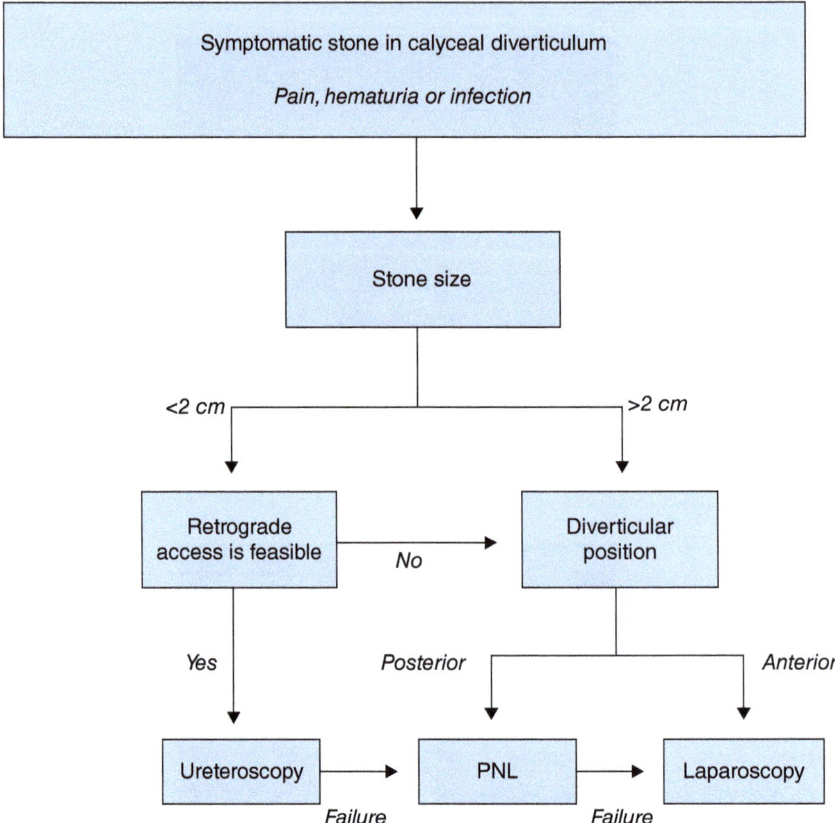

Figure 23.3 Algorithm for managing renal stones located in calyceal diverticula.

Simple nephrectomy

Patients who present with large stones in a non-functioning kidney after appropriate relief of obstruction has been performed may require nephrectomy or partial nephrectomy. Laparoscopic rather than open nephrectomy is now considered the gold standard approach, reserving open nephrectomy for more complex surgery such as xanthogranulomatous pyelonephritis where the laparoscopic approach may be complicated due to perinephric infection and inflammation, severe fibrosis, and adhesions [5,24].

Ureteric calculi

Laparoscopic or open surgical ureteric stone removal may be considered in rare cases when ESWL, URS, and percutaneous URS have failed or are unlikely to be successful. When expertise is available, laparoscopic surgery should be the preferred option before proceeding to open surgery [7].

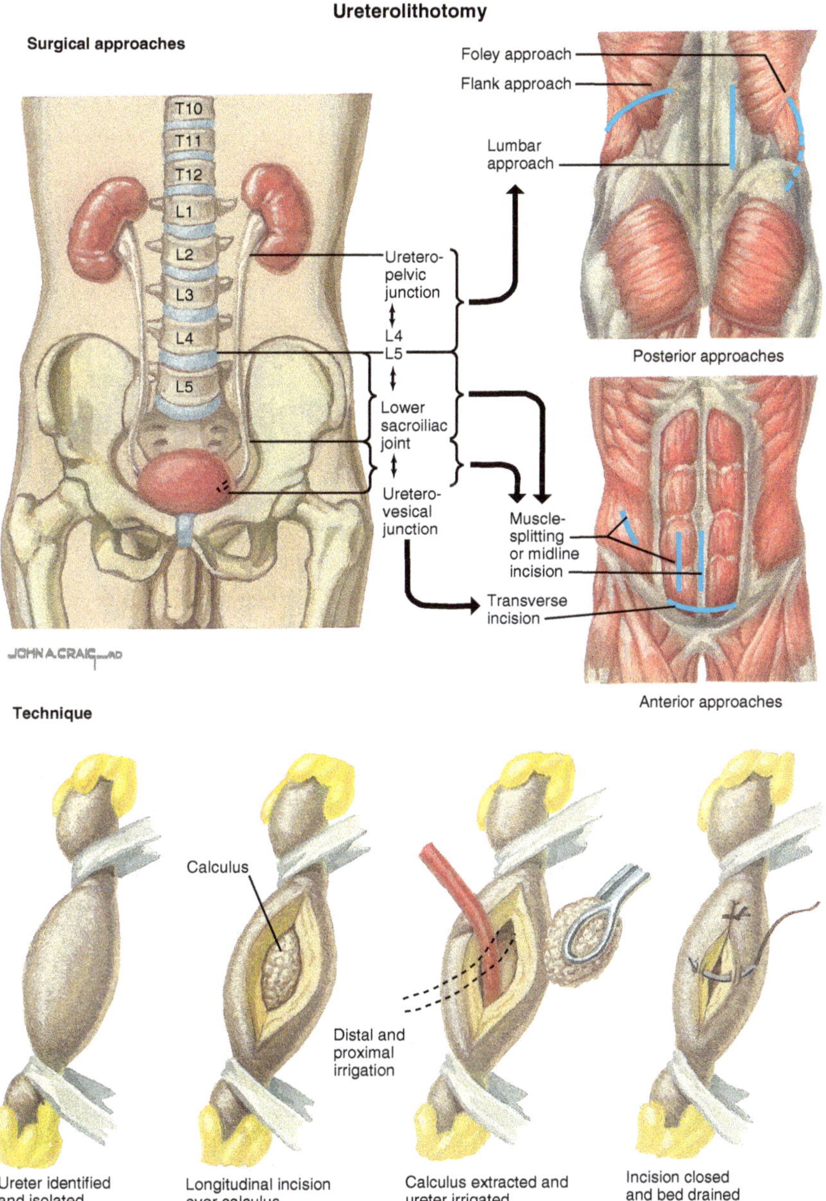

Figure 23.4 Open ureterolithotomy. Source: www.netterimages.com. Netter illustration used with permission of Elsevier, Inc. All rights reserved.

Ureterolithotomy

Laparoscopic ureterolithotomy can be performed transperitoneally or retroperitoneally, depending on stone location and surgeon experience. Large stones are easily identified in most cases; for smaller calculi, preoperative or intraoperative imaging is neccessary.

After identification of the stone, the ureter is temporarily occluded proximally and distally of the stone to prevent it shifting. A longitudinal incision of the ureter for stone removal is preferred by most surgeons (Figure 23.4). Closure of the ureter should be performed using an intracorporeal suture after inserting a double J stent. Some authors state, however, that a suture is not necessary when a ureteral stent is used. Moreover, some surgeons advocate not placing a stent after suturing. In all cases, however, a retroperitoneal drain should be inserted to prevent the possibility of urinoma (Table 23.2) [25,26].

In contrast to ureterscopy and ESWL, laparoscopic ureterolithotomy is associated with fewer surgical procedures and higher success rates with stone-free rates ranging from 90% to 97%. However, more postoperative pain, longer surgical procedures, and a longer hospital stay ranging from 2 to 7 days with an average of 3–4 days are typically seen [26,27,28,29,30]. Although it is associated with the highest success rates for large proximal ureteral calculi, laparoscopic ureterolithotomy remains, generally, a second-line procedure, primarily due to the increased invasiveness over endourological techniques. More contemporary studies have reported the feasibility of laparoendoscopic single-site (LESS) ureterolithotomy which may offer cosmetic advantages although it is more technically challenging [31,32].

Bladder calculi

Vesicolithiasis is classified as primary bladder stones which exist during childhood and are associated with nutritional deficiencies or form secondarily in the bladder because of urinary stasis due to bladder outlet obstruction, neurogenic bladder, a diverticulum, infection, or foreign bodies. Occasionally, a stone which passes from the upper tract to the bladder can then fail to pass, often due to bladder outlet obstruction. In the course of considering surgical approaches, evaluation and treatment of contributing etiologies should also be addressed (nutritional, obstructive, anatomical or functional) [33].

Open cystolithotomy

Once commonly performed, open cystolithotomy has been replaced by transurethral or percutaneous cystolithopexy with the introduction of more effective stone-breaking modalities such as ultrasonic, ballistic or laser lithotripsy. Among these, the holmium:YAG laser is used transurethrally to fragment the stone and is considered the new gold standard. However, open cystolithotomy can be offered in cases of very large stones not amenable to endoscopic modalities. It is fast, effective and tolerable with stone-free rates exceeding 90%. In addition, open surgery is still widely used for treating pediatric vesicolithiasis. The drawback of open cystolithotomy is that it requires longer catheter drainage and cosmetically is less attractive, as well as the increased morbidity of an incision in the lower abdomen [34,35,36,37].

Table 23.2 Summary of open and laparoscopic ureteric and bladder calculi surgeries

Surgery	Favorable approach	Indications	Reported complications	Technical tips
Ureterolithotomy	Lap	• When less invasive modalities have failed (ESWL, URS or percutaneous ureterolithotomy) • Large, impacted stones (>15 mm) mainly in proximal or middle ureter • Multiple ureteral stones • Concurrent conditions requiring abdominal surgery	• Hemorrhage • Stone migration • Bowel injury • Ureter avulsion • Wound and retroperitoneal hematoma • Fever/UTI • Ileus • Urinary leakage • Urinoma • Ureteral stricture	• Intraoperative fluoroscopy or ultrasound helps to locate the stone • Occlusion of the ureter proximal and distal to the stone prevents stone migration • Use flexible nephroscope in case of stone migration • Place double J stent through the ureteric incision or endoscopically after stone removal • Close the ureterotomy incision with absorbable sutures
Cystolithotomy	Open	• Large >4 cm or multiple bladder stones not amenable to endoscopic removal • Bladder stone associated with very large prostate necessitating open prostatectomy • Pediatric patients • Endoscopic or percutaneous access is contraindicated due to previous reconstructive surgery	• Hemorrhage • Urinary leakage	• Close the bladder in two layers in watertight fashion • Avoid opening the bladder close to bladder neck

ESWL, extracorporeal shock wave lithotripsy; Lap, laparoscopic; URS, ureteroscopy; UTI, urinary tract infection.

Key points

- Current advances in endourological procedures and ESWL (ESWL) have minimized the role of open stone surgery in the management of patients with urinary calculi.
- Only 1–5% of urinary stones are performed by open or laparoscopic surgery.

Renal calculi

- Percutaneous nephrolithotomy remains the first-line treatment for large renal stones more than 2 cm.
- Laparoscopic pyelolithotomy is an effective treatment modality for stone extraction, especially in the setting of UPJ repair where pyeloplasty is needed.
- Robot-assisted laparoscopic pyelolithotomy with pyeloplasty is promising. Due to its advanced ergonomics and visualization, complex reconstruction of the collecting system is much easier to perform.
- Anatrophic nephrolithotomy has been replaced by PNL for treating staghorn calculi. It offers high stone-free rates in a single operation exceeding 90% for large complex renal stones.
- Laparoscopic diverticulectomy is a feasible option for treating stones in calyceal diverticula, mainly for anteriorly located diverticula with thin overlying renal parenchyma.
- Calyceal diverticulum and stone size, location of diverticulum and the length and width of the diverticular neck are paramount in selecting the appropriate approach.
- Laparoscopic simple nephrectomy is considered the gold standard approach for stone in non-functioning kidneys.
- Open nephrectomy is sometimes required for more complex stone surgery such as xanthogranulomatous pyelonephritis.

Ureteric calculi

- Laparoscopic ureterolithotomy removal may be considered in rare cases when ESWL, URS, and percutaneous URS have been unsuccessful.

Bladder calculi

- Open cystolithotomy has been replaced by transurethral or percutaneous cystolithopexy with the introduction of more effective stone-breaking modalities.

References

1. Paik ML, Wainstein MA, Spirnak JP, Hampel N, Resnick MI. Current indications for open stone surgery in the treatment of renal and ureteral calculi. J Urol 1998; 159(2): 374–9.
2. Matlaga BR, Assimos DG. Changing indications of open stone surgery. Urology 2002; 59(4): 490–3; discussion 493–4.
3. Chaussy CG, Fuchs GJ. Current state and future developments of noninvasive treatment of human urinary stones with extracorporeal shock wave lithotripsy. J Urol 1989; 141(3 Pt 2): 782–9.
4. Honeck P, Wendt-Nordahl G, Krombach P, et al. Does open stone surgery still play a role in the treatment of urolithiasis? Data of a primary urolithiasis center. J Endourol 2009; 23(7): 1209–12.

5. Kijvikai K. The role of laparoscopic surgery for renal calculi management. Ther Adv Urol 2011; 3(1): 13–18.
6. Preminger G, Assimos D, Lingeman J, et al. Staghorn calculi. American Urological Association Guidelines, 2005.
7. Türk C, Petrik A, Sarica K, Seitz C. Urolithiasis. Euoropean Association of Urology Guidelines, 2012.
8. Wignall GR, Canales BK, Denstedt JD, Monga M. Minimally invasive approaches to upper urinary tract urolithiasis. Urol Clin North Am 2008; 35(3): 441–54.
9. Al-Hunayan A, Khalil M, Hassabo M, Hanafi A, Abdul-Halim H. Management of solitary renal pelvic stone: laparoscopic retroperitoneal pyelolithotomy versus percutaneous nephrolithotomy. J Endourol 2011; 25(6): 975–8.
10. Lee JW, Cho SY, Yeon JS, et al. Laparoscopic pyelolithotomy: comparison of surgical outcomes in relation to stone distribution within the kidney. J Endourol 2013; 27(5): 592–7.
11. Borges R, Azinhais P, Retroz E, et al. Coagulum pyelolithotomy "revisited" by laparoscopy: technique modification. Urology 2012; 79(6): 1412.
12. Mason BM, Hoenig D. Carbon dioxide based nephroscopy: a trick for laparoscopic pyelolithotomy. J Endourol 2008; 22(12): 2661–3.
13. Badalato GM, Hemal AK, Menon M, Badani KK. Current role of robot-assisted pyelolithotomy for the management of large renal calculi: a contemporary analysis. J Endourol 2009; 23(10): 1719–22.
14. Assimos DG. Anatrophic nephrolithotomy. Urology 2001; 57(1): 161–5.
15. Lam HS, Lingeman JE, Barron M, et al. Staghorn calculi: analysis of treatment results between initial percutaneous nephrostolithotomy and extracorporeal shock wave lithotripsy monotherapy with reference to surface area. J Urol 1992; 147(5): 1219–25.
16. Deger S, Tuellmann M, Schoenberger B, Winkelmann B, Peters R, Loening SA. Laparoscopic anatrophic nephrolithotomy. Scand J Urol Nephrol 2004; 38(3): 263–5.
17. Giedelman C, Arriaga J, Carmona O, et al. Laparoscopic anatrophic nephrolithotomy: developments of the technique in the era of minimally invasive surgery. J Endourol 2012; 26(5): 444–50.
18. Zhou L, Xuan Q, Wu B, et al. Retroperitoneal laparoscopic anatrophic nephrolithotomy for large staghorn calculi. Int J Urol 2011; 18(2): 126–9.
19. Simforoosh N, Aminsharifi A, Tabibi A, et al. Laparoscopic anatrophic nephrolithotomy for managing large staghorn calculi. BJU Int 2008; 101(10): 1293–6.
20. Wyler SF, Bachmann A, Jayet C, Casella R, Gasser TC, Sulser T. Retroperitoneoscopic management of caliceal diverticular calculi. Urology 2005; 65(2): 380–3.
21. Waxman SW, Winfield HN. Laparoscopic management of caliceal diverticulum. J Endourol 2009; 23(10): 1731–2.
22. Miller SD, Ng CS, Streem SB, Gill IS. Laparoscopic management of caliceal diverticular calculi. J Urol 2002; 167(3): 1248–52.
23. Ramakumar S, Segura JW. Laparoscopic surgery for renal urolithiasis: pyelolithotomy, caliceal diverticulectomy, and treatment of stones in a pelvic kidney. J Endourol 2000; 14(10): 829–32.
24. Hemal AK, Goel A, Kumar M, Gupta NP. Evaluation of laparoscopic retroperitoneal surgery in urinary stone disease. J Endourol 2001; 15(7): 701–5.
25. Hruza M, Schulze M, Teber D, Gozen AS, Rassweiler JJ. Laparoscopic techniques for removal of renal and ureteral calculi. J Endourol 2009; 23(10): 1713–18.

26. Hammady A, Gamal WM, Zaki M, Hussein M, Abuzeid A. Evaluation of ureteral stent placement after retroperitoneal laparoscopic ureterolithotomy for upper ureteral stone: randomized controlled study. J Endourol 2011; 25(5): 825–30.
27. Karami H, Javanmard B, Hasanzadeh-Hadah A, et al. Is it necessary to place a Double J catheter after laparoscopic ureterolithotomy? A four-year experience. J Endourol 2012; 26(9): 1183–6.
28. Lopes Neto AC, Korkes F, Silva JL, et al. Prospective randomized study of treatment of large proximal ureteral stones: extracorporeal shock wave lithotripsy versus ureterolithotripsy versus laparoscopy. J Urol 2012; 187(1): 164–8.
29. Basiri A, Simforoosh N, Ziaee A, Shayaninasab H, Moghaddam SM, Zare S. Retrograde, antegrade, and laparoscopic approaches for the management of large, proximal ureteral stones: a randomized clinical trial. J Endourol 2008; 22(12): 2677–80.
30. Leonardo C, Simone G, Rocco P, Guaglianone S, Pierro G, Gallucci M. Laparoscopic ureterolithotomy: minimally invasive second line treatment. Int Urol Nephrol 2011; 43(3): 651–4.
31. Lee JY, Han JH, Kim TH, Yoo TK, Park SY, Lee SW. Laparoendoscopic single-site ureterolithotomy for upper ureteral stone disease: the first 30 cases in a multicenter study. J Endourol 2011; 25(8): 1293–8.
32. Wen X, Liu X, Huang H, et al. Retroperitoneal laparoendoscopic single-site ureterolithotomy: a comparison with conventional laparoscopic surgery. J Endourol 2012; 26(4): 366–71.
33. Philippou P, Moraitis K, Masood J, Junaid I, Buchholz N. The management of bladder lithiasis in the modern era of endourology. Urology 2012; 79(5): 980–6.
34. Teichman JM, Rogenes VJ, McIver BJ, Harris JM. Holmium:yttrium-aluminum-garnet laser cystolithotripsy of large bladder calculi. Urology 1997; 50(1): 44–8.
35. Wollin TA, Singal RK, Whelan T, Dicecco R, Razvi HA, Denstedt JD. Percutaneous suprapubic cystolithotripsy for treatment of large bladder calculi. J Endourol 1999; 13(10): 739–44.
36. Richter S, Ringel A, Sluzker D. Combined cystolithotomy and transurethral resection of prostate: best management of infravesical obstruction and massive or multiple bladder stones. Urology 2002; 59(5): 688–91.
37. Papatsoris AG, Varkarakis I, Dellis A, Deliveliotis C. Bladder lithiasis: from open surgery to lithotripsy. Urol Res 2006; 34(3): 163–7.

CHAPTER 24

Multimodality Therapy: Mixing and Matching of Surgical Techniques for the Treatment of Stone Disease

Nir Kleinmann,[1] *Kelly A. Healy,*[2] *and Demetrius H. Bagley*[2]

[1]Sheba Medical Center, Tel Hashomer, Israel

[2]Thomas Jefferson University, Philadelphia, PA, USA

Do's and don'ts box

- Pre-SWL stenting should not be used routinely. It should be reserved for selected cases, mainly stones larger than 2 cm.
- The combination of PCNL and SWL should be reserved for unique cases, wherein access to certain calyces is not feasible. PCNL should be the last step, in order to clear the remaining fragments and achieve stone-free state.
- The combination of laparoscopy and endoscopy should be utilized in cases of concomitant anatomic anomaly in order to treat the deformity as well as the stone in a single procedure.
- Pre-ureteroscopy stenting should only be considered in selected cases with a large stone burden.
- Combined antegrade and retrograde stone treatment is used for stones inaccessible percutaneously during PCNL.

Introduction

Challenging stone problems can benefit from a combination of surgical modalities. These techniques are complementary to each other and can effectively treat the stones with minimal additional complications. This chapter reviews the current literature and describes different multimodal stone treatments. The treatment decision should be based upon the patient's anatomy, stone features, and surgeon preference.

Urinary Stones: Medical and Surgical Management, First Edition. Edited by Michael Grasso and David S. Goldfarb.

Shock wave lithotripsy with a ureteral stent

Shock wave lithotripsy (SWL) was first introduced into the urological armamentarium in 1980 [1]. Some consider it as the first-line treatment for renal and proximal ureteral stones [2]. However, a major disadvantage associated with this technique is the inability to retrieve stone fragments. Consequently, retained fragments need to pass out of the urinary tract spontaneously [3]. The outcomes vary significantly and depend on various factors, including patient body habitus as well as stone size, position, and composition [4,5,6]. When fragments fail to pass, post-SWL complications may occur, such as hydronephrosis, infection, acute renal colic, and renal failure [7]. In 4–8% of cases, a large leading stone cannot pass out of the ureter, and additional stone fragments accumulate proximally to form a steinstrasse [8]. This can lead to irreversible loss of renal function or ureteral stricture disease [9].

To prevent steinstrasse, some authors have suggested preprocedural insertion of a double pigtail ureteral stent, but this has been an area of controversy [10,11,12]. Opponents have argued that stent insertion is an invasive procedure with associated morbidity and risks, including the need for general anesthesia and the added costs of treatment. Importantly, approximately 80% of patients suffer from stent-related symptoms, including irritative lower urinary tract symptoms (LUTS) (76%) along with flank and suprapubic pain (19–32%), sexual dysfunction (32%), hematuria (25%), and incontinence [13,14]. These symptoms are largely attributed to the presence of a foreign body in the urinary bladder, which irritates the mucosa [15]. In addition, there is a potential risk of complications related to instrumentation of the urinary tract, such as ureteral perforation (11%), failure of stent placement (20%), urinary tract infection (UTI), stent migration or encrustation, as well as vesicoureteral reflux. Moreover, an additional procedure is required for stent removal [16].

Shen et al. performed a comprehensive meta-analysis of the recent literature to evaluate the utility of ureteral stent insertion prior to SWL. The study included eight randomized controlled trials (RCT) and a total of 876 patients, which were divided into stented (453) and non-stented groups (423) [17]. The overall stone-free rate was reported to be 80–92.1%. Collectively, these studies indicated that the use of ureteral stents prior to SWL does not improve stone-free rate [11,18,19,20,21,22, 23,24] (Figure 24.1). Of the eight RCTs, only five (62.5%) reported on the presence or absence of steinstrasse following SWL. Overall, there was no significant difference in the incidence of steintrasse after SWL between the two groups. After stratifying based on stone location (renal versus ureteral), subgroup analysis of four studies failed to demonstrate any difference in risk of steinstrasse between stented and non-stented patients [11,18,19,20]. Only one study reported a higher incidence of steintrasse in the non-stented group [21]. Among a total of 400 patients, 38 (9.5%) developed steinstrasse, including 12 (6%) from the stented group and 26 (13%) from the non-stented group ($p<0.05$).

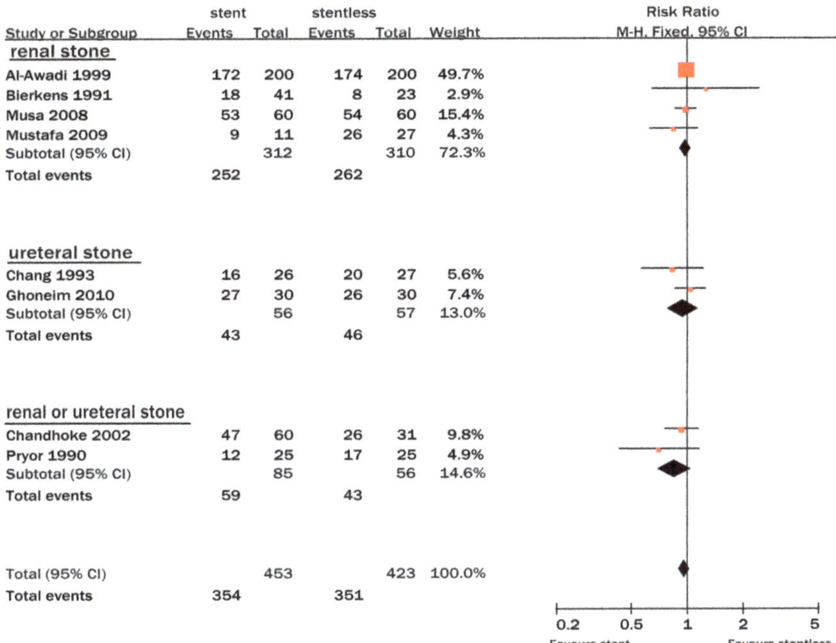

Figure 24.1 Stone-free rate in patients with and without stent before ESWL. Source: Shen P, Jiang M, Yang J et al. 2011 [17]. Reproduced with permission of Elsevier.

Furthermore, there is no convincing evidence that insertion of a ureteral stent prior to SWL decreases the risk of postoperative fever or UTI [11,18,20]. The incidence of hematuria was also similar between the stented and non-stented groups [18,22,23]. Pain (suprapubic, flank, bladder, and penile pain) and the need for analgesia did not differ between the groups [11,18,19,21,22,23]. In contrast, several reports showed that stenting before SWL significantly increases LUTS [18,19,23]. The stented and non-stented groups were found to be equivalent in terms of need for ancillary treatment, with rates reported between 7% to 17%.

In a survey of practice patterns conducted among 1029 American urologists, Hollowell et al. found that stent use before SWL for renal pelvic stones was highly dependent on stone size: 25% for 10 mm stones, 57% for 15 mm stones, and 87% for 20 mm stones [25]. Thus, most American urologists tend to use stents for stones greater than 20 mm and occasionally for those less than 10 mm. For stones between 10 mm to 20 mm, there appears to be no general consensus in practice patterns about the usefulness of stenting [25]. In a prospective randomized study, Chandhoke and colleagues have addressed this question [20]. The authors divided 97 patients undergoing SWL with a solitary renal stone size of 10–20 mm or ureteral stone smaller than 20 mm into three groups: group 1 (no stent), group 2 (4.7F stent), and group 3 (7F stent). Overall stone-free and retreatment rates were 80% and 7%, respectively. No significant differences were found between the three groups. However, emergency room visits and hospitalization rates were significantly lower in the stented patients compared to the non-stented patients (7% versus 22%, respectively, $p<0.05$) [20]. This might be of importance in the US, where Medicare does not cover expenses for hospital readmission.

In summary, insertion of a double pigtail ureteral stent prior to SWL does not result in higher stone-free rates, lower incidence of pain, hematuria, fever or UTI. In contrast, it is significantly associated with more LUTS. Better designed stents may presumably have more effect on preventing steinstrasse and decrease the incidence of stent-related LUTS. According to both the American Urological Assocation (AUA) and European Association of Urology (EAU) guidelines, routine stenting is not recommended as part of SWL [6,26]. This should be reserved for selected cases, mainly for large stone size and in cases of infection, although this is considered a contraindication to SWL. More high-quality RCTs are needed to better define this issue with special attention to stone composition, size, and location.

Combination of shock wave lithotripsy and percutaneous nephrolithotomy

Staghorn calculi are branched stones that occupy a large portion of the collecting system, typically filling the renal pelvis and involving several or all of the calyces. These calculi are usually the result of an infection and are composed of mixtures of magnesium ammonium phosphate (struvite) and/or calcium carbonate apatite. However, recent evidence suggests that metabolic stones are comprising an increasing proportion of staghorn calculi [27]. Several methods have been suggested to define a staghorn stone in terms of the extent of the involved calyces or to calculate the overall stone burden [28,29,30,31,32]. Still, there is no current clear definition. The term "partial staghorn" calculus is frequently used to describe a branched stone that occupies part but not all of the collecting system, whereas the term "complete staghorn" calculus refers to a stone that occupies virtually the entire collecting system. The designation does not relate to specific volume criteria.

Considering the natural history of untreated staghorn calculi, complete stone clearance is imperative. If left untreated, staghorn calculi may result in obstruction of the involved kidney, deterioration of renal function, end-stage renal disease, or even life-threatening urosepsis [33,34]. Moreover, residual stone fragments may serve as a nidus for recurrent UTIs or further stone propagation [35,36].

In addition to achieving a stone-free status, treatment aims to minimize complications and subsequent unplanned procedure rates.

Currently, PCNL is considered the first-line treatment for most patients with staghorn calculi due to its superior efficacy and acceptable morbidity [37]. Alternative treatment options include:

- combinations of PCNL and SWL
- staged ureteroscopic laser lithotripsy
- SWL monotherapy
- open surgery

Based on the original Nephrolithiasis Guidelines Panel in 1994, combination therapy of PCNL and SWL was initially recommended as the treatment of choice for patients with staghorn calculi [38]. This technique involves an initial percutaneous debulking, to remove a large stone volume, followed by SWL of residual stones which cannot be accessed endoscopically. Finally, percutaneous nephroscopy is utilized to retrieve any remaining fragments. As such, this combination approach is referred to as "sandwich therapy" and allows the removal of a large stone volume and provides an accurate assessment of the stone-free status.

Meretyk et al. conducted a RCT of PCNL and SWL combination therapy versus SWL monotherapy in 50 kidneys (23 and 27 renal units, respectively) and found a significantly higher stone-free rate for the combination therapy group (74% versus 22%, respectively, p=0.0005) [39]. In addition, over 50% of the patients in the SWL monotherapy group had a total residual stone burden exceeding 16mm compared to only 8% of those in the combination group. Furthermore, SWL monotherapy was associated with a significantly higher complication rate compared to combination therapy, with 56% and 9% septic events respectively. Combination therapy was also shown to be superior in terms of ancillary procedures (4% versus 30%, p=0.03) and overall treatment length (1 versus 6 months, p=0.0006). However, patients undergoing PCNL and SWL combination therapy had significantly greater narcotic requirements compared to those undergoing SWL [39].

Advancements in technique and instrumentation have improved PCNL outcomes and, consequently, limited the role of sandwich therapy in the treatment of staghorn calculi. Most renal calyces can now be effectively reached by accurate and carefully selected renal accesses, multiple accesses, and by the use of flexible nephroscopes during PCNL alone [40]. The use of the holmium laser with flexible fibers for intracorporeal lithotripsy enables the urologist to treat these hard-to-reach stones. Additionally, better grasping devices and baskets aid in clearing stone fragments.

In 2005, the AUA Guidelines Panel conducted a meta-analysis on the treatment of staghorn calculi including 32 articles in which 776 patients underwent PCNL, 365 underwent combination therapy, and 392 underwent SWL monotherapy. In contrast to a prior review conducted by this panel in 1994, the more recent analysis found that PCNL alone resulted in higher stone-free rates compared to combination therapy (78% versus 66%, respectively) or SWL monotherapy (54%). Again, these findings contradict the previous 1994 guidelines [38], which showed stone-free rates of 81% for the combination therapy. This discrepancy likely stems from the above-mentioned improvements in percutaneous techniques and technology. Additionally, at the time when the original guidelines were written, the majority of the studies analyzed were based on a combination therapy approach in which PNL was the final procedure, whereas the current guidelines include a number of studies in which SWL was the final procedure, which yields lower stone-free rates. Therefore, the AUA guidelines state that percutaneous nephroscopy should be the final part of a combination therapy sequence because it is the most sensitive method of detecting residual fragments and achieving a stone-free state [37].

In addition to superior stone clearance, the 2005 panel also found that PCNL requires fewer total procedures compared to the other treatment approaches. While PCNL required a mean of 1.9 total procedures, combination therapy and SWL required 3.3 and 3.6 total procedures, respectively (Table 24.1). The panel found a similar risk of overall complications between the treatment modalities, ranging from 13% to 19%. The transfusion rate was also shown to be equivalent in comparisons of PCNL and combination therapy (18% and 17%, respectively).

Table 24.1 Staghorn calculi treatment – overall outcomes. Modified from AUA guidelines on management of staghorn calculi

	PNL	Combination PNL and SWL	SWL	Open Surgery
	Median probability (95% CI)	**Median probability (95% CI)**	**Median probability (95% CI)**	**Median probability (95% CI)**
Stone-free rate	78% (74–83%)	66% (60–72%)	54% (45–64%)	71% (56–84%)
Procedures per patient	**Weighted mean**	**Weighted mean**	**Weighted mean**	**Weighted mean**
Primary	1.3	3.0	2.8	1.0
Secondary	0.4	0.0	0.2	0.2
Adjunctive	0.2	0.3	0.6	0.2
Acute complications	**Median probability (95% CI)**	**Median probability (95% CI)**	**Median probability (95% CI)**	**Median probability (95% CI)**
Transfusion	18% (14–24%)	17% (10–26%)	Insufficient data	Insufficient data
Death	0% (0–1%)	0% (0–2%)	Insufficient data	Insufficient data
Overall significant complications	15% (7–27%)	14% (9–20%)	19% (11–30%)	13% (4–27)%)

CI, confidence interval; PNL, percutaneous nephrolithotomy; SWL, shock wave lithotripsy.

Source: Preminger GM, Assimos DG, Lingeman JE et al. 2005 [37]. Reproduced with permission of Elsevier.

In summary, the PCNL-based procedure has emerged as the treatment of choice for staghorn calculi based on high stone-free rates and the need for fewer total procedures. It is considered a safe approach with an acceptably low morbidity. The combination with SWL should be reserved for unique cases, wherein access to certain calyces is not feasible. However, this situation is becoming increasingly rare due to the currently available improved endoscopic technology. Often, it may be followed by a secondary PCNL, as it allows for better clearance of remaining stone fragments.

Laparoscopy combined with endoscopy

In recent years, laparoscopy and robotic surgeries have gained popularity in a wide variety of urological procedures. Advancements in endourology, however, have limited their role in the treatment of urolithiasis. Nevertheless, whenever underlying anatomical anomalies co-exist with urolithiasis, a combination of laparoscopy and endoscopy has been shown to be an effective surgical approach which reduces the overall number of procedures. Several studies have reported laparoscopic and robotic pyeloplasty for ureteropelvic junction (UPJ) obstruction with concomitant pyelolithotomy for nephrolithiasis [41,42,43,44,45,46,47].

The procedure involves an initial dismembering of the UPJ, followed by removal of calculi from the renal pelvis with a rigid grasper. A flexible nephroscope is subsequently inserted through a laparoscopic port and is used to clear calyceal stones with a basket or to pulverize stones with holmium:YAG laser. This approach was shown to result in high stone-free rates exceeding 75–100% and relief of obstruction in 90–100%, whereby it is associated with low complication rates. The combination of laparoscopy and endoscopy was also reported to obtain access during PCNL in cases of pelvic and horseshoe kidneys in order to avoid injury to adjacent organs. The bowel was laparoscopically mobilized and the kidney was exposed. Access was then achieved after the injection of contrast through an open-ended catheter and by the combination of fluoroscopy and direct vision [48,49].

Ureteroscopy before renal transplantation

Due to lack of kidney donors and long wait lists, more than 75% of medical centers are now considering patients with nephrolithiasis as candidates for donor nephrectomy [50]. However, this may result in ureteral obstruction [51].

In order to avoid that, the combination of *ex vivo* ureteroscopy (ExURS) was described in donor nephrectomy patients with nephrolithiasis before renal transplantation [52,53]. Immediately after nephrectomy, the kidney was placed in ice, flushed, and perfused. Either a semi-rigid or flexible ureteroscope was used. The kidney was manipulated with the surgeon's hand to align the stone-containing calyx with the same axis of the ureteroscope whenever a semi-rigid ureteroscope was used. The stones were removed using a Nitinol basket or treated with holmium laser lithotripsy and basket extraction. Operative time ranged between 3 and 45 min, and stones ranged in size from 1 to 12 mm. Stone-free rate was 89–100%. No intraoperative complications were encountered. The authors concluded that ExURS is a safe procedure for the treatment of nephrolithiasis prior to renal transplantation.

Pre-ureteroscopy ureteral stenting

In some circumstances, access to the upper urinary tract cannot be obtained due to anatomical factors, such as ureteral strictures or tightness. One of the options for overcoming this obstacle is to passively dilate the ureter by placement of a ureteral stent for 1–2 weeks prior to definitive treatment [54,55]. Several authors, however, have suggested that a combination of preoperative ureteral stent insertion and ureteroscopy may offer benefit even in normal-caliber ureters; the dilation of the ureter allows easier access to the upper urinary tract, which is necessary in certain cases, especially when dealing with a large stone burden [56]. Additionally, a dilated ureter can accommodate a larger ureteroscope or access sheath.

However, a number of retrospective studies found conflicting evidence with regard to stone-free rates (SFR) using this approach [57,58,59]. Netsch et al. reviewed 286 patients (143 stented versus 143 non-stented). SFR was higher for the stented group (95.1%) compared to the non-stented group (86.7%, $p<0.013$) [57]. In contrast, Shields and colleagues studied the SFR in a group of 221 patients. The authors did find a small, but not significant ($p<0.254$), difference between the stented and non-stented groups (88.7% versus 83.1%, respectively). SFR was negatively associated with stone size ($p=0.020$), total stone number ($p=0.001$), and cumulative stone burden ($p<0.001$) [59].

Although prestenting involves an additional procedure, it was found to decrease the overall number of procedures for stones larger than 1 cm ($p=0.001$). Operative time was 93.3 ± 39.9 min for the stented group and 123.6 ± 59.8 min for the non-stented group ($p=0.008$) [58]. Preoperative stenting was also shown to decrease the cost of ureteroscopy from $27,806 to $17,706 ($p<0.01$) for stones larger than 1 cm.[60]

In summary, pre-ureteroscopy stenting should only be considered in selected cases with a large stone burden.

Combined antegrade and retrograde treatment (Figure 24.2)

Traditionally, PCNL has been considered the treatment of choice for large and/or complex renal calculi. Since its initial description by Fernström and Johansson in 1976 [61], advances in endoscopic instrumentation and technique have led to decreased complications and improved surgical outcomes. Despite the liberal use of flexible nephroscopy to treat calyceal branches of complex staghorn calculi, access to the entire intrarenal collecting system through one percutaneous tract can be technically difficult. Consequently, 20–58% of cases require multiple tracts for complete stone clearance [62,63,64]. However, multiple-puncture PCNL is associated with increased blood loss and increased renal parenchymal damage, as well as increased postoperative pain [65]. Instead, retrograde ureteroscopy can be employed concomitantly with PCNL to treat calculi not otherwise accessible through a single percutaneous tract, which are typically located in a calyx parallel to the access tract or in a superior calyx. Furthermore, retrograde intrarenal surgery facilitates the irrigation of renal cavities and prevents stone migration into the ureter during lithotripsy [66].

Using a combined above-and-below approach, stones encountered with the ureteroscope in unfavorable locations relative to the access tract can be treated *in situ* with holmium laser or electrohydraulic lithotripsy. Alternatively, a basket may be utilized to relocate stones from otherwise inaccessible sites and present them to the rigid nephroscope for extraction or fragmentation. In doing so, the urologist may exploit the advantages of ureteroscopy and PCNL. Stones that are difficult to reach percutaneously may be accessed and, in some cases, treated ureteroscopically. At the same time, PCNL can be utilized to debulk large stone burdens.

The usefulness of a simultaneous antegrade and retrograde endoscopic approach to upper urinary tract pathology was first reported in 1988 by Lehman and Bagley [67]. Three female patients with large renal and extensive ureteral calculi were treated with simultaneous percutaneous and rigid ureteroscopy. Access was achieved in a modified prone position. As flexible ureteroscopy became available, the ureter and urethra could be

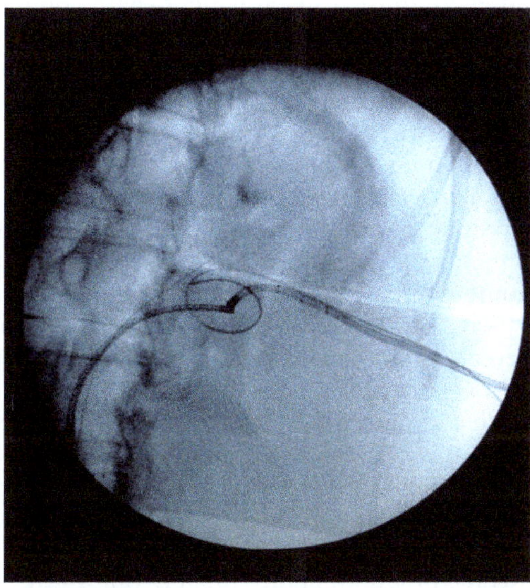

Figure 24.2 Fluoroscopy demonstrating the simultaneous combination of antegrade and retrograde endoscopy.

accessed in both males and females in the prone position using a split-leg modification. The prone split-leg position offers easy access to the flank for PCNL as well as retrograde access for ureteroscopy. Nord et al. in 1991 used the prone split-leg position in 10 patients and found it to be easily adaptable in both sexes and with both flexible and rigid endoscopes [68]. Subsequently, Grasso et al. in 1993 evaluated their experience with simultaneous upper tract access using a two-team approach in a larger retrospective study of 126 patients [69]. Of these, the majority of patients were placed in the prone split-leg position (111/126, 88.1%). While one team debulked the staghorn stone burden accessible percutaneously, another team treated otherwise inaccessible stone components ureteroscopically in a retrograde fashion. The remainder of the patients (15/126, 11.9%) were deemed treatable in a predominantly retrograde fashion and, therefore, placed in dorsal lithotomy position with flank roll elevation. Utilizing these two positions for simultaneous above-and-below access, the authors found improved efficiency in treating upper tract pathologies. Importantly, the authors highlight that the two-team approach for simultaneous procedures requires two skilled endoscopists as well as equipment and careful attention to room set-up.

Recently, there has been wider renewed interest in combined percutaneous and ureteroscopic stone surgery. Landman et al. in 2003 reported their initial experience with PCNL for complete or partial staghorn calculi using a combined antegrade and retrograde approach [70]. In this small series, the entire procedure was performed with patients in the prone split-leg position. Total stone clearance was achieved in a single session with only one percutaneous access tract in the majority of patients (7/9, 78%).

Subsequently, Marguet et al. in 2005 combined the use of flexible ureteroscopy and PCNL to treat seven patients with complex renal calculi [71]. First, retrograde access was obtained and satellite stones in peripheral calces were fragmented *in situ* with holmium laser lithotripsy. Alternatively, using a basket, the stone burden was translocated into the renal pelvis for intracorporeal lithotripsy or easier percutaneous access. Patients were then placed prone for percutaneous lithotripsy using a single tract. Five out of seven patients (71.4%) were stone free, while the remaining two patients had small asymptomatic residual calculi measuring <3 mm. Compared with multiple-puncture PCNL, mean blood loss was significantly less in patients undergoing combined flexible ureteroscopy and PCNL (345 mL versus 79 mL, $p<0.05$). Notably, mean operative duration was not significantly different despite the need for repositioning with the combined approach (166 min versus 142 min, $p=0.36$).

Various alternative supine positions have been proposed for percutaneous access, which can also provide easy retrograde access. Scoffone and colleagues described their experience with endoscopic combined intrarenal surgery (ECIRS) utilizing a Galdakao-modified supine Valdivia (GMSV) position [66]. A total of 127 patients underwent combined PCNL and retrograde ureteroscopy, of whom approximately one-third had staghorn or multiple calculi. Of these, retrograde ureteroscopy was deemed necessary in 42 (33%) patients due to stones in calyces inaccessible percutaneously or due to ureteral calculi. Overall mean stone size was 2.38 cm (range 1.1–4.0 cm). The majority of patients (125, 98.4%) had one percutaneous tract placed. Stone-free status was achieved in 81.9% (104 patients) after one treatment and 87.4% (111 patients) after a second early treatment using the same percutaneous access with acceptable morbidity. These rates compare favorably with stone-free rates between 67% and 95.5% in contemporary PCNL series which commonly use multiple tracts [37,72,73]. The authors concluded that ECIRS in the GMSV position is a safe and effective approach with high stone-free rates and a short learning curve.

Lezrek et al. in 2011 employed the split-leg modified lateral decubitus position for PCNL with simultaneous retrograde access [74]. The patient was maintained in this position for the entire procedure, which resulted in decreased operating room time. After the initial 20 patients, stone clearance rates reached equivalence with the prone position. The added advantage was being able to perform additional procedures such as internal urethrotomy, transurethral resection of the prostate, endopyelotomy, and endopyeloplasty, without any change in position.

Moraitis et al. in 2012 assessed the Bart's modified lateral position for simultaneous antegrade and retrograde access in 45 patients with complex upper urinary tract pathologies, including significant stone burden in the setting of UPJ obstruction, ureteral stricture, encrusted ureteral stent, or urinary diversion [75]. Purported advantages of this position include wide flank exposure and, in turn, a large surface area for selection of puncture site(s), enhanced control, and a wide angle for manipulation of antegrade instruments. Mean stone surface area was 300 mm^2 (range 20–433). Total stone clearance was achieved in 36 patients (80%) using a single combined procedure and, in the vast majority of patients (93%), only one access tract. Moreover, all patients with UPJ and ureteral strictures were successfully recanalized. Overall stone-free rate was 91% at the first postoperative follow-up visit.

Synchronous unilateral PCNL and contralateral ureteroscopy has proven to be safe, efficient, and efficacious for patients who present with bilateral discordant stone burdens. The main advantages of a single procedure include decreasing the number of anesthesia sessions and achieving stone clearance from both upper tracts with only one postoperative recovery period. In a retrospective study of 26 patients, Mason et al. evaluated concurrent PCNL with contralateral ureteroscopy in the prone split-leg position [76]. Of these, 81% (21/26) of patients were stone free following one procedure. All cases that required a second-look PCNL or URS (5/26, 19%) were rendered stone free, for an overall 100% stone-free rate. Complication rates were equivalent to patients treated with unilateral PCNL and ureteroscopy in contemporary series. The authors advocate bilateral postoperative drainage.

In summary, the combination of antegrade PCNL and retrograde ureteroscopy is a valuable tool in the endourologist's armamentarium which facilitates access to the entire intrarenal collecting system. Therefore, it is particularly useful for complex renal calculi that would otherwise require multiple percutaneous tracts. A two-team approach maximizes the efficiency of the procedure but requires two experienced endoscopists as well as preprocedural planning.

References

1. Chaussy C, Brendel W, Schmiedt E. Extracorporeally induced destruction of kidney stones by shock waves. Lancet 1980; 13: 1265–8.
2. Arrabal-Polo MA, Arrabal-Martín M, Miján-Ortiz JL, et al. Treatment of ureteric lithiasis with retrograde ureteroscopy and holmium: YAG laser lithotripsy vs extracorporeal lithotripsy. BJU Int 2009; 104: 1144–7.
3. Buchholz N, Meier-padel S, Rutishauser G. Minor residual spontaneous fragments after extracorporeal lithotripsy: shockwave clearance or risk factor for recurrent stone formation? J Endourol 1997; 11: 227–32.
4. Argyropoulos AN, Tolley DA. Optimizing shock wave lithotripsy in the 21st century. Eur Urol 2007; 52: 344–52.
5. Kim FJ, Rice KR. Prediction of shockwave failure in patients with urinary tract stones. Curr Opin Urol 2006; 16: 88–92.
6. Tiselius HG, Ackermann D, Alken P, et al. Guidelines on urolithiasis. Eur Urol 2010; 40: 28.
7. Salem S, Mehrsai A, Zartab H, et al. Complications and outcomes following extracorporeal shock wave lithotripsy: a prospective study of 3,241 patients. Urol Res 2010; 38: 135–42.
8. Kim SC, Oh CH, Moon YT, Kim KD. Treatment of steinstrasse with repeat extracorporeal shock wave lithotripsy: experience with piezoelectric lithotriptor. J Urol 1991; 145: 489–91.
9. Grasso M, Loisides P, Beaghler M, Bagley D. The case for primary endoscopic management of upper urinary tract calculi: I. A critical review of 121 extracorporeal shock-wave lithotripsy failures. Urology 1995; 45: 363–71.
10. Kirkali Z, Esen A, Akan G. Place of double-J stents in extracorporeal shock wave lithotripsy. Eur Urol 1993; 23: 460–2.
11. Bierkens AF, Hendrikx AJ, Lemmens WA, Debruyne FM. Extracorporeal shock wave lithotripsy for large renal calculi: the role of ureteral stents. A randomized trial. J Urol 1991; 145: 699–702.
12. Preminger GM, Kettelhut M, Elkins S, et al. Ureteral stenting during extracorporeal shock wave lithotripsy: help or hindrance? J Urol 1989; 142: 32–6.
13. Joshi HB, Stainthorpe A, MacDonagh RP, et al. Indwelling ureteral stents: evaluation of symptoms, quality of life and utility. J Urol 2003; 169: 1065–9.
14. Miyaoka R, Monga M. Ureteral stent discomfort: etiology and management. Indian J Urol 2009; 25: 455–60.
15. Dunn MD, Portis AJ, Kahn SA, et al. Clinical effectiveness of new stent design: randomized single-blind comparison of tail and double-pigtail stents. J Endourol 2000; 14: 195–202.
16. Mokhmalji H, Braun PM, Martinez Portillo FJ, et al. Percutaneous nephrostomy versus ureteral stents for diversion of hydronephrosis caused by stones: a prospective, randomized clinical trial. J Urol 2001; 165: 1088–92.
17. Shen P, Jiang M, Yang J, et al. Use of ureteral stent in extracorporeal shock wave lithotripsy for upper urinary calculi: a systematic review and meta-analysis. J Urol 2011; 186: 1328–35.

18. Ghoneim IA, El-Ghoneimy MN, El-Naggar AE, et al. Extracorporeal shock wave lithotripsy in impacted upper ureteral stones: a prospective randomized comparison between stented and non-stented techniques. Urology 2010; 75: 45–50.
19. Mustafa M, Ali-el-dein B. Stenting in extracorporeal shockwave lithotripsy; may enhance the passage of the fragments! J Pak Med Assoc 2009; 59: 141–3.
20. Chandhoke PS, Barqawi AZ, Wernecke C, Chee-Awai RA. A randomized outcomes trial of ureteral stents for extracorporeal shock wave lithotripsy of solitary kidney or proximal ureteral stones. J Urol 2002; 167: 1981–3.
21. Al-Awadi KA, Abdul Halim H, Kehinde EO, Al-Tawheed A. Steinstrasse: a comparison of incidence with and without J stenting and the effect of J stenting on subsequent management. BJU Int 1999; 84: 618–21.
22. Musa AA. Use of double-J stents prior to extracorporeal shock wave lithotripsy is not beneficial: results of a prospective randomized study. Int Urol Nephrol 2008; 40: 19–22.
23. Pryor J, Jenkins A. Use of double-pigtail stents in extracorporeal shock wave lithotripsy. J Urol 1990; 143: 475–8.
24. Chang S, Kuo H, Hsu T. Shock wave lithotripsy for obstructed proximal ureteral stones. A prospective randomized study comparing in situ, stent bypass and below stone catheter with irrigation. Eur Urol 1993; 24: 177–84.
25. Hollowell CM, Patel R V, Bales GT, Gerber GS. Internet and postal survey of endourologic practice patterns among American urologists. J Urol 2000; 163: 1779–82.
26. The Management of Ureteral Calculi: Diagnosis and Treatment Recommendations. AUA Guidelines 2010: 34–5.
27. Viprakasit DP, Sawyer MD, Herrell SD, Miller NL. Changing composition of staghorn calculi. J Urol 2011; 186: 2285–90.
28. Lam HS, Lingeman JE, Barron M, et al. Staghorn calculi: analysis of treatment results between initial percutaneous nephrostolithotomy and extracorporeal shock wave lithotripsy monotherapy with reference. J Urol 1992; 147: 1219–25.
29. Lam HS, Lingeman JE, Russo R, Chua GT. Stone surface area determination techniques: a unifying concept of staghorn stone burden assessment. J Urol 1992; 148: 1026–9.
30. Griffith D, Valiquette L. PICA/burden: a staging system for upper tract urinary stones. J Urol 1987; 138: 253–7.
31. Rocco F, Mandressi A, Larcher P. Surgical classification of renal calculi. Eur Urol 1984; 10: 121–3.
32. Di Silverio F, Gallucci M, Alpi G. Staghorn calculi of the kidney: classification and therapy. Br J Urol 1990; 65: 449–52.
33. Rous S, Turner W. Retrospective study of 95 patients with staghorn calculus disease. J Urol 1977; 118: 902–4.
34. Koga S, Arakaki Y, Matsuoka M, Ohyama C. Staghorn calculi – long-term results of management. Br J Urol 1991; 68: 122–4.
35. Beck EM, Riehle RA Jr. The fate of residual fragments after extracorporeal shock wave lithotripsy monotherapy of infection stones. J Urol 1991; 145: 6–9.
36. Streem SB, Yost A, Dolmatch B. Combination "sandwich" therapy for extensive renal calculi in 100 consecutive patients: immediate, long-term and stratified results from a 10-year experience. J Urol 1997; 158: 342–5.
37. Preminger GM, Assimos DG, Lingeman JE, et al. AUA guideline on management of staghorn calculi: diagnosis and treatment recommendations. J Urol 2005; 173: 1991–2000.

38. Segura JW, Preminger GM, Assimos DG, et al. Clinical Guidelines Panel summary report on the management of staghorn calculi. The American Urological Association Nephrolithiasis Clinical Guidelines Panel. J Urol 1994; 151: 1648–51.
39. Meretyk S, Gofrit ON, Gafni O, et al. Complete staghorn calculi: random prospective comparison between extracorporeal shock wave lithotripsy monotherapy and combined with percutaneous nephrostolithotomy. J Urol 1997; 157: 780–6.
40. Lam HS, Lingeman JE, Mosbaugh PG, et al. Evolution of the technique of combination therapy for staghorn calculi: a decreasing role for extracorporeal shock wave lithotripsy. J Urol 1992; 148: 1058–62.
41. Whelan JP, Wiesenthal JD. Laparoscopic pyeloplasty with simultaneous pyelolithotomy using a flexible ureteroscope. Can J Urol 2004; 11: 2207–9.
42. Ramakumar S, Lancini V, Chan DY, et al. Laparoscopic pyeloplasty with concomitant pyelolithotomy. J Urol 2002; 167: 1378–80.
43. Srivastava A, Singh P, Gupta M, et al. Laparoscopic pyeloplasty with concomitant pyelolithotomy – is it an effective mode of treatment? Urol Int 2008; 80: 306–9.
44. Stein RJ, Turna B, Nguyen MM, et al. Laparoscopic pyeloplasty with concomitant pyelolithotomy: technique and outcomes. J Endourol 2008; 22: 1251–5.
45. Nadu A, Schatloff O, Morag R, et al. Laparoscopic surgery for renal stones: is it indicated in the modern endourology era? Int Braz J Urol 2009; 35: 9–17.
46. Mufarrij PW, Woods M, Shah OD, et al. Robotic dismembered pyeloplasty: a 6-year, multi-institutional experience. J Urol 2008; 180: 1391–6.
47. Atug F, Castle EP, Burgess S V, Thomas R. Concomitant management of renal calculi and pelvi-ureteric junction obstruction with robotic laparoscopic surgery. BJU Int 2005; 96: 1365–8.
48. Mousavi-Bahar SH, Amir-Zargar MA, Gholamrezaie HR. Laparoscopic assisted percutaneous nephrolithotomy in ectopic pelvic kidneys. Int J Urol 2008; 15: 276–8.
49. Tahmaz L, Ozgok Y, Zor M, et al. Laparoscopy-assisted tubeless percutaneous nephrolithotomy in previously operated ectopic pelvic kidney with fragmented J-J stent. Urol Res 2009; 37: 257–60.
50. Ennis J, Kocherginsky M, Schumm LP, et al. Trends in kidney donation among kidney stone formers: a survey of US transplant centers. Am J Nephrol 2009; 30: 12–18.
51. Klingler HC, Kramer G, Lodde M, Marberger M. Urolithiasis in allograft kidneys. Urology 2002; 59: 344–8.
52. Schade GR, Wolf JS, Faerber GJ. Ex-vivo ureteroscopy at the time of live donor nephrectomy. J Endourol 2011; 25: 1405–9.
53. Olsburgh J, Thomas K, Wong K, et al. Incidental renal stones in potential live kidney donors: prevalence, assessment and donation, including role of ex vivo ureteroscopy. BJU Int 2013: 111: 784–92.
54. Hubert KC, Palmer JS. Passive dilation by ureteral stenting before ureteroscopy: eliminating the need for active dilation. J Urol 2005; 174: 1079–80.
55. Jones BJ, Ryan PC, Lyons O, et al. Use of the double pigtail stent in stone retrieval following unsuccessful ureteroscopy. Br J Urol 1990; 66: 254–6.
56. Kawahara T, Ito H, Terao H, et al. Preoperative stenting for ureteroscopic lithotripsy for a large renal stone. Int J Urol 2012; 19: 881–5.
57. Netsch C, Knipper S, Bach T, et al. Impact of preoperative ureteral stenting on stone-free rates of ureteroscopy for nephroureterolithiasis: a matched-paired analysis of 286 patients. Urology 2012; 80: 1214–19.

58. Chu L, Sternberg KM, Averch TD. Preoperative stenting decreases operative time and reoperative rates of ureteroscopy. J Endourol 2011; 25: 751–4.
59. Shields JM, Bird VG, Graves R, Gómez-Marín O. Impact of preoperative ureteral stenting on outcome of ureteroscopic treatment for urinary lithiasis. J Urol 2009; 182: 2768–74.
60. Chu L, Farris CA, Corcoran AT, Averch TD. Preoperative stent placement decreases cost of ureteroscopy. Urology 2011; 78: 309–13.
61. Fernström I, Johansson B. Percutaneous pyelolithotomy. A new extraction technique. Scand J Urol Nephrol 1976; 10: 257–9.
62. Lam HS, Lingeman JE, Mosbaugh PG, et al. Evolution of the technique of combination therapy for staghorn calculi: a decreasing role for extracorporeal shock wave lithotripsy. J Urol 1992; 148: 1058–62.
63. Lashley DB, Fuchs EF. Urologist-acquired renal access for percutaneous renal surgery. Urology 1998; 51: 927–31.
64. Munver R, Delvecchio FC, Newman GE, Preminger GM. Critical analysis of supracostal access for percutaneous renal surgery. J Urol 2001; 166: 1242–6.
65. Stoller M, Wolf JS Jr, St Lezin MA. Estimated blood loss and transfusion rates associated with percutaneous nephrolithotomy. J Urol 1994; 152: 1977–81.
66. Scoffone CM, Cracco CM, Cossu M, et al. Endoscopic combined intrarenal surgery in Galdakao-modified supine Valdivia position: a new standard for percutaneous nephrolithotomy? Eur Urol 2008; 54: 1393–403.
67. Lehman T, Bagley DH. Reverse lithotomy: modified prone position for simultaneous nephroscopic and ureteroscopic procedures in women. Urology 1988; 32: 529–31.
68. Nord RG, Cubler-Goodman A, Bagley DH. Prone split-leg position for simultaneous retrograde ureteroscopic and percutaneous nephroscopic procedures. J Endourol 1991; 5: 13–16.
69. Grasso M, Nord RG, Bagley DH. Prone split leg and flank roll positioning: simultaneous antegrade and retrograde access to the upper urinary tract. J Endourol 1993; 7: 307–10.
70. Landman J, Venkatesh R, Lee DI, et al. Combined percutaneous and retrograde approach to staghorn calculi with application of the ureteral access sheath to facilitate percutaneous nephrolithotomy. J Urol 2003; 169: 64–7.
71. Marguet CG, Springhart WP, Tan YH, et al. Simultaneous combined use of flexible ureteroscopy and percutaneous nephrolithotomy to reduce the number of access tracts in the management of complex renal calculi. BJU Int 2005; 96: 1097–100.
72. Shoma AM, Eraky I, El-Kenawy MR, El-Kappany HA. Percutaneous nephrolithotomy in the supine position: technical aspects and functional outcome compared with the prone technique. Urology 2002; 60: 388–92.
73. Manohar T, Jain P, Desai M. Supine percutaneous nephrolithotomy: effective approach to high-risk and morbidly obese patients. J Endourol 2007; 21: 44–9.
74. Lezrek M, Ammani A, Bazine K, et al. The split-leg modified lateral position for percutaneous renal surgery and optimal retrograde access to the upper urinary tract. Urology 2011; 78: 217–20.
75. Moraitis K, Philippou P, El-Husseiny T, et al. Simultaneous antegrade/retrograde upper urinary tract access: Bart's modified lateral position for complex upper tract endourologic pathologic features. Urology 2012; 79: 287–92.
76. Mason BM, Koi PT, Hafron J, et al. Safety and efficacy of synchronous percutaneous nephrostolithotomy and contralateral ureterorenoscopy for bilateral calculi. J Endourol 2008; 22: 889–93.

CHAPTER 25

Management of Complications Associated with Various Lithotripsy Techniques

Angela M. Cottrell and Andrew J. Dickinson
Derriford Hospital, Plymouth Hospitals NHS Trust, Plymouth, UK

Do's and don'ts box

Extracorporeal shock wave lithotripsy

- Identify contraindications to treatment.
- Check urine prior to treatment and treat infection accordingly.
- Look for features suggestive of steinstrasse following treatment.
- Consider liaising with cardiology prior to treatment in patients with cardiac pacemakers and internal defibrillators.

Percutaneous nephrolithotomy

- Preoperative cross-sectional imaging is important to evaluate stone burden and intrarenal collecting system anatomy, and identify co-morbidities which may increase the risk of trauma to adjacent structures.
- Prophylactic antibiotics should be administered perioperatively.
- Tract bleeding can be managed conservatively in most patients. When arterial bleeding is encountered, resuscitation followed by selective angio-embolization is most often successful.
- Renal drainage must be ensured postoperatively, with either an internal stent or nephrostomy, to minimize the risk of extravasation and urinoma, as well as to help facilitate healing.

Ureterorenoscopy

- A safety guidewire should be employed when access is difficult.
- Endoscopic basketing of a stone too large to pass should be avoided, while blind fluoroscopic basketing is contraindicated.
- Prestenting can decrease the risk of perioperative complications.
- Impacted calculi increase the risk of a complicated endoscopy and therefore extra care should be taken.
- The end result of ureteroscopic lithotripsy should be sand and easily passable fragments.

Urinary Stones: Medical and Surgical Management, First Edition. Edited by Michael Grasso and David S. Goldfarb.

Introduction

Urologists have a broad armamentarium with which to treat calculi in the urinary tract. These include extracorporeal shock wave lithotripsy (ESWL), percutaneous nephrolithotomy (PCNL), ureterorenoscopy (URS), and stone fragmentation. Whilst these techniques are highly effective, each method has its own risk of complications. This chapter describes common and serious complications of current stone management techniques and offers management strategies to the urologist to deal with such events.

Extracorporeal shock wave lithotripsy

Extracorporeal shock wave lithotripsy is a widely available treatment for both renal and ureteric calculi that is efficacious and minimally invasive, commonly being performed in an outpatient setting. Despite these advantages, it is not without contraindications and complications. In certain groups of patients, ESWL may not be appropriate and even contraindicated.

Contraindications include:
- bleeding diatheses
- pregnancy
- abdominal aortic aneurysm.

Relative contraindications include:
- skeletal malformations
- obesity.

Safety of extracorporeal shock wave lithotripsy

Complications of ESWL may be early, related to the direct effect of shock waves on the kidney or adjacent structures; sepsis related, or secondary to the direct fragmentation of calculi and passage of fragments. Late complications may be as a result of the effects of shock waves on renal or adjacent tissue and the fate of residual fragments. To minimize the risks of ESWL, preventive steps should be taken such as ensuring the patient has no contraindications and a recognition of co-morbidities and risk factors that make complications more likely.

Early complications include:
- hematoma (symptomatic/asymptomatic)
- hematuria
- sepsis
- steinstrasse
- renal colic
- cardiac arrhythmia
- gastrointestinal.

Late complications include:
- hypertension
- decreased renal function.

Hematoma

It has been demonstrated that ESWL elicits histological changes of the parenchyma of the kidney causing endothelial change in the renal vasculature [1]. These histological changes may lead clinically to renal hematoma and hematuria. Renal hematomas may be symptomatic or asymptomatic. Whilst the rate of symptomatic hematoma is low, radiological detection is higher. One study found 4.1% of patients had a subcapsular or perinephric hematoma identified on ultrasound imaging post ESWL treatment, but only 0.7% of patients in this series were found to be symptomatic [2]. In patients undergoing computed tomography (CT) or magnetic resonance imaging (MRI) investigation following ESWL, up to 25% may demonstrate hematoma [3,4].

A number of patient risk factors for renal hematoma following ESWL have been suggested, including pre-existing hypertension, obesity, renal disease, increased age, presence of cardiovascular disease, and diabetes [2,5]. It is appropriate therefore prior to ESWL to recognize these risks and optimize accordingly. Technical factors, such as rate and intensity of shock waves given, seem to play a smaller part in the risk of development of hematoma. The majority of hematoma following ESWL can be adequately managed conservatively, monitoring vital signs, analgesia, and transfusion if necessary.

Infectious complications

Bacteriuria and sepsis can complicate treatment with ESWL. Bacteria may be present in the urine and within the stone itself and therefore ESWL may lead to sepsis following stone fragmentation. The rate of bacteriura may range from 5% to 14% following treatment [6,7]. Whilst the risk of sepsis is low, it is increased in patients with staghorn or struvite stones (2.1% compared with 17.3%) [7]. The presence of urinary tract obstruction and concurrent instrumentation of the urinary tract may also increase the risk of sepsis.

In order to reduce the risk of infective complications, urine should be tested and cultured prior to treatment and postponed if necessary. Whilst the routine use of antibiotic prophylaxis in patients with sterile urine is controversial, one meta-analysis showed a relative risk reduction of urinary tract infection by 0.45 (95% confidence interval 0.22–0.93) ($p=0.0005$) using antibiotic prophylaxis (reducing a post-treatment rate of urinary tract infection from 5.7% to 2.1%) [8].

Steinstrasse

Steinstrasse (literally 'stone street') is a complication of ESWL whereby stone fragments descend and accumulate in the ureter. Steinstrasse may cause symptoms such as pain, fever or vomiting suggestive of obstruction but may also be silent in up to 15% [9]. The rate of steinstrasse is approximately 5–6% [9,10]; risk factors include increased size of stone (>2 cm) and higher energy of shock waves applied at the start of treatment [9,10].

Whilst pre-procedure insertion of a ureteric stent may decrease the rate of acute presentation, it does not prevent the development of steinstrasse or need for subsequent intervention [11].

With regard to the management of steinstrasse, approximately half may be managed expectantly with a combination of careful observation or medical expulsion therapy [11]. Where this fails, due to pain, obstruction or sepsis, intervention may be necessary in the form of ESWL to leading fragment, percutaneous drainage and/or staged antegrade and retrograde ureteroscopy [9].

Cardiac arrhythmias

Arrhythmias may be a common complication of ESWL, identified in 8.8–59% of those undergoing treatment [12,13]. Whilst these arrhythmias may range from minor atrial to ventricular ectopics, cardiac arrest has been described [12]. Although these arrhythmias may largely be clinically insignificant, temporary cessation of treatment or ECG-synchronized ESWL (in which the shock wave release is timed with the refractory phase of the cardiac cycle) can lead to resolution of such arrhythmias and ESWL treatment can be continued [13]. In patients with severe cardiovascular disease or complex arrhythmias, ECG monitoring may be prudent and in addition, ECG-synchronized ESWL can facilitate the continuation of ESWL treatment by reducing the rate of arrhythmias [12,13].

Extracorporeal shock wave lithotripsy should be performed with care in those with implantable pacemakers or defibrillator devices as reprogramming can occur. Whilst this may not lead to immediate morbidity, it is recommended that devices should be tested by cardiac technicians following ESWL treatment [13].

Hypertension

It has been postulated that ESWL may lead to hypertension later in life. Review of the literature has found contradictory results so no conclusion can be reached [14].

Percutaneous nephrolithotomy

Percutaneous nephrolithotomy is a stone extraction technique that has increased in popularity since the 1970s. PCNL is the first-line treatment for stones larger than 20 mm in the renal pelvis or upper pole calyces and those greater than 15 mm in the lower pole [14]. PCNL achieves excellent stone-free rates but it does not come without complications. Prior to performing PCNL, patients' characteristics and contraindications of treatment should be considered.

Contraindications include:

- anticoagulation
- untreated urinary tract infection
- atypical bowel interposition
- tumor in access area
- pregnancy [14]
- patient factors: anatomy (e.g. pelvic kidney, horseshoe kidney).

Complications of percutaneous nephrolithotomy

Complications may be related to access of the kidney (and formation of tract), treatment of stone or sepsis. Percutaneous renal access may lead to complications including bleeding or trauma to adjacent structures (e.g. bowel or pleura).

- Access-related complications: bleeding, damage to adjacent structures
- Complications related to treatment of stone: extravasation
- Sepsis-related complications: fever, sepsis
- Clinically significant residual stone

Bleeding complications

Percutaneous puncture of the renal collecting system to access a stone may lead to bleeding, as the kidney is a highly vascular organ. Significant bleeding that requires blood transfusion was seen in 2.5–5.7% of PCNL procedures described in two recent series [15,16]. Clinically significant bleeding is most often managed with conservative measures, with less than 1% requiring selective arterial embolization of a bleeding vessel [15,17,18].

Risk factors for significant bleeding associated with PCNL include puncture site, anterior being greater than posterior, and multiple punctures which increases the risk with each new tract [17]. Treatment of a large complex stone burden, such as a branching staghorn calculus, increases the risk of bleeding [15]. Greater surgical experience and centers where this procedure is performed commonly decrease the risk in general [17]. The method of tract dilation (e.g. balloon dilation versus passage of sequential dilators – radial dilating force versus shearing force) and the associated risk of bleeding are controversial. One study found a transfusion rate of 25% with serial dilation versus 10% with balloon [19], while other studies have found the converse (7.5% transfusion rate with balloon versus 4.9% with sequential dilator [20]). The general rule of balloon dilating into a hydronephrotic system with room for the balloon to expand, while employing graduated dilators in the setting of a complete staghorn, will help minimize bleeding in general.

Straight percutaneous access tracts are superior to a serpiginous route into the kidney. An initial straight needle puncture into a calyx with minimal angulation will decrease the risk of bleeding. Placing and access in a prone patient, for example, into an anterior calyx, can be associated with tract bleeding on dilation as the parenchymal defect extends into the posterior calyx. For these reasons, posterior calyces are best for prone positioned access, while anterior calyces can be accessed in lateral or supine patients.

Management of bleeding

The kidney carries a rich blood supply and therefore a certain amount of bleeding post puncture can be expected and only a minority requires transfusion. Bleeding post PCNL is usually managed conservatively. Venous tract bleeding is far more common than arterial injuries, and responds well to prompt conservative maneuvers. The insertion of a large-bore nephrostomy tube, with subsequent clamping and administration of diuretic, will stop most venous sinus bleeding. This maneuver facilitates an increase in intrarenal pressure above central venous pressure, filling the defect with clot temporarily. The nephrostomy is left clamped transiently, later being set to gravity and draining as urokinase acts on the clot. The insertion of a Kaye tract tamponade tube was a mainstay historically in this setting, but is rarely employed primarily and has a role only when the aforementioned maneuvers are unsuccessful. It is based on a nephrostomy catheter surrounded by a tract compression balloon, with a second distal balloon to maintain intrarenal access. Being a poor drainage catheter, when employed it commonly requires conversion to a better drainage catheter in a staged fashion.

If tract bleeding persists the origin is most often arterial, with delayed tract bleeding commonly representing an arteriovenous fistula. Renal angiography is key to identifying and treating the source. Selective arterial embolization is universally successful in this setting [17].

When bleeding is severe and less invasive measures unsuccessful, surgical exploration may be required. Emergency nephrectomy is rarely indicated. One large series defined complications of PCNL where 0.2% of patients required emergency nephrectomy [18]. In another series, 3/3878 (0.07%) underwent exploration, one requiring suturing of bleeding point, one nephrectomy, with one mortality [17].

Trauma to adjacent structures

The kidney being anatomically appropriate to access percutaneously, there is an inherent risk of damage to adjacent structures while gaining tract access. Although risks are low (0.4% in a recent series [16]), it is essential to identify risk factors and describe treatment modalities, thus minimizing morbidity.

Pleural injury

The proximity of the diaphragm to the superior pole of the kidney increases the risk of transpleural access with concurrent hydrothorax, pneumothorax, and potentially hemothorax. A recent series describes this risk of 1.8% of hydrothorax in patients undergoing PCNL [16]. Supracostal punctures above the 12th rib increase this risk to approximately 10%, while above the 11th rib the rate increases to approximately 50% [21]. The risk of transpleural access is minimized by performing puncture below the level of the 12th rib, employing ultrasonography guidance with full expiration, and with a more lateral approach.

Intraoperative assessment commonly will define a transpleural access. Intraoperative fluoroscopy defines either a pneumo- or hydrothorax. Intraoperative thoracocentesis, with or without placement of a small-caliber pigtail thoracostomy, is often all that is required.

Trauma to hollow viscus

The colon lies in close proximity to the left kidney and therefore carries a greater risk of being traversed during percutaneous puncture. CT evaluation in the prone position identified colon lying posterior to the kidney in 11.9–26.2% of patients [22]. Colonic perforation rate is low, around 0.3% [17]. One series describes all perforations being retroperitoneal and two-thirds occurring on the left side [17]. The greatest risk is in the diabetic patient population, and in those with long-standing constipation and chronic colonic dilation (e.g. spinal cord injured, meningomyelocele, etc.).

Risk factors for colonic puncture also include renal ectopy and anomalies. Intraoperative signs of a transcolon access include gas and fecal material drainage. Since the majority of transcolon access tracts reflect a retroperitoneal perforation, conservative management is most often successful. Firstly, withdrawal of the nephrostomy tube from the kidney with positioning in the colon defect creates a controlled fistula (i.e. colostomy tube), which after a period of maturation over a few weeks can be removed without sequelae. Maintaining separate renal drainage with the insertion of an internal double pigtail stent is also essential. In the rare case where conservative management fails, a temporary bowel diversion is thus required [17].

A rare complication of percutaneous puncture is access into the duodenum employed for right-sided PCNL. As opposed to colonic perforations where the access is through the posterior colon and then into the kidney, duodenal injuries occur from past pointing, thus placing the catheter through the kidney into the duodenum. If this reflects only a needle or guidewire perforation, and is recognized before tract dilation, it can be managed conservatively by withdrawing and maintaining transient nasogastric drainage. However, if a tract is dilated into the duodenum, separated drainage is challenging and definitive repair is often required.

Extravasation

During PCNL, irrigation fluid may extravasate from a perforation of the collecting system or from overdistension, particularly when an operative sheath is not being employed to decompress the system. The rate of extravasation can be as high as 3.4–7.2% [16]. Small perforations during PCNL are common, with minimal change in serum electrolytes when sterile saline irritant is employed. Significant extravasation can be identified by medial displacement of the kidney during fluoroscopy or a discrepancy between inflow and outflow of irrigation fluid [23]. Drainage is essential to minimize problems from extravasation. Proper positioning of a nephrostomy and internal drainage obviates the need for other interventions in this setting [21].

Infectious complications and sepsis

Transient perioperative fever is commonly observed in up to one-third of patients undergoing PCNL (range 10.5–16% [15,16]), with this most often reflecting atelectasis secondary to the subcostal location of the nephrostomy. Urosepsis, however, is an infrequent morbidity, with death related to sepsis reported in 0.3% of PCNL treatments [21]. Pre-existing risk factors for sepsis include the presence of positive urine culture preoperatively, infectious struvite calculi, immunosuppression, presence of a long-standing nephrostomy with intrarenal colonization, and poorly controlled diabetes.

The presence of a negative urine culture does not completely remove the risk of fever and sepsis associated with PCNL. In one series 8.8% of patients experiencing an infectious complication post PCNL had a negative preoperative culture, compared to 18.8% in those with a positive culture [24]. With regard to antibiotics, a short course preoperatively may be superior to a longer course, particularly in those with struvite stone where longer preoperative treatment may confer resistance. Even in the presence of sterile urine, antibiotic prophylaxis prior to treatment has been shown to decrease the rate of postoperative urinary tract infection (UTI) [23]. Further steps to reduce the risk of sepsis during the procedure include minimizing operative time, maintaining low irrigation pressure, and ensuring adequate postoperative drainage.

Ureteropyeloscopic lithotripsy

Ureterorenoscopy (URS) is based on the access of the intrarenal collecting system and ureter by means of complimentary semi-rigid or actively deflectable flexible endoscope, employed to facilitate intraluminal lithotripsy. Within the ureter, URS remains a first-line treatment for the majority of stones, especially when ureteric stenting is required to obtain drainage of an obstructed system. For calculi in the kidney, URS is an excellent option, particularly those with lower pole, and in those with modest sized non-infectious calculi [14].

Technological advances have lead to a significant decrease in size of the ureteroscope. These endoscopes have distal tips less than 8F, thus significantly decreasing the risk of ureteric wall trauma with both access and intraluminal lithotripsy. Actively deflectable, flexible ureteroscopes allow for complete intrarenal access, facilitating the placement of a powerful lithotrite like the holmium laser throughout the collecting system. Visualization has also improved with the application of digital imaging in this setting.

As technology and surgical expertise improve, the majority of renal tract calculi may be appropriate for ureteroscopic management, including patients in whom other modalities such as PCNL or ESWL may be less appropriate, such as the obese or anticoagulated.

Contraindications

There are few contraindications to URS; the procedure is performed with either general or regional anesthetic. Anatomical parameters including ureteral tortuosity and renal ectopy should be defined preoperatively or with a retrograde ureteropyelogram to help define access strategies, but rarely preclude the passage of the endoscope.

Complications

Evolution in the technologies described above has led to a change in complications reported due to URS. Semi-rigid ureteroscopes are largely used to treat distal ureteric calculi and flexible ureteroscopes permit access to mid and proximal ureteric calculi. These technological advances have also facilitated the treatment of a larger, more complex stone burden, which may have historically been reserved for ESWL or PCNL. Historically, the complication rate decreased over time at the earlier stages of adoption (both semi-rigid and flexible URS). A recent systematic review of flexible URS for larger stones is included for comparison [24].

Minor complications of URS include those without long-term effects or those causing minimal or transient postoperative complications. These include bleeding, UTI or false passage formation. Major complications may require a further procedure or close monitoring or have significant postoperative sequelae, such as ureteric perforation, avulsion and stricture or cardiopulmonary complications. The European Association of Urology reports an overall complication rate of 9–25%, with major complications being infrequent at a rate of 1% [14]. Severe complications, defined as the need for cardiovascular support or treatment of sepsis, are rare, with a mortality rate of 0.06% [30].

A recent systematic review of complications following treatment of larger calculi by flexible ureteroscopy illustrates complication rates in current practice with an excellent stone-free rate of 93.7% [24]. Major complications were defined as those requiring further procedures or close monitoring. With a mean stone size of 2.5 cm, minor complications were reported in 5.3% of procedures and major complications in 4.8%. This was further subdivided into a group of intermediate stones (2–3 cm) and larger stones (greater than 3 cm). There were no major complications reported in the intermediate sized stone group and 14.3% minor complications. For larger stones (>3 cm), major complications were seen in 11.5%, minor in 15.4%.

Complications may be related to the passage of the endoscope, retrieval of calculi or sepsis.

- Endoscope access: mucosal trauma, false passage, hematuria, ureteric perforation – minor and major

- Retrieval of calculi
- Technological failure
- Sepsis
- Stricture
- Ureteric avulsion

Passage of the endoscope: bleeding, false passage, and perforation

The passage of a ureteroscope may be associated with ureteral trauma, leading to hematuria and mucosal injury (e.g. abrasion, formation of false passage, perforation, and/or extravasation). Some degree of transient hematuria is associated with endoscopic instrumentation of the urinary tract, while significant bleeding is rare and is reported in less than 1% of procedures (Table 25.1). Mucosal trauma can risk false passage formation and difficult visualization of the ureteric lumen leading to cessation of the procedure, but major perforation (greater than the diameter of a guidewire = 1 mm) is seen in less than 1%. Ureteric perforation ranges from simple guidewire puncture (most common) to larger perforation leading to extravasation. Perforation of the ureter is significantly associated with a longer operative time, particularly in those systems in which a stone is impacted or in which access is difficult [31]; therefore early recognition of problems is essential and measures to minimize trauma should be taken.

Smaller perforations or false passages can be managed by the passage of a double J stent to facilitate drainage of urine and allow for healing of the ureter. Where perforations are large, early recognition is extremely important to enable diversion of urine by means of nephrostomy (thus reducing the risk of urinoma formation) and to minimize late complications such as stricture. A nephrostomy will facilitate drainage of the kidney and also provide a means for subsequent imaging to delineate injury and plan further treatment if required.

Urinary tract infection and sepsis

Instrumentation of the ureter and kidney carries the risk of sepsis and therefore antibiotic prophylaxis is recommended, with UTIs being treated completely prior to URS [14]. A meta-analysis of complications of URS found an incidence of UTI and sepsis of 2–4% [32]. Prophylactic antibiotic use, prior treatment of infection, and careful technique are prudent practice to minimize infective complications.

Avulsion of the ureter

Avulsion of the ureter is a serious complication leading to considerable morbidity. Reassuringly, ureteric avulsion is rare; recent series of both rigid and flexible URS range from 0% to 0.17% [24,33,34]. Ureteric avulsion may occur when retrieving a calculus in a stone basket using excess

Table 25.1 Complications of ureterorenoscopy

	Blute [25]	Abdel-Razzak [26]	Harmon [27]	Grasso [28]	Jiang [29]	Aboumarzouk [24]
Year	1988	1992	1997	1998	2007	2012 (FURS)
Number of patients	346	290	209	580	697	445
Minor (%)	**8.5**	**21**	**5.5**	**8.2**		**4.8**
Colic/pain	–	9.0	3.5	5.5		
False passage	0.9	–	–	0.4		–
Fever	6.2	6.9	2.0	1.4		0.8
Bleeding minor	0.5	2.0	0	0.7		0.25
Bleeding prolonged	0.3	1.0	0	0.2		–
Extravasation	0.6	1.0	0	–		–
Urinary tract infection	–	1.0	–	1.6		1.26
Pyelonephritis	–	–	–	0.5		0.25
Acute urinary retention	–	–	–	–		0.25
Major (%)	**7.5**	**2.4**	**2.0**	**0.8**	**1.8**	**5.3**
Perforation	4.6	1.7	1.0	0.0	1.1	0
Stricture	1.4	0.7	0.5	0.5	0.7	–
Avulsion	0.6	0	0	0	0	0
Urosepsis	0.3	0	0	0		0.25
Steinstrasse	–	–	–	–	–	1.26
Subcapsular hematoma	–	–	–	–	–	1.0
Prostatitis	–	–	–	–	–	0.25
Clot retention	–	–	–	–	–	0.25
Cardiovascular accident/ deep vein thrombosis/ myocardial infarction						0.25

force. Upper ureteric calculi and impacted calculi carry a particular risk of ureteric avulsion.

Usually ureteric avulsion is recognized immediately intraoperatively, but late presentation of fever and/or loin pain in a complicated patient should carry a high index of suspicion of ureteric avulsion. Ureteric avulsion can be managed successfully by reimplanation. Where the avulsion is low, the distal ureter may be reimplanted into the bladder, and where more length is required, a psoas hitch may be used to facilitate a tension-free repair. Mid-ureteric avulsions may be managed by means of a Boari flap and reimplantation. Avulsion of the proximal ureter may provide a more challenging repair as the standard method of proximal ureteric repair of trans-ureteroureterostomy is contraindicated in renal stone disease. A small bowel interposition or autotransplantation to a pelvic position is a management option in this scenario but nephrectomy may be necessary if renal function is impaired.

Stricture formation

An important late complication of URS (and indeed impacted calculus) is formation of ureteric stricture. The risk of stricture formation following ureteroscopy is fortunately low, approximately 0.1% [14]. Perioperative factors may increase the risk of stricture formation, such as mucosal trauma, perforation, need for dilation, and impaction of stone [33]. In these cases, postoperative imaging is advised to identify late strictures. One series followed this management strategy and performed postoperative imaging in complicated cases. No cases of silent obstruction were missed and a stricture rate of 5.3% was reported (0% in those procedures with no perioperative concerns) [35].

Management of ureteric stricture following URS is dependent on stricture size and location. Short-term options may include insertion of a double J stent, or endourological procedures may be appropriate for short strictures and include incision of stricture with knife or laser. Ureteric reimplantation may be necessary in the case of complex or long strictures. Where stricture has led to obstruction and loss of renal function, nephrectomy may be appropriate.

Minimizing complications

The technique of ureterorenoscopy has a learning curve and patients undergoing a procedure performed by a urologist specializing in endourology experienced a lower risk of complications [31]; similarly a hospital with a high volume of procedures reports a significantly lower number of severe complications [30].

Particular care should be taken in treating those with co-existing morbidities and the elderly, as the severe complication rate is significantly higher.

Small fragments less than 3 mm in diameter are likely to pass by themselves. Perseverance in order to fragment further (thus increasing operative time) leads to a significant increase in complications [31,34] and therefore should be avoided. Early recognition of failure to progress during ureteroscopy should be considered, and stenting and completion at a later date are prudent to reduce potential complications.

References

1. Karlsen SJ, Smevik B, Hovig T. Acute morphological changes in canine kidneys after exposure to extracorporeal shock waves. A light and electron microscopic study. Urol Res 1991; 19(2): 105–15.
2. Dhar NB, Thornton J, Karafa MT, et al. A multivariate analysis of risk factors associated with subcapsular hematoma formation following electromagnetic shock wave lithotripsy. J Urol 2004; 172(6 Pt 1): 2271.
3. Kaude JV, Williams CM, Millner MR, et al. Renal morphology and function immediately after extracorporeal shock-wave lithotripsy. Am J Roentgenol 1985; 145(2): 305–13.
4. Rubin JI, Arger PH, Pollack HM, et al. Kidney changes after extracorporeal shock wave lithotripsy: CT evaluation. Radiology 1987; 162(1 Pt 1): 21–4.
5. Kostakopoulos A, Stavropoulos NJ, Macrychoritis C, et al. Subcapsular hematoma due to ESWL: risk factors. A study of 4,247 patients. Urol Int 1995; 55(1): 21–4.
6. Müller-Mattheis VG, Schmale D, Seewald M, et al. Bacteremia during extracorporeal shock wave lithotripsy of renal calculi. J Urol 1991; 146(3): 733–6.
7. Dinçel C, Ozdiler E, Ozenci H, et al. Incidence of urinary tract infection in patients without bacteriuria undergoing SWL: comparison of stone types. J Endourol 1998; 12(1): 1–3.
8. Pearle MS, Roehrborn CG. Antimicrobial prophylaxis prior to shock wave lithotripsy in patients with sterile urine before treatment: a meta-analysis and cost-effectiveness analysis. Urology 1997; 49(5): 679–86.
9. Sayed MA, el-Taher AM, Aboul-Ella HA, et al. Steinstrasse after extracorporeal shockwave lithotripsy: aetiology, prevention and management. BJU Int 2001; 88(7): 675–8.
10. Lucio J 2nd, Korkes F, Lopes-Neto AC, et al. Steinstrasse predictive factors and outcomes after extracorporeal shockwave lithotripsy. Int Braz J Urol 2011; 37(4): 477–82.
11. Ather MH, Shrestha B, Mehmood A. Does ureteral stenting prior to shock wave lithotripsy influence the need for intervention in steinstrasse and related complications? Urol Int 2009; 83(2): 222–5.
12. Zeng ZR, Lindstedt E, Roijer A, et al. Arrhythmia during extracorporeal shock wave lithotripsy. Br J Urol 1993; 71(1): 10–16.
13. Zanetti G, Ostini F, Montanari E, et al. Cardiac dysrhythmias induced by extracorporeal shockwave lithotripsy. J Endourol 1999; 13(6): 409–12.
14. Turk C, Knoll T, Petrik A, et al. Guidelines on Urolithiasis. European Association of Urology, 2012.
15. Armitage JN, Irving SO, Burgess NA, et al. Percutaneous nephrolithotomy in the United Kingdom: results of a prospective data registry. Eur Urol 2012; 61(6): 1188–93.
16. De la Rosette J, Assimos D, Desai M, et al. The Clinical Research Office of the Endourological Society Percutaneous Nephrolithotomy Global Study: indications, complications, and outcomes in 5803 patients. J Endourol 2011; 25(1): 11–17.
17. El-Nahas AR, Shokeir AA, El-Assmy AM, et al. Post-percutaneous nephrolithotomy extensive hemorrhage: a study of risk factors. J Urol 2007; 177(2): 576–9.
18. Keoghane SR, Cetti RJ, Rogers AE, et al. Blood transfusion, embolisation and nephrectomy after percutaneous nephrolithotomy (PCNL). BJU Int 2013; 111(4): 628–32.

19. Davidoff R, Bellman GC. Influence of technique of percutaneous tract creation on incidence of renal hemorrhage. J Urol 1997; 157: 1229–31.
20. Lopes T, Sangam K, Alken P, et al. The Clinical Research Office of the Endourological Society Percutaneous Nephrolithotomy Global Study: tract dilation comparisons in 5537 patients. J Endourol 2011; 25: 755–62.
21. Chalasani V, Bissoon D, Bhuvanagir AK, et al. Should PCNL patients have a CT in the prone position preoperatively? Can J Urol 2010; 17(2): 5082–6.
22. Wein A, Kavoussi L, Novick A, et al. *Campbell-Walsh Urology*, 10th edn. Philadelphia: Elsevier-Saunders, 2012.
23. Negrete-Pulido O, Gutierrez-Aceves J. Management of infectious complications in percutaneous nephrolithotomy. J Endourol 2009; 23(10): 1757–62.
24. Aboumarzouk O, Monga M, Kata S, et al. Flexible ureteroscopy and laser lithotripsy for stones >2cm: a systematic review and meta-analysis. J Endourol 2012; 26(10): 1257–63.
25. Blute ML, Segura JW, Patterson DE. Ureteroscopy. J Urol 1988; 139: 510.
26. Abdel-Razzak OM, Bagley DH. Clinical experience with flexible ureteropyeloscopy. J Urol 1992; 148: 1788.
27. Harmon WJ, Sershon PD, Blute ML, et al. Ureteroscopy: current practice and long-term complications. J Urol 1997; 157: 28–32.
28. Grasso M. Ureteropyeloscopic treatment of ureteral and intrarenal calculi. Urol Clin North Am 2000; 27: 623–31.
29. Jiang H, Wu Z, Ding Q, et al. Ureteroscopic treatment of ureteral calculi with holmium:YAG laser lithotripsy. J Endourol 2007; 21(2): 151–4.
30. Sugihara T, Yasunaga H, Horiguchi H, et al. A nomogram predicting severe adverse events after ureteroscopic lithotripsy: 12,372 patients in a Japanese national series. BJU Int 2013; 111(3): 459–66.
31. Schuster T, Hollenbeck B, Faerber G, et al. Complications of ureteroscopy: analysis of predictive factors. J Urol 2001; 166: 538–40.
32. Preminger G, Tiselius H-G, Assimos D, et al. 2007 Guideline for the management of ureteral calculi. J Urol 2007; 178: 2418–34.
33. El-Nahas AR, El-Tabey NA, Eraky I, et al. Semirigid ureteroscopy for ureteral stones: a multivariate analysis of unfavorable results. J Urol 2009; 181(3): 1158–62.
34. Tanriverdi O, Silay MS, Kadihasanoglu M, et al. Revisiting the predictive factors for intra-operative complications of rigid ureteroscopy: a 15-year experience. Urol J 2012; 9(2): 457–64.
35. Adiyat K, Meuleners R, Monga M. Selective postoperative imaging after ureteroscopy. Urology 2009; 73: 490–3.

Index

Illustrations are comprehensively referred to from the text. Therefore, significant items in illustrations (figures and tables) have only been given a page reference in the absence of their concomitant mention in the text referring to that illustration.

Urinary Stones: Medical and Surgical Management, First Edition. Edited by Michael Grasso and David S. Goldfarb.

www.ingramcontent.com/pod-product-compliance
Ingram Content Group UK Ltd.
Pitfield, Milton Keynes, MK11 3LW, UK
UKHW052225270726
14059UKWH00003B/114

9 781118 405437